# Case Studies from Primary Care Settings

## NOTICE

Medicine is an ever-changing science. As new research and clinical experience broaden our knowledge, changes in treatment and drug therapy are required. The editors and the publisher of this work have checked with sources believed to be reliable in their efforts to provide information that is complete and generally in accord with the standards accepted at the time of publication. However, in view of the possibility of human error or changes in medical sciences, neither the editors nor the publisher nor any other party who has been involved in the preparation or publication of this work warrants that the information contained herein is in every respect accurate or complete, and they are not responsible for any errors or omissions or for the results obtained from use of such information. Readers are encouraged to confirm the information contained herein with other sources. For example and in particular, readers are advised to check the product information sheet included in the package of each drug they plan to administer to be certain that the information contained in this book is accurate and that changes have not been made in the recommended dose or in the contraindications for administration. This recommendation is of particular importance in connection with new or infrequently used drugs.

# Case Studies from Primary Care Settings

EDITORS

## Marie L. Talashek, Ed.D., R.N., C.S.
Associate Professor
College of Nursing
University of Illinois at Chicago
Chicago, Illinois

## Laina M. Gerace, Ph.D., R.N.
Associate Professor and Director
College of Nursing
Rockford Regional Program
University of Illinois at Chicago
Rockford, Illinois

## Arlene Miller, Ph.D., R.N., C.S.
Assistant Professor
College of Nursing
University of Illinois at Chicago
Chicago, Illinois

## Marie Lindsey, Ph.D., R.N., C.S.
Clinical Assistant Professor
College of Nursing
University of Illinois at Chicago
Chicago, Illinois

McGRAW-HILL
Health Professions Division

New York   St. Louis   San Francisco   Auckland   Bogotá   Caracas
Lisbon   London   Madrid   Mexico City   Milan   Montreal
New Delhi   San Juan   Singapore   Sydney   Tokyo   Toronto

# McGraw-Hill

A Division of The **McGraw·Hill** Companies

**Case Studies from Primary Care Settings**

Copyright © 1998 by *The McGraw-Hill Companies, Inc.* All rights reserved.
Printed in the United States of America. Except as permitted under the
United States Copyright Act of 1976, no part of this publication may be
reproduced or distributed in any form or by any means, or stored in a data
base or retrieval system, without the prior written permission of the publisher.

1 2 3 4 5 6 7 8 9 0   DOCDOC   9 9 8

ISBN 0-07-105487-1

This book was set in Korinna by V&M Graphics Incorporated.
The editors were John J. Dolan, Susan R. Noujaim and Muza Navrozov.
The production supervisor was Heather A. Barry.
The cover was designed by Marsha Cohen/Parallelogram.
The index was prepared by Geraldine Beckford.
R. R. Donnelley & Sons was printer and binder.

This book is printed on recycled, acid-free paper.

**Library of Congress Cataloging-in-Publication Data**

Case studies from primary care settings / editors, Marie L. Talashek
... [et al.].
   p.   cm.
  Includes bibliographical references and index.
  ISBN 0-07-105487-1
  1. Primary nursing—Case studies.   2. Primary care (Medicine)—
Case studies.   I. Talashek, Marie L.
  [DNLM: 1. Therapeutics.   2. Primary Health Care.   WB 300 C337
1998]
RT90.7.C366   1998
610—dc21
DNLM/DLC
for Library of Congress

# Contents

# Contributors*

Jill S. Anderson, Ph.D., R.N.,
C.S. [14]
Clinical Nurse Consultant
Department of Psychiatry
University of Illinois at Chicago
Chicago, Illinois

Terese M. Bertucci, M.S., R.N.,
C.S., C.D.E. [32]
Nurse Practitioner
Rush Prudential Anchor HMO
Chicago, Illinois

Linda Ehrlich, Ph.D.(c), R.N., C.S.
[37]
Clinical Nurse Specialist
University of Chicago
Chicago, Illinois

Linda Farrand, Ph.D., R.N., C.S.
[3, 10, 15]
Clinical Assistant Professor
College of Nursing
Urbana-Champaign Regional Program
University of Illinois at Chicago
Urbana, Illinois

Susan A. Fontana, Ph.D., R.N.,
C.S. [18, 24, 27]
Associate Professor and Coordinator
Family Nurse Practitioner Program
School of Nursing
University of Wisconsin at Milwaukee
Milwaukee, Wisconsin

Patricia A. Furnace, M.S., R.N.,
C.S. [8, 12, 20, 35]
Clinical Assistant Professor
Peoria Regional Program
College of Nursing
University of Illinois at Chicago
Peoria, Illinois

Laina M. Gerace, Ph.D., R.N. [14,
16, 17, 19, 31, 36, 40, 41]
Associate Professor and Director
College of Nursing
Rockford Regional Program
University of Illinois at Chicago
Rockford, Illinois

Diane Graybill Pineda, M.S., R.N.,
C.S. [34]
Family Nurse Practitioner
Alivio Medical Center
Chicago, Illinois

Eugenie F. Hildebrandt, Ph.D.,
R.N., C.S. [37, 42]
Assistant Professor
School of Nursing
University of Wisconsin at Milwaukee
Milwaukee, Wisconsin

Dorothy Kent, M.S.N., R.N.,
C.P.N.P. [5, 39]
Pediatric Nurse Practitioner
Great Lakes Naval Hospital
Great Lakes, Illinois

*The number in brackets following the contributor name refers to chapter(s) written or
co-written by the contributor.*

**Marie Lindsey, Ph.D., R.N., C.S.**
[1, 11, 13, 21, 22, 23, 25, 29,
30, 32, 33, 38]
Clinical Assistant Professor
College of Nursing
University of Illinois at Chicago
Chicago, Illinois

**Ann M. McCormick, M.S., R.N.,
C.S., C.C.R.N.** [4]
Nurse Practitioner
Chicago, Illinois

**Judith McDevitt, Ph.D., R.N., C.S.**
[13, 21]
Assistant Professor of Nursing
School of Nursing
University of Wisconsin at Milwaukee
Milwaukee, Wisconsin

**Arlene Miller, Ph.D., R.N., C.S.** [6,
7, 8, 12, 26, 28, 31, 35, 36, 40,
41, 42]
Assistant Professor
College of Nursing
University of Illinois at Chicago
Chicago, Illinois

**Sharon E. Muran, M.S., R.N.,
C.S., C.O.H.N.-S.** [30]
Executive Director
IntegraCare, LLC
Deerfield, Illinois

**Jeanne M. Ondyak, B.S., R.N.**
[10, 15]
Family Nurse Practitioner Candidate
Naperville, Illinois

**Janice M. Phillips, Ph.D., R.N.** [28]
Assistant Professor
Department of Acute
and Long-term Care
American Cancer Society Professor
of Oncology Nursing
University of Maryland at Baltimore
School of Nursing
Baltimore, Maryland

**Marilyn Scott, R.N.** [29]
Family Nurse Practitioner
Mile Square Health Center
Chicago, Illinois

**Marlene G. Smith, Ph.D.(c), R.N.,
C.S.** [2, 6]
Clinical Instructor
College of Nursing
University of Illinois at Chicago
Chicago, Illinois

**Cheryl A. Sullivan, M.S.N., R.N.**
[17]
Instructor
St. Anthony College of Nursing
Rockford, Illinois

**Bernard P. Tadda, M.S., R.N.,
C.S.** [11, 22, 38]
Family Nurse Practitioner
Moline, Illinois

**Marie L. Talashek, Ed.D., R.N.,
C.S.** [1, 2, 3, 4, 5, 9, 16, 18, 19,
20, 23, 24, 27, 33, 39]
Associate Professor
College of Nursing
University of Illinois at Chicago
Chicago, Illinois

**Lorrita Verhey, M.S., C.S., R.N.,**
[7, 34]
Clinical Instructor
College of Nursing
University of Illinois at Chicago
Chicago, Illinois

**Ricki S. Witz, M.S., C.S., R.N.,**
[9, 25]
Urbana Regional Program
College of Nursing
University of Illinois-Urbana
Urbana, Illinois

**JoEllen Wilbur, Ph.D., R.N., C.S.**
[26]
Associate Professor
College of Nursing
University of Illinois at Chicago
Chicago, Illinois

# Acknowledgments

We owe our gratitude to the many people who assisted and encouraged us in compiling this book of case studies. A clinical book is realized only with the support of those who practice in advanced practice nursing roles. We are grateful to all contributors. Especially we thank our colleagues, both clinical faculty and practitioner, who contributed such rich clinical case material. Their names and affiliating agencies are listed on a separate page. We thank the experts in nursing and medicine who provided feedback relevant to case studies from their specialty areas. We also recognize the support of the U.S. Department of Health and Human Services Training Grant (PHS NU00334-01, JoEllen Wilbur, P.I.). One of its objectives was to expand the use of case studies in the FNP program at the University of Illinois–Chicago (UIC). Some of the cases in this book expanded cases developed during the training grant. We also thank the UIC, College of Nursing graduate students, who gave us helpful insight and astute feedback by "working through" the simulated cases.

Further, we thank those who provided such fine technical support: Mark Mershon for his excellent photography and media support; and Jeanne Ondyak, Mirabel Corral, and Carol Taylor for their careful attention to formatting details and a myriad of other chores. Their dedication was invaluable to the project.

Gratitude is also extended to Dr. Lucy Marion, Chair of the Department of Public Health, Mental Health and Administrative Nursing for her leadership and encouragement.

The Editors

# Preface

This book has been designed to identify and enhance your level of knowledge requisite for managing patient problems in primary care settings. The book has been arranged across the life span, from infancy through older adult, ending with a section of family case studies.

Cases can be studied in two ways. After reading the background information and answering the first question, look up the correct answers sequentially (A–E) as you choose an answer, or answer the entire question and then check for each correct answer. It is important to read the rationale for each choice, because important information is included in each choice. However, answers do not include data required for answering subsequent questions. Either method will help to identify your level of knowledge for managing each case in primary health care settings. Understanding the rationale for the correct answers will help you to provide comprehensive and efficient care.

The book is intended for primary care practitioners and students in clinical settings.

## Case Studies from Primary Care Settings

# I

# INFANT AND TODDLER

# Introduction

*Marie L. Talashek*

Primary care providers are partners with parents in achieving high levels of wellness and normal development for infants and toddlers. Preventing illnesses and injuries through immunizations and parental education, screening patients for diseases and developmental lags, and the timely identification and treatment of illnesses helps children reach their optimum level of health and development.

The American Academy of Pediatrics recommends 10 visits for health supervision during the first 3 years of life. Each visit should include the following:

1. A history of health and wellness since the last visit should be taken.
2. A complete physical examination should be given.
3. Graphing of length, weight, and head circumference for developmental progress should be done.
4. Vision and hearing screening should be done.
5. Developmental assessment using the Denver II (gross motor skills, fine motor skills, language and social responses) and emotional and cognitive development should be completed.
6. Immunization status should be brought into compliance.
7. Appropriately timed screening with purified protein derivative (PPD), urinalysis, hematocrit or hemoglobin, and lead screening should be done.
8. Anticipatory guidance should be given.

According to Erikson, a child is in the psychosocial developmental stage of trust versus mistrust during the first year of life and in the stage of autonomy versus shame and doubt during the second year. Parents need to gain confidence in their ability as parents and provide a safe, nurturing environment for their baby. According to Piaget, infancy is the sensory-motor period of cognitive development, with year one culminating in the emergence of anticipatory and intentional behavior, and year two in the beginnings of sym-

3

bolic representation and internal experimentation rather than external trial and error. Understanding normal developmental milestones helps parents provide an environment that will foster development.

Anticipatory guidance during the first 3 years includes information on developmental and behavioral norms, diet, elimination, sleep, discipline, and safety. These are covered in all health care visits because growth and developmental changes occur rapidly during the first 3 years of life. The parent can take advantage of emerging development to encourage new behaviors in a timely manner such as toilet training, drinking from a cup, and moving from the breast or bottle as the primary source of nutrition to solids. Safety should also be addressed in a timely manner, because accidents are the number one cause of death in children older than 6 months of age. Pointing out the importance of car seats and smoke alarms at the initial appointment is appropriate. During subsequent appointments, linking emerging gross motor skills to the necessary environmental accommodations for safety will help prevent household accidents. Parent-child interactions should be carefully assessed to prevent or identify child neglect and abuse. Timely anticipatory guidance will encourage the development of successful parenting skills so that infants and toddlers can be healthy and happy.

The first illness is often experienced during this developmental phase. Parental competence in coping with a child's initial illness is indicative of continued parental coping ability. Illness episodes provide opportunities for health supervision and anticipatory guidance for children who are behind in the recommended schedule of visits. Immunizations, other procedures, and anticipatory guidance can be brought up to date during minor illness episodes.

Cases were chosen for this section for the following reasons: they have a high rate of occurrence during the first 3 years of life (otitis); age-related variations are important considerations when ruling out pathology (torsional deformities); they illustrate common preventable problems (anemia); and they give an asymptomatic presentation of an illness with long-term consequences (lead exposure).

## REFERENCES

Centers for Disease Control and Prevention. (1996). Immunization of adolescents: Recommendations of the Advisory Committee on Immunization Practices, the American Medical Association. *Morbidity Mortality Weekly Report 45,* No. RR-13, pp. 3–9.

Committee on Practice and Ambulatory Medicine. (1995). Recommendations for preventive pediatric health care. *Pediatrics 92*(6), 751.

Deloian, B. (1996). Developmental management of infants. In C. Burns, N. Barber, M. Brady, A. Dunn (eds.), *Pediatric Primary Care: A Handbook for Nurse Practitioners,* 81–100. Philadelphia: W. B. Saunders.

Erikson, E. (1963). *Childhood and Society.* New York: Norton.

Murray, R., Zentner, J. (1997). *Health Assessment and Promotion Strategies through the Life Span,* 6th ed. Stamford, CT: Appleton and Lange.

Pulaski, M. A. (1971). *Understanding Piaget: An Introduction to Children's Cognitive Development.* New York: Harper & Row Publishers.

U.S. Preventive Services Task Force. (1996). *Guide to Clinical Services,* 2d ed. Baltimore: Williams & Wilkins.

Woolf, S., Jonas, S., Lawrence, R. (eds.). (1996). *Health Promotion and Disease Prevention in Clinical Practice.* Baltimore: Williams & Wilkins.

# 1

# Otitis

*Marie L. Talashek*
*Marie Lindsey*

Caroline T., a 5-month-old infant, was last seen in the clinic for her 4-month well-child visit. She is accompanied by her mother. Records indicate that her immunization status is up to date without adverse reactions (hepatitis B vaccine was received at 2 days and at 1 month of age; diphtheria-pertussis-tetanus, polio, and *Haemophilus influenzae* b were received at 2 and 4 months of age). At the 4-month visit, Mrs. T. was instructed to introduce rice cereal mixed with breast milk into Caroline's diet. She had been receiving breast milk every 3 to 4 h during the day and every 5 to 6 h during the night. Growth and developmental progress have been normal. The office nurse took a rectal temperature today; it is 38.6°C (101.8°F). Caroline is fussy, and Mrs. T. is anxious, as this is her baby's first illness.

## CHIEF COMPLAINT

"Caroline awoke crying during the night. She's been fussy ever since. She usually calms right down once I pick her up."

## HISTORY OF PRESENT ILLNESS

Caroline went to bed at her usual time, but did not nurse as long as usual and was not interested in her cereal. She has not wanted to nurse for more than a minute at a time since the middle of the night. Caroline felt warm, but her mother was too nervous to take her temperature, even though she was instructed in the procedure at the 1-month well-child visit. When asked if Caroline had been pulling at her ears, her mother said, "She has been flailing her arms around her head, but I didn't realize that she may have been reaching for her ears."

QUESTION 1. Which of the following are required to complete the history of present illness? (Select all that apply.)
A. Stool changes
B. Urinary output
C. Discharge from the ear
D. Nasal discharge
E. Review of systems

QUESTION 2. Important additional subjective data include which of the following? (Select all that apply.)
A. Bottle propping
B. Exposure to cigarette smoke
C. Family history of allergies or acute otitis media (AOM)
D. Mother's ability to cope with the illness, including her support system

## OBJECTIVE DATA

General:     A well-developed, moderately ill, crying infant.
Skin:        Clear without diaper rash, good turgor.
Head/neck:   No lymphadenopathy, fontanelles flat.
Eyes, ears,  Conjunctiva clear; external ears no lesions or tenderness,
nose, throat: canals clear, tympanic membranes (see Fig. 1-1); nose no
             discharge; mouth mucous membranes pink, edentulous;
             pharynx pink without exudate.
Abdomen:     Symmetrically rounded, bowel sounds present and slightly
             increased in all four quadrants. Loose greenish yellow stool in
             the diaper.

QUESTION 3. Which one of the following best describes the tympanic membrane (TM) in Fig. 1-1?
A. Wax obscures the canals.
B. TM is erythematous; light reflex is diminished; and bony landmarks are obscured.
C. TM is pearly grey, with light reflex at 4 o'clock.
D. TM has hyperemic vessels with amber-colored fluid below the bony landmarks.

QUESTION 4. What additional objective data or procedures are needed? (Select all that apply.)
A. Complete blood count (CBC)
B. Weight and length
C. Lung sounds
D. Palpation of mastoid process
E. Pneumatic otoscopy

## ASSESSMENT

QUESTION 5. Which one of the following is the appropriate diagnosis?
A. Serous otitis media
B. Acute otitis media with diarrhea

C. Gastroenteritis
D. Bullous myringitis

## PLAN

**QUESTION 6.** Which one of the following is the first-line drug of choice for treating this infant?
A. Augmentin
B. Erythromycin
C. Amoxicillin
D. Ampicillin
E. Antihistamine

**QUESTION 7.** Which of the following data should be discussed with the mother? (Select all that apply.)
A. Medication instructions
B. Course of the illness
C. Prevention of AOM
D. Confidence in mother's ability to care for the ill infant

## ANSWERS

**QUESTION 1.** Which of the following are required to complete the history?
A. *YES.* Diarrhea and vomiting are often systemic reactions to AOM.
B. *YES.* Urinary output must be monitored as a measure of hydration, especially if diarrhea and vomiting are also present.
C. *YES.* Discharge from the ear may be present when the tympanic membrane is ruptured. It is important that fluid is not introduced into the ear canal as a result of removing cerumen.
D. *YES.* Rhinorrhea indicates an upper respiratory infection, which often precedes AOM.
E. *NO.* A complete review of systems is not necessary. A good *focused* analysis of symptoms based on the presenting complaint was done and revealed some classic signs of AOM: irritability, pain (ear pulling in an infant), and fever. Although these symptoms are not always present, AOM is often preceded by rhinorrhea, which can impair eustachian tube drainage. The infant was seen 1 month ago, and this visit should be focused on the presenting complaint.

**QUESTION 2.** Important subjective data include which of the following?
A. *YES.* Bottle propping or taking a bottle to bed can cause milk to be forced into the infant's short eustachian tube, resulting in AOM. Conversely, breastfeeding is protective against otitis media.
B. *YES.* Cigarette smoke is an irritant to the upper airways that sometimes causes inflammation. Infants 12 to 18 months of age who are exposed to passive smoke are at risk for persistent middle ear effusion.
C. *YES.* Family history of allergies or AOM may indicate that the infant has familial allergic rhinitis. AOM is common in such children.

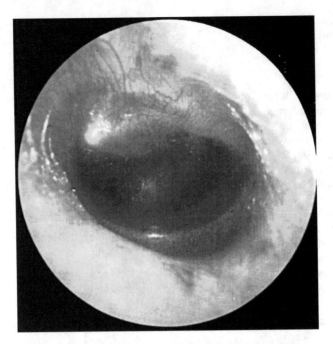

FIGURE 1-1.  Tympanic membrane when observed with an
otoscope (see Color Plate 1). John Bain, Philip Carter,
Richard Morton (eds.). *Colour Atlas of Mouth, Throat, and
Ear Disorders in Children,* 1985. Norwell, MA: Kluwer
Academic Publishers. With kind permission from Kluwer
Academic Publishers.

D.  *YES.* It is important to assess the mother's ability to cope with an ill
child, as this is her first experience. If she copes well with this illness,
she will be more likely to manage subsequent illnesses well.

QUESTION 3. Which one of the following best describes the tym-panic
membrane in Fig. 1-1?
A.  *NO.* Visualization of the tympanic membrane is not obscured by wax.
B.  *YES.* The TM is erythematous, the light reflex is diminished, and bony
landmarks are obscured.
C.  *NO.* The TM is not pearly grey, nor is the light reflex visualized at 4
o'clock.
D.  *NO.* Amber-colored fluid is not visualized below the bony landmarks.

QUESTION 4. What additional objective data or procedures are needed?
A.  *NO.* A CBC is generally done only with recurring cases of AOM.
B.  *YES.* Weight and length are needed to assess hydration and to prescribe
the appropriate drug dosage. If a family is slow to come for care,
growth can also give an indication of the length and effect of an illness.
C.  *YES.* Lung sounds should be assessed, because AOM and other respiratory infections can occur simultaneously.

D.  *YES.* Mastoiditis is a complication of AOM that has not been treated. It is rare in infants and children under 2 years of age, but palpation of the mastoid process should be part of the routine exam for investigating ear infections.

E.  *YES.* Pneumatic otoscopy is the best diagnostic tool for AOM when it is done properly. Tympanic membranes can be red because of fever or crying, and bony landmarks are not always visible in healthy infants. It is very important that the ear speculum be of a size that enables it to seal the canal without touching the inner two-thirds of the canal, which is very tender. All areas of the tympanic membrane should be checked for mobility. A retracted tympanic membrane will not move when the bulb is squeezed, and a bulging one will not move when the collapsed bulb is released.

**QUESTION 5.** Which of the following is the appropriate diagnosis?

A.  *NO.* It is not serous otitis media because there is no observable fluid level behind the TM.

B.  *YES.* AOM with diarrhea is correct.

C.  *NO.* Gastroenteritis is an associated symptom with the diagnosis of AOM.

D.  *NO.* The signs of bullous myringitis are multiple hemorrhagic bullae on the medial external canal wall and the posterior aspect of the TM.

**QUESTION 6.** Which one of the following is the first-line drug of choice for treating this infant?

A.  *NO.* While Augmentin (amoxicillin plus clavulanate) is an effective treatment for AOM, it is more expensive than amoxicillin. Therefore, it is not usually used as a first-line therapy unless the patient lives in geographic areas known for amoxicillin-resistant organisms such as the ß-lactamase-producing *Hemophilus influenzae* and *Moraxella catarrhalis*. Augmentin may be used as a second-line therapy if the patient doesn't respond to amoxicillin. The Augmentin dose is 40 mg/kg per day in three divided doses for 10 days.

B.  *NO.* Erythromycin is more expensive than amoxicillin; thus, it is not usually first-line therapy. However, the combination erythromycin-sulfisoxazole (Pediazole) is a good choice for children allergic to the pencillins. If used for this purpose, the dose is 50 mg/kg, given every 12 h.

C.  *YES.* Antibiotic therapy to cover *Streptococcus pneumoniae, H. influenzae,* and *M. catarrhalis* is needed. The first-line drug of choice is amoxicillin 40 mg/kg per day in three divided doses every 8 h for 10 days.

D.  *NO.* Ampicillin is not first-line therapy because dosing is four times a day rather than the three times a day dosing of amoxicillin. It is more likely to cause diarrhea, and is not absorbed as well in the gut as is amoxicillin.

E.  *NO.* The use of antihistamines and decongestants has not been proven to prevent or resolve otitis media. Therefore, they should not be ordered unless the child has concurrent allergic rhinitis.

**QUESTION 7.** Which of the following data should be discussed with the mother?

A. *YES.* The mother must know exactly how to administer the medication in order for the infection to be resolved quickly and to prevent antibiotic-resistant organisms from developing. The mother should be instructed in the amount of medication to be given and the times to administer it. She should understand the importance of continuing to administer antibiotics for the entire course of treatment (10 days). Many people discontinue medications once symptoms are alleviated. Mrs. T. must be instructed to give acetaminophen every 4 to 6 h for fever, and to phone the clinic if Caroline has a fever that is not controlled with the acetaminophen, or if she develops an allergic rash. Furthermore, she must be instructed regarding the difference between an allergic rash and diaper rash and instructed to use Desitin if a diaper rash occurs.

B. *YES.* She should understand that Caroline will improve within 24 to 48 h *if* she administers the medication correctly. If she does so, and Caroline does not improve within that time frame, the mother should be instructed to call for further instructions.

C. *YES.* AOM can be prevented by avoiding bottle propping, cigarette smoke, and contacts with other people with upper respiratory infections. AOM can have sequelae such as hearing impairment leading to delayed speech and should be prevented if possible.

D. *YES.* This is the mother's first experience of dealing with a sick infant, and she is clearly anxious about it. It is important to assess whether the patient teaching is sufficient to instill confidence in her ability to care for the ill infant.

## REFERENCES

Berman, S., Chan, K. (1997). Ear, nose, and throat. In W. W. Hay, J. R. Groothis, A. R. Hayward, M. J. Levin (eds.), *Current Pediatric Diagnosis and Treatment,* 13th ed., 403–411. Stamford, CT: Appleton & Lange.

Boynton, R. W., Dunn, E. S., Stephens, G. R. (1992). *Manual of Ambulatory Pediatrics,* 3d ed., 324–327. Philadelphia: J. B. Lippincott.

Janwetz, E. (1995). Penicillins and cephalosporins. In B. G. Katzung (ed.), *Basic and Clinical Pharmacology,* 680–692. Norwalk, CT: Appleton & Lange.

Macknin, M. (1993). Acute otitis media. In R. A. Dershewitz (ed.), *Ambulatory Pediatric Care,* 2d ed., 290–294. Philadelphia: J. B. Lippincott.

# 2

# In-Toeing

*Marie L. Talashek*
*Marlene G. Smith*

Jimmy J., a 24-month-old African American male, is accompanied to the free inner-city clinic by his mother. She is an excellent historian and brings up-to-date health records with her. Jimmy was seen at the Health Department clinic for his 2-year checkup last month, when health supervision, as recommended by the American Academy of Pediatrics, was completed and all findings were normal. Jimmy, an only child, has always lived in public housing with his mother. He has received well-child care at the Health Department and was seen at the County Hospital emergency room once for an ear infection.

## CHIEF COMPLAINT

"Jimmy continues to be flat-footed and pigeon-toed. They told me he'd grow out of it, but I'm not certain he has."

## HISTORY OF PRESENT ILLNESS

Jimmy started to walk at 12 months of age, and his mother noted in-toeing shortly thereafter. Ms. J. believes that the in-toeing has gradually lessened, but she is still concerned about it and about his flat feet.

## PAST MEDICAL HISTORY

Ms. J. states that Jimmy was a full-term infant and that he has never been hospitalized. He received antibiotics once for an ear infection at 9 months of age.

**QUESTION 1.** Necessary additional subjective data include which of the following? (Select all that apply.)
   **A.** Complete review of systems
   **B.** Foot position during early infancy
   **C.** Sitting and sleeping positions
   **D.** Family history of in-toeing
   **E.** Walking history/problems

## PHYSICAL FINDINGS

A focused physical exam was completed to identify in-toeing. The lower extremities and feet have full range of motion and strength bilaterally. When running and walking, Jimmy appears flat-footed, but his feet are not pronated. When he stands on his toes, an arch appears. His angle of gait is observed, and his feet turn in slightly more than normal (see Fig. 2-1 for an example of normal gait). Hip external and internal rotation are both normal (see Figs. 2-2 and 2-3 for evaluation procedure). You observe the position of his knees relative to his feet and his internal malleoli relative to his external malleoli (see Fig. 2-4 for position for evaluation). His knees point ahead, his feet turn in slightly, and his external malleoli are positioned slightly in front of his internal malleoli.

**QUESTION 2.** In-toeing may be related to problems at which of the following sites? (Select all that apply.)
   **A.** Hips
   **B.** Knees
   **C.** Tibial shafts
   **D.** Feet

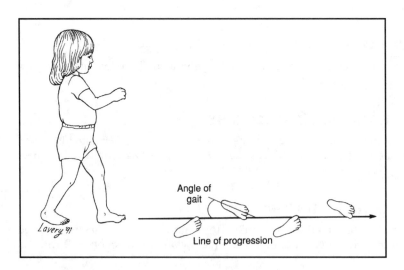

**FIGURE 2-1.** Angle of gait. [Staheli, L. T. (1977). Torsional deformity. *Pediatr Clin North Am 24,* 802.] With permission.

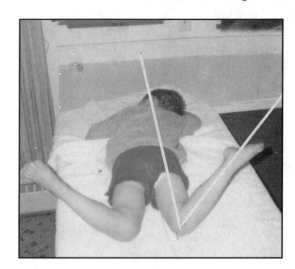

FIGURE 2-2. Internal
femoral rotation.
(M. L. Talashek,
personal photograph,
September 1997.)

## ASSESSMENT

QUESTION 3. Based on the findings, what is the diagnosis?
A. Femoral neck anteversion
B. Metatarsus adductus
C. Bilateral internal tibial torsion
D. Bilateral internal tibial torsion with flat feet
E. Muscle imbalance

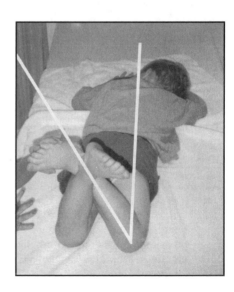

FIGURE 2-3.   External femoral
rotation. (M. L. Talashek, personal
photograph, September 1997.)

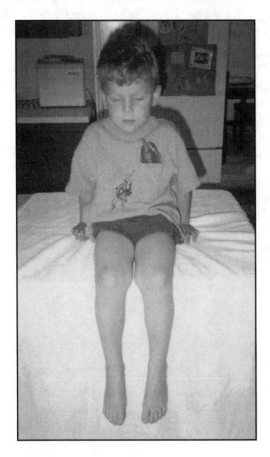

FIGURE 2-4.   Evaluation position. (M. L. Talashek, personal photograph, September 1997.)

## PLAN

QUESTION 4. What is the intervention at this time?
  A. X-ray the lower extremities.
  B. Refer to an orthopedist for splinting.
  C. Recommend high shoes with a good arch.
  D. Educate the mother about sleeping and sitting positions.

## ANSWERS

QUESTION 1. Necessary additional subjective data include which of the following?
  A. *NO*. A complete review of systems is not necessary. A good focused analysis of the orthopedic variation, including age of presentation, progression, and any noted mobility limitations, will be adequate to differentiate self-limiting developmental variations from those that require interventions.

B. *YES.* In-toeing (metatarsus adductus) during infancy is usually related to intrauterine positioning and resolves on its own or with gentle stretching of the forefoot by caregivers during the first month of life. For those feet that are rigid (cannot be corrected past the midline) or for in-toeing that has not resolved by 4 to 6 months of age, orthopedic intervention with serial casting is necessary. If the condition is not recognized until after age 2, surgical intervention may be necessary.

C. *YES.* Some children sleep with their haunches up toeing in and/or sit in a W position. This can exacerbate internal femoral torsion and increase in-toeing.

D. *YES.* Knowledge of a strong family history of in-toeing provides data for planning whether or not to intervene. If in-toeing continues into adulthood, the potential for self-correction in the toddler may not be as good.

E. *YES.* In-toeing associated with torsional deformities does not usually interfere with ambulation. All young children stumble and fall regardless of the position of their feet. However, it is important to find out whether the child walked at an appropriate age without problems to assess potential for neuromuscular problems.

**QUESTION 2.** In-toeing may be related to problems at which of the following sites?

A. *YES.* Increased femoral neck anteversion and/or femoral torsion at the hip is the most common cause of in-toeing diagnosed after 3 years of age.

B. *YES.* The position of the knees compared to the feet during ambulation helps to diagnose the site of the torsion.

C. *YES.* Tibial shafts are often twisted internally, with resultant in-toeing. This is usually diagnosed when the child begins to walk.

D. *YES.* The entire foot is turned in with femoral torsion, femoral neck anteversion, or tibial torsion, but only the forefoot is turned in with metatarsus adductus. The collection of objective data is directed toward identifying the cause of the in-toeing. It is possible to have more than one of these conditions without in-toeing. For example, a child could have internal femoral torsion with external tibial torsion.

**QUESTION 3.** Based on the findings, what is the diagnosis?

A. *NO.* Jimmy has almost equal external and internal hip rotation (45°), which is normal for this age. A diagnosis of femoral anteversion is made when internal rotation is 30° more than external rotation. This is the primary cause of in-toeing after 3 years of age; Jimmy is only 2 years old. Thus femoral anteversion is ruled out.

B. *NO.* In metatarsus adductus, only the forefoot is turned in. Jimmy has full range of motion in his foot, and his entire foot is slightly turned in. Therefore metatarsus adductus is ruled out.

C. *YES.* Jimmy has bilateral internal tibial torsion. His lateral malleoli are slightly anterior to his medial malleoli. Normally the medial malleoli are 10 to 15° anterior to the lateral malleoli. When Jimmy is seated, his knees are straight ahead and his feet turn in slightly, indicating a problem below the knee. Therefore, the diagnosis is tibial torsion. However, the degree of rotation is minimal, and his mother reported that the in-toeing had become less.

D. *NO.* Toddlers often appear flat-footed because of a fat pad. An arch appeared when Jimmy stood on tiptoe and when his feet dangled over the edge of the table. Flatfoot (pes planus) has been ruled out.

E. *NO.* Muscle imbalance would be evident during walking and running. Jimmy has minor in-toeing observed both at rest and walking, and lower extremity strength was equal bilaterally.

QUESTION 4. What is your intervention at this time?

A. *NO.* There is no reason to x-ray the extremities. The physical exam gave adequate information to arrive at the diagnosis of internal tibial torsion. An x-ray would expose the child to unnecessary radiation and would be costly.

B. *NO.* Referral to an orthopedist is both unnecessary and costly. Splinting is reserved for children who have more than 40° variations that have persisted after ambulating for 6 months. Family history and sleeping in a knee-chest position are also considered.

C. *NO.* There is no evidence that orthopedic shoes are beneficial. Well-fitting tennis shoes and going barefoot in the house are appropriate.

D. *YES.* Educate Ms. J. to allay her concerns. She is a conscientious mother, and knowledge will discourage unnecessary visits to health care providers. The best way to accommodate this is to show her each maneuver and explain the findings as the physical exam is done. Review the information with her at the conclusion of the exam and inform her that the findings are normal in regard to flat feet. Have her encourage Jimmy to sit in a tailor position rather than a W.

## REFERENCES

Burns, C. (1996). Musculoskeletal disorders. In C. Burns, N. Barber, M. Brady, A. Dunn (eds.), *Pediatric Primary Care*, 769–791. Philadelphia: W. B. Saunders.

Neinstein, L. S. (1996). *Adolescent Health Care: A Practical Guide*, 3d ed. Baltimore: Williams & Wilkins.

Seidel, H. M., Ball, J. W., Dains, J. E., Benedict, G. W. (1995). *Mosby's Guide to Physical Examination*, 3d ed. St. Louis: Mosby.

# 3

# Anemia

*Marie L. Talashek*
*Linda Farrand*

Tommy C., a 9-month-old African American male, is accompanied to the rural health clinic by his mother. Tommy, an only child, was last seen at the clinic for his 6-month health maintenance examination; he has not received health care since that visit. His migrant farm worker parents have been working in another state since that time. Tommy's mother shares child care with three other young mothers so that she can continue to work in the fields. Tommy smiles, coos, and plays with his mother's keys during the interview.

## CHIEF COMPLAINT

"Tommy is a fussy eater. He seems to only want his bottle."

## HISTORY OF PRESENT ILLNESS

Tommy consumes 32 oz of cow's milk in 24 h. He had iron-fortified formula until 7 months of age. After that, the parents could not easily access a women, infants, and children (WIC) nutritional site to receive the cereal because they were traveling from job to job. He completed the box of iron-fortified cereal he received at his 6-month WIC visit, and has been offered mashed table foods for the past 2 months. He has never taken vitamins. The mother denies pica, diarrhea, and exposure to infections. Review of systems is noncontributory. His laboratory values at his 6-month WIC visit were: hemoglobin (Hb) 11 g/dL, hematocrit (HCT) 33%, and blood lead level 2 μ/dL.

## PAST MEDICAL HISTORY

Birth:          Normal vaginal delivery; APGARs 7 and 10; length 21 in, weight 8 lb.
Immunizations:  Up to date, denies reactions.
Medications:    None.

Allergies:                        No known allergies.
Hospitalizations/injuries:  None.
Development:                 Sat up at 7 months; normal Denver Developmental
                                    Screening Tool (Denver II) at 6 months.

## PHYSICAL FINDINGS

Vital signs:      Temperature (ear) 36.7°C (98°F); length 29 in, weight 24 lb,
                      head circumference 45 cm.
General:          Chubby infant.
Skin:              Dark brown with good turgor.
Head:             Normocephalic, posterior fontanelle nonpalpable, anterior
                      fontanelle 1 cm.
Face:              Symmetrical.
Eyes:              Pupils equal, round, react to light; symmetrical corneal light
                      reflex; conjunctivae pale; red light reflex bilaterally.
Ears:              Normal shape and placement, canal clear, tympanic
                      membrane pearly grey with good light reflex and mobility
                      bilaterally, landmarks visualized.
Nose:              No drainage, patent, membranes slightly pale.
Oropharynx:    Mucosa slightly pale, four teeth, positive gag reflex, pink
                      tongue.
Neck:             Full range of motion, no lymphadenopathy.
Lungs:            Clear to percussion and auscultation.
Heart:             Apical pulse 110 with regular rhythm; $S_1$ $S_2$, no splitting, no
                      thrills.
Abdomen:       Rounded, bowel sounds in all four quadrants, no masses.
                      Femoral pulses equal bilaterally.
Genitalia:        Noncircumcised penis, foreskin retracts, testes descended
                      bilaterally, no inguinal hernia.
Anus:             Patent with good tone.
Back:             Straight.
Extremities:     Straight and symmetrical bilaterally with good tone,
                      strength, and equal skin creases.
Hips:              Abduction at 90°, flexion equal with knees touching the table.
Development:  Denver II normal for age.
Lab:               HCT 27%, Hb 9 mg/dL, blood lead level 9 µg/dL.

QUESTION 1. What additional historical information is required? (Select all
that apply.)
  A. Change in stools
  B. Chemical exposure
  C. Urinary frequency
  D. Family history
  E. Fatigue and irritability

QUESTION 2. What additional physical findings are helpful for determining
the cause of the low HCT and Hb? (Select all that apply.)
  A. Primitive reflexes
  B. Petechiae or purpura

C. Splenomegaly
D. Heart murmur

**QUESTION 3.** What initial laboratory tests are required at this time? (Select all that apply.)
A. Complete blood count (CBC) with differential
B. Liver profile
C. Blood smear
D. Reticulocyte count

**QUESTION 4.** If laboratory results indicate a low mean corpuscular value (MCV) and normal reticulocyte count, what is the next step, considering the history and physical findings? (Select all that apply.)
A. Investigate for blood loss
B. Order a platelet count
C. Initiate a trial of therapeutic iron
D. Do nutritional counseling

**QUESTION 5.**
If a course of therapeutic iron is initiated and there is no change in the reticulocyte count within 5 days, what other conditions are potential causes of the decreased MCV? (Select all that apply.)
A. Elevated lead level
B. Thalassemia
C. Bleeding or hemolysis
D. Poor compliance
E. Chronic inflammatory disease

**QUESTION 6.** A serum iron (Fe), total iron-binding capacity (TIBC), and ferritin are ordered to rule out thalassemia and chronic inflammatory disease. Which of the following are supportive of nutritional iron deficiency?
A. Decreased Fe, increased TIBC, decreased ferritin
B. Increased Fe, normal TIBC, increased ferritin
C. Decreased Fe, decreased TIBC, increased ferritin
D. Decreased Fe, decreased TIBC, decreased ferritin

## ASSESSMENT

The diagnosis is nutritional iron deficiency anemia.

## PLAN

**QUESTION 7.** The plan should include which of the following? (Select all that apply.)
A. Elemental iron 2 mg/kg per day in three divided doses
B. Iron-fortified formula
C. Recheck hemoglobin in 1 month
D. Continue elemental iron for 2 months after hemoglobin returns to normal
E. Refer to WIC for further nutritional counseling

## ANSWERS

QUESTION 1. What additional historical information is required?

A. *YES.* It is important to identify gastrointestinal bleeding, which can result from the consumption of whole milk in an infant under 12 months of age. Stools would be black and tarry. Stool changes are also likely with an intestinal parasitic infection.

B. *YES.* Chemical exposure can occur with fertilizers and weed killers. Tommy may have been exposed because his parents are migrant farm workers. Chemicals as well as some drugs can cause hemolysis and/or bone marrow depression.

C. *NO.* Skin turgor is good and there is no indication of a urinary tract infection.

D. *YES.* Family history is very important because many anemias are hereditary. Sickle cell disease and glucose-6-phosphate dehydrogenase (G6PD) deficiency are most common among African Americans. Thalassemias, though more common among those with Asian and Mediterranean heritage, also occur in African Americans. Mixed heredity is not always indicated on the records or recognizable, so ethnicity should not be assumed. A family history of anemia, drug and toxin exposure, jaundice, gallbladder disease, chronic diseases, and bleeding tendencies should be elicited.

E. *YES.* Fatigue and irritability may be present in moderate or severe iron deficiency, along with pallor and decreased motor development; however, mild iron deficiency is generally asymptomatic.

QUESTION 2. What additional physical findings are helpful for determining the cause of the low HCT and Hb?

A. *NO.* Primitive reflexes are not related to anemia, and most should disappear by 6 months of age.

B. *YES.* Petechiae or purpura are signs of leukemia, aplastic anemia, and hemolytic uremic syndrome.

C. *YES.* Splenomegaly may be present in leukemia, hereditary spherocytosis, liver disease, sickle syndromes, and chronic or recurrent infection.

D. *YES.* Heart murmurs are a common finding in moderate and severe anemia.

QUESTION 3. What initial laboratory tests are required at this time?

A. *YES.* The CBC will allow one to narrow the diagnosis by using the MCV to determine whether the anemia is microcytic, normocytic, or macrocytic. The MCV measures red corpuscle volume. In iron deficiency anemia the erythrocytes will be smaller in size, which is reflected in a low MCV. The white blood cell count and differential can provide information about acute infections (increased immature neutrophils indicate bacterial infection), hemolysis, hemorrhage, or cancer.

B. *NO.* A liver profile provides limited information for diagnosing and differentiating anemia.

C. *YES.* The peripheral blood smear is used to determine cellular iron status and the degree of hemoglobinization. Cells are categorized as hyperchromic, normochromic, and hypochromic (i.e., more to less hemoglobinization). Because of a decrease of cellular hemoglobin content in iron deficiency anemia, the red corpuscles will appear pale or hypochromic. Hemolysis can be identified by finding spherocytes, red cell fragmentation, or sickle forms.

D. *YES.* The reticulocyte count is usually elevated with hemolytic diseases. Reticulocytes are immature red cells; increased circulating reticulocytes indicate rapid red cell production. Increased reticulocytes are expected in response to iron therapy in the treatment of iron deficiency anemia.

**QUESTION 4.** If laboratory results indicate a low MCV and normal reticulocyte count, what is the next step, considering the history and physical findings?

A. *NO.* The reticulocyte count would be elevated with blood loss.

B. *NO.* Qualitative or quantitative abnormalities in platelets are related to bleeding disorders.

C. *YES.* Iron deficiency is the most common cause of microcytic anemia between 6 and 24 months of age. The normal reticulocyte count rules out hemolytic anemia. The history of whole milk ingestion for the past 2 months, negative family history for inherited conditions such as thalassemia, and normal physical findings except for pale mucosa and conjunctivae support nutritional-related iron deficiency.

D. *YES.* Nutritional counseling is required. Iron-fortified formula should replace cow's milk, and intake should be limited to 26 oz in 24 h. Iron-fortified cereals and increased solids should be included in Tommy's diet.

**QUESTION 5.** If a course of therapeutic iron is initiated and there is no change in the reticulocyte count within 5 days, what other conditions are potential causes of the decreased MCV?

A. *NO.* The blood lead level was 9 $\mu$g/dL. Tommy should be rescreened at 24 months.

B. *YES.* Thalassemia could present with decreased MCV and normal or decreased reticulocytes.

C. *NO.* Bleeding or hemolysis would result in increased reticulocytes.

D. *YES.* Poor compliance is very likely, because of the cost of iron-fortified formula and the availability of cow's milk. Mrs. C. does not provide all of the child care, and the other mothers may not be giving Tommy the therapeutic iron.

E. *YES.* Chronic inflammatory disease is possible with those laboratory findings. However, your physical findings do not indicate illness.

**QUESTION 6.** A serum Fe, TIBC, and ferritin are ordered to rule out thalassemia and chronic inflammatory disease. Which of the following are supportive of nutritional iron deficiency?

A. *YES.* This is the classic picture of iron deficiency related to nutrition. Serum iron is the concentration of iron bound to transferrin. The TIBC measures the amount of iron that transferrin can still bind. Ferritin is the form of iron stored in the tissues; it is the best indicator of iron stores.

**B.** *NO.* Increased serum iron and ferritin with a normal TIBC indicates thalassemia minor. The blood smear will indicate hypochromia and target cells and possibly basophilic stippling. The diagnosis is supported with hemoglobin electrophoresis findings of decreased Hb $A_1$ (adult) and increased Hb $A_2$, and/or increased Hb F (fetal). In thalassemia major there is marked iron deficiency, with the smear indicating fragmented red cells and many target cells. Serum iron and ferritin are often elevated.
**C.** *NO.* Decreased serum iron and TIBC and increased ferritin are associated with chronic inflammatory disease.
**D.** *NO.* Decreased serum iron and decreased ferritin along with a decreased TIBC would not be a finding. There is an inverse relationship between circulating serum iron and the TIBC, as circulating iron binds to the cell when possible.

**QUESTION 7.** The plan should include which of the following?
**A.** *NO.* The correct dosage of elemental iron is 4 to 6 mg/kg per day in three divided doses. It should not be given with meals because food interferes with absorption. Rather, it should be given with orange juice, as this increases absorption.
**B.** *YES.* Tommy should have iron-fortified formula until he is 12 months of age.
**C.** *YES.* The Hb should be checked after 1 month of treatment to see if the level has returned to normal.
**D.** *YES.* Iron therapy should continue for 2 additional months. The life of an erythrocyte is 90 days; therefore, it will take 3 months of treatment before the body's iron stores are returned to normal.
**E.** *YES.* Further nutritional counseling may increase compliance with nutritional recommendations. WIC can also provide the iron-fortified formula and cereal.

## REFERENCES

Lane, P., Nuss, R., Ambruso, D. (1997). Hematologic disorders. In W. Hay, J. Groothuis, A. Hayward, M. Levin (eds.), *Current Pediatric Diagnosis and Treatment*, 13th ed., 732–780. Stamford, CT: Appleton & Lange.

Swartz, M. (1996). Hematological diseases. In C. E. Burns, N. Barber, M. A. Brady, A. M. Dunn (eds.), *Pediatric Primary Care: A Handbook for Nurse Practitioners*, 529–549. Philadelphia: W. B. Saunders.

U.S. Department of Health and Human Services. Centers for Disease Control and Prevention (February, 1997). *Screening Young Children for Lead Poisoning: Guidance for State and Local Public Health Officials* (Draft). Washington, D.C.

# 4

# Lead Exposure

*Ann M. McCormick*
*Marie L. Talashek*

Tatiana J., an 18-month-old African American girl, has been seen episodically at the clinic for illness visits. She has never been seen for routine well-child care. However, records show that she is up to date with her immunizations, having received them from mobile immunization vans sponsored by the city. Tatiana is covered by Medicaid. She is accompanied by her father.

## CHIEF COMPLAINT

"The school sent us here because Tatiana's brother has lead poisoning. They say she needs a lead test."

## HISTORY OF PRESENT ILLNESS

During routine lead testing at a Head Start preschool, Tatiana's brother was found to have an elevated lead level. Her father does not know how high the lead level was, but states that his son is not on medication. Her father states that Tatiana has been well. Tatiana has never received lead or hemoglobin testing. She lives with her parents and 4-year-old brother in an inner-city neighborhood.

QUESTION 1. Based on Tatiana's risk factors, what would be the recommended age for her first lead screening?
  A. Six months
  B. One year
  C. Two years
  D. At school entry

**QUESTION 2.** What additional historical information is necessary? (Select all that apply.)
  A. Parents' occupational history
  B. Age of her home and of those homes frequently visited
  C. Folk remedies used by the family
  D. Condition of her home and of those regularly visited
  E. Hobbies of family members

**QUESTION 3.** The most common symptoms of low-level lead poisoning include which of the following?
  A. Gastrointestinal symptoms: abdominal pain, vomiting, decreased appetite, constipation
  B. Neurological symptoms: inattention, irritability, headache, hyperactivity, lethargy
  C. Usually no symptoms are present
  D. Developmental problems: developmental delay, failure to thrive, school problems
  E. Respiratory symptoms: tachypnea, shortness of breath

## PHYSICAL FINDINGS

| | |
|---|---|
| General: | Happy, playful African American toddler. |
| Vital signs: | Height 32 in, weight: 24 lb, head circumference 18½ in. |
| Head, eyes, ears, nose, throat: | Fontanelles closed; pupils equal, round, react to light and accommodate (PERRLA); extraocular movements intact (EOMI), consensual reflex equal bilaterally, red reflex present. Tympanic membranes (TMs) pink, light reflex present, throat pink, 2+ tonsils, no lesions or exudate. No obvious caries. |
| Neck: | Lymph nodes nonpalpable. |
| Lungs: | Clear to auscultation and percussion. |
| Cardiovascular: | $S_1 S_2$ without murmurs or extra sounds, 2+ peripheral pulses. |
| Abdomen: | Soft, nontender, no masses or organomegaly. Normoactive bowel sounds in all four quadrants. |
| Neurological: | 2+ DTRs, cranial nerves II–XII intact, gait age-appropriate. |
| Musculoskeletal: | Muscle strength good and equal bilaterally. Slightly bowlegged. No hip click. Back without scoliosis, tufts, or dimpling. |
| Developmental: | Denver II age-appropriate. |

**QUESTION 4.** In a child with low-level lead poisoning, what are the most common findings on initial physical exam?
  A. Usually no physical findings
  B. Dark lines along the gums
  C. Skin rash
  D. Hyperactivity
  E. Wheezing

**QUESTION 5.** Because of the long-term effects of lead poisoning, special attention should be paid to which system during the physical exam?
  A. Cardiovascular
  B. Neurological
  C. Genitourinary
  D. Musculoskeletal

## ASSESSMENT

Initial assessment is a well child with good growth and development. A week after her checkup, Tatiana's venous lead level result is 22 $\mu$g/dL.

**QUESTION 6.** According to Centers for Disease Control and Prevention (CDC) 1997 guidelines, what is the lowest blood lead level to indicate lead poisoning?
  A. 10 $\mu$g/dL
  B. 20 $\mu$g/dL
  C. 25 $\mu$g/dL
  D. 45 $\mu$g/dL
  E. 70 $\mu$g/dL

## PLAN

Recheck of the blood lead level
Investigation of sources of lead exposure
Schedule for well-child care at age 2

**QUESTION 7.** What are other important considerations for cases like Tatiana's? (Select all that apply.)
  A. Contact the local public health authority.
  B. Assign Tatiana's family to case management.
  C. Check lead screening status during illness episodes.
  D. Conduct parent education.
  E. Notify the CDC.

**QUESTION 8.** When should Tatiana's blood lead level be rechecked?
  A. Immediately
  B. In 2 months
  C. At age 2 years
  D. At school entry

**QUESTION 9.** Besides a recheck of Tatiana's lead level, the plan of care should include which of the following? (Select all that apply.)
  A. Hemoglobin
  B. Investigation of the home environment
  C. Chelation therapy with succimer
  D. Investigation of Tatiana's habits
  E. Nutritional history

QUESTION 10. While laws for protecting children from lead poisoning vary among states and public health authorities, what are all landlords'/homeowners' obligations under current *federal* law?
   A. Landlords may not rent and homeowners may not sell units with peeling lead-based paint to families with children under 6 years of age.
   B. Landlords and homeowners of buildings built before 1978 must disclose any knowledge of the presence of lead-based paint to potential renters/ buyers and give them an informational booklet on lead poisoning.
   C. Landlords and homeowners are required to eliminate all lead-based paint from their property before renting to a new tenant or selling the property.
   D. A landlord is legally responsible for any child who becomes lead poisoned while residing in one of the landlord's units.
   E. It is the buyer's or renter's responsibility to be aware and take precautions to protect his or her children from lead poisoning.

## ANSWERS

QUESTION 1. Based on Tatiana's risk factors, what would be the recommended age for her first lead screening?
   A. *NO.* Six months was the previous recommendation for beginning testing of high-risk children. As a result of low yields, the current recommendation is to begin testing at 1 year for high-risk children. The CDC recommends that public health authorities use local data to choose either universal screening, screening based on housing data, screening based on membership in a high-risk group, or screening based on a questionnaire. The goal of having the state or local public health authority establish its own policy is to decrease the number of low-risk children who are tested and increase the amount of money available for increased screening and follow-up of high-risk children.
   B. *YES.* High-risk children should begin testing at age 1. Although universal screening is no longer recommended, poor children are at increased risk of lead poisoning, and the CDC recommends universal screening for all children in federally funded well-child programs, unless it can be proven that they are not at risk. The NHANES III Phase 2 (1991–1994) showed that 11.2 percent of black children had lead poisoning as compared to 2.3 percent of white children.
   C. *NO.* High-risk children with a normal lead level at age 1 should be retested at age 2. If they test negative (<10 μg/dL), they do not need to be retested yearly. Lead levels peak at 18 months.
   D. *NO.* A high-risk child should be screened at school entry if he or she has never been screened in the past. However, it is recommended that screening begin at age 1 and be repeated at 2 for high-risk children.

QUESTION 2. What additional historical information is necessary?
   A. *YES.* Both the occupations and hobbies of adults in the house can cause lead poisoning.
   B. *YES.* In 1978, use of paint with 0.06 percent or greater of lead by weight was banned for housing. Lead paint is still available for indus-

TABLE 4-1  Traditional Medicines and Folk Remedies
That Increase Risk for Lead Poisoning

| | | | |
|---|---|---|---|
| Azarcon | Greta | Liga | Poying tan |
| Bali goli | Hai ge fen | Mai ge fen | Rueda |
| Coral | Kandu | Pay-loo-ah | X-yoo-fa |
| Ghasard | Kohl | | |

trial use and has, at times, found its way into residential housing. Parents should be questioned as to the source of their paint. Housing built before 1950 is the most dangerous. Lead carbonate was the most significant lead compound used in paint, and housing built before 1950 contained 92 percent of all lead carbonate ever used in paint. After 1950, lead concentrations in paint were much lower. Twenty-seven percent of the housing in the United States was built before 1950. The CDC recommends testing children for lead if 27 percent or more of the housing stock in an area was built before 1950.

   **C.** *YES.* Children may be at risk for lead poisoning from traditional medicines (see Table 4-1), Asian cosmetics, ceramic cookware, and imported food in lead-soldered cans.

   **D.** *YES.* Lead paint is the chief source of lead poisoning in children. Living in or regularly visiting housing built before 1978 that is being remodeled increases the risk for lead poisoning. Any chipping or peeling paint poses risk to children age 6 and under who may ingest the paint flakes. Well-maintained housing does not pose the same risk. Any housing built prior to 1978 will release lead during the remodeling process. This lead can remain airborne for as long as 6 months. As it settles, it can be ingested by small children during their normal hand to mouth activity.

   **E.** *YES.* Both the occupations and hobbies of adults in the house (such as car repair and soldering) can cause lead poisoning.

**QUESTION 3.** The most common symptoms of low-level lead poisoning include which of the following?

   **A.** *NO.* Patients with low levels of lead poisoning are usually asymptomatic. Gastrointestinal symptoms, including abdominal pain, vomiting, decreased appetite, and constipation, are symptoms of high-level lead poisoning. However, even children with lead levels over 70 $\mu$g/dL (the highest category of lead poisoning) may present with no symptoms.

   **B.** *NO.* Neurological symptoms are present only with high-level lead poisoning.

   **C.** *YES.* There are usually no symptoms with low-level lead poisoning.

   **D.** *NO.* Developmental problems will not usually be apparent on an initial screen; however, developmental delay has been found with lead levels as low as 10 $\mu$g/dL. Recent studies have found that these delays persist as long as 10 years after lead poisoning, and so they are presumed to be lifelong effects. The developmental effects can be very subtle. For example, children with a lead level of 10 $\mu$g/dL may have a 5-point drop in IQ scores compared with unpoisoned children.

   **E.** *NO.* There are no respiratory symptoms associated with lead poisoning.

QUESTION 4. In a child with low-level lead poisoning, what are the most common findings on initial physical exam?
  A. *YES.* As with symptoms, there are usually no physical findings in low-level lead poisoning. Children are more likely to have physical findings with lead levels over 70 µg/dL, but even these children may have normal physical findings.
  B. *NO.* Dark lines along the gums (lead lines) are symptoms of high-level lead poisoning.
  C. *NO.* Skin rash is not a symptom of lead poisoning.
  D. *NO.* However, hyperactivity can be a symptom of high-level lead poisoning.
  E. *NO.* Wheezing is not a symptom of lead poisoning.

QUESTION 5. Because of the long-term effects of lead poisoning, special attention should be paid to which system during the physical exam?
  A. *NO.* The primary effect of lead poisoning is not on the cardiovascular system, although lead poisoning is a risk factor for hypertension.
  B. *YES.* Lead poisoning does its greatest damage to a child's neurological system. In low-level lead poisoning, these long-term effects manifest themselves primarily as decreased intelligence and developmental delay.
  C. *NO.* The primary effect of lead poisoning is not on the genitourinary system, although lead poisoning is a risk factor for renal failure.
  D. *NO.* Lead poisoning does not affect the musculoskeletal system. However, lead is stored in the long bones, and these stores can be released into the blood during chelation therapy, sometimes causing the blood lead level to remain unchanged or even to rise. For this reason, chelation is reserved for higher lead levels (over 45 µg/dL).

QUESTION 6. According to CDC 1997 guidelines, what is the lowest blood lead level to indicate lead poisoning?
  A. *YES.* According to the CDC, 10 µg/dL is the lowest blood lead level to indicate lead poisoning. This is considered to be low-level lead poisoning. There is no physiologic need for lead, and therefore there is no "normal" level for lead in the blood. Animal studies have revealed lead to be detrimental at minute levels. Though there has been much research in humans, scientists have been unable to find a threshold below which lead does not produce a negative effect. There are researchers who advocate lowering the threshold for lead poisoning further.
  B. *NO.* At lead levels between 10 µg/dL and 20 µg/dL, management consists of education and investigation of sources of lead poisoning. At 20 µg/dL a complete medical evaluation is also necessary.
  C. *NO.* Prior to 1991, 25 µg/dL was considered to be the lowest blood lead level to indicate lead poisoning. As recently as the 1960s, only children with lead levels above 60 µg/dL were considered to be lead poisoned. As our knowledge of the effects of lead has grown, the lead level defined as toxic has been drastically lowered.
  D. *NO.* A lead level over 45 µg/dL is an urgent situation and should be treated within 48 h. At this level, chelation therapy is usually recommended along with assessment and remediation of the child's environment.

E. *NO.* A lead level of 70 μg/dL or more is considered a medical emergency, usually requiring hospitalization. Medical treatment and assessment and remediation of the environment must begin immediately.

**QUESTION 7.** What are other important considerations for cases like Tatiana's?

A. *YES.* Many local health authorities have lead programs that will do site visits for environmental investigation, send public health nurses out for home visits, assist with follow-up, and advise on complex cases. Housing agencies may help by bringing action against landlords; providing temporary safe, lead-free housing; and providing legal advice. Many services are available for children with developmental delays. It is essential to be knowledgeable about local resources.

B. *YES.* The CDC recommends that any child with a blood lead level ≥20 μg/dL or two levels 15 to 19 μg/dL at least 3 months apart should be in case management. Tatiana's family should be referred to case management so that both children receive consistent follow-up. The best case management programs are composed of multidisciplinary teams including the health care provider, community health nurse, environmental specialist, housing specialist, social services, and the case management coordinator. Case management is typically done by the local health department; however, do not assume that this is the case. Any provider conducting screening must be responsible for follow-up.

C. *YES.* As part of a high-risk group (African American, low-income, inner-city), Tatiana should have received lead testing at age 1. Children who do not keep well-child appointments can be tested when they present for an illness visit. It is estimated that only one-third of high-risk children are tested for lead. In a recent study, only slightly more than half of the members of the American Academy of Pediatrics participating in the study were aware of current guidelines on lead testing.

D. *YES.* Parent education on lead poisoning should begin prenatally and should be part of early childhood visits. Parent education should include the meaning of a lead test, the effect of lead on a developing child, sources of lead poisoning, importance of good nutrition, the timing and frequency of lead tests, and the need to test any other children in the house.

E. *NO.* Reporting requirements vary among state and local health authorities. There is no current obligation to notify the CDC.

**QUESTION 8.** When should Tatiana's blood lead level be rechecked?

A. *NO.* It would be too early to see a reduction in Tatiana's lead level. However, a child with a lead level above 45 μg/dL for whom chelation therapy is being considered should have the lead level rechecked. This is done to prevent initiation of potentially hazardous therapy based on a false positive result. If the initial lead level was performed on capillary blood, any high results should be rechecked using venous blood (see Table 4-2). Because of lead in the environment, capillary lead levels are especially prone to false positive results. This can be avoided with scrupulous attention to technique.

TABLE 4-2 Timetable for Confirming Elevated Capillary
Blood Lead Levels with a Venous Blood Lead Level

| Capillary Lead Level, μg/dL | Venous Lead Level |
|---|---|
| 10–19 | 3 months |
| 20–44 | 1 month–1 week |
| 45–59 | 48 h |
| 60–69 | 24 h |
| >70 | Immediately |

SOURCE: U.S. Department of Health and Human Services. Centers for
Disease Control and Prevention. (November 1997). *Screening Young
Children for Lead Poisoning: Guidance for State and Local Public
Health Officials.* Washington, D.C.

B.  *YES.* The CDC recommends retesting children every 1 to 2 months if
they have lead levels over 15 μg/dL. Children with lead levels greater
than 45 μg/dL should be tested monthly in conjunction with case management and medical treatment.
C.  *NO.* A child with an elevated lead level should be tested every 1 to 2
months. Lead levels should be rechecked at age 2 in high-risk children, but only if their lead level was normal at age 1.
D.  *NO.* A child with an elevated lead level should be tested every 1 to 2
months; however, high-risk children should be tested at school entry if
they have not been previously tested.

QUESTION 9. Besides a recheck of Tatiana's lead level, the plan of care
should include which of the following?
A.  *YES.* Lead poisoning can cause iron deficiency anemia, and iron deficiency anemia can increase both lead absorption and lead toxicity.
Treatment is with iron supplementation in addition to decreasing Tatiana's
lead level.
B.  *YES.* Lead paint is the major cause of lead poisoning. In addition to an
evaluation of the home, other homes where the child spends a lot of
time, day care centers, and schools should be evaluated. Homes built
before 1950 and homes built before 1978 that are being renovated
pose the greatest risk to the child. Chipping or peeling paint is the
primary source of lead poisoning in children. Good housekeeping
decreases the amount of lead in a home. If a child has moved recently,
it is also helpful to evaluate a previous home or homes, especially if no
source of lead poisoning is found in the current environment. Investigation of the occupations and hobbies of all adults in the house and
use of traditional medications and cosmetics is also part of a home
investigation. Water can be a source of lead in the home, as lead can
leach out of water pipes containing lead solder. Letting the taps run for
5 min first thing in the morning is sufficient to remove most of this lead.
Although there are many sources of lead in the environment, it is
important to remember that lead paint is the chief culprit in almost all
cases of childhood lead poisoning.

**C.** *NO.* The American Academy of Pediatrics now recommends chelation therapy for a lead level of 45 μg/dL or when symptomatic. Previous recommendations for chelation of lead levels as low as 25 μg/dL have been changed. There has been no evidence that chelation therapy is beneficial for low levels of lead, and the risk of side effects is great. Succimer is the only oral chelating agent. It is approved for lead levels over 45 μg/dL and can be given on an outpatient basis.

**D.** *YES.* The amount of mouthing activity is a risk factor for lead poisoning, as is pica. Attention should also be paid to the child's play and eating areas. Where is food eaten? What are the child's handwashing habits? Does the child play on the floor, where concentration of lead dust is highest? Lead paint content is high in window wells, a common play area. Does the child play outside a lot, and what is the condition of the exterior of the house? Also, play areas near expressways and major highways have increased lead in the soil as a result of the fallout from leaded gasoline. Lead does not decompose or settle into the ground, but stays in the top 2 or 3 in. Play areas and parks built on landfills may also contain high levels of lead in the soil.

**E.** *YES.* Deficiencies of calcium and iron and a diet high in fat increase lead absorption. More absorption of lead occurs on an empty stomach.

**QUESTION 10.** While laws for protecting children from lead poisoning vary among state and public health authorities, what are all landlords'/homeowners' obligations under current federal law?

**A.** *NO.* Local laws vary, but this is not the current federal law.

**B.** *YES.* This is the current federal law.

**C.** *NO.* This is not the current federal law, and would be cost-prohibitive given that 27 percent of the housing stock in this country was built before 1950.

**D.** *NO.* A landlord who does not disclose the presence of lead-based paint may be held liable, but enforcement varies according to locality.

**E.** *NO.* This is not the law, but it is always a good idea!

## REFERENCES

American Academy of Pediatrics Committee on Drugs. (1995). Treatment guidelines for lead exposure in children. *Pediatrics 96*, 155–160.

Needleman, H. L., Gatsonis, C. A. (1990). Low-level lead exposure and the IQ of children: A meta-analysis of modern studies. *JAMA 263(5)*, 673–678.

Schwartz, J. (1994). Low-level lead exposure and children's IQ: A meta-analysis and search for a threshold. *Environ Res 65*, 42–55.

U.S. Department of Health and Human Services. (1991). *Preventing Lead Poisoning in Young Children.* Washington D.C.

U.S. Department of Health and Human Services. (November 1997). *Screening Young Children for Lead Poisoning: Guidance for State and Local Public Health Officials.* Washington D.C.

U.S. Department of Housing and Urban Development. (1996). *Lead: Requirements for Disclosure of Known Lead-based Paint and/or Lead-based Paint Hazards in Housing; Final Rule.* Washington D.C.

# II

# PRESCHOOL

# Introduction

*Marie L. Talashek*

Primary care providers for preschoolers should facilitate family activities that encourage the development of positive health behaviors that children can continue throughout their lives. Development is not as rapid during this time; rather, children become more adept at activities such as walking, talking, and interacting with others.

The American Academy of Pediatrics recommends annual visits from 3 through 5 years of age. Each visit should include the following:

1. History of health and wellness since the last visit should be taken.
2. A complete physical examination should be given.
3. Height and weight and, beginning at age 3, blood pressure should be graphed.
4. Vision and hearing should be assessed.
5. Immunization status should be brought into compliance with the state's school admission criteria, and diphtheria-pertussis-tetanus (DTP or DTaP), poliovirus (OPV), measles-mumps-rubella (MMR), and varicella zoster virus vaccines should be administered if these have not been given.
6. Screening with purified protein derivative (PPD), urinalysis, and hematocrit or hemoglobin should be done once during this period, and lead screening should be done for all at-risk preschoolers.
7. Anticipatory guidance should be given.
8. Referral for a dental examination is made at the 3-year visit and children need one every 6 months thereafter. Caries are common in the primary teeth of children between 4 and 8 years of age. It is important to intervene early so that children do not lose their primary teeth prematurely, leading to space problems.

According to Erikson, preschool children are in the developmental stage of initiative vs. guilt. Children are naturally inquisitive, imaginative, and enthusiastically busy. Parents should be encouraged to praise children for these characteristics, and to limit punishment to those things that may pose a danger to the child. Children are in the Piagetian preoperational period. Symbolic play with verbal representation is the norm, and preschoolers begin to see more than one aspect of an event as they expand their intellectual abilities.

Anticipatory guidance includes accident prevention, because accidents are the number one cause of death for preschoolers. Neighborhood and home safety should be stressed, keeping in mind the expanding capabilities of the child, in order to prevent falls, drowning, and poisoning. Other safety interventions include practicing responses to a fire alarm and using seat belts. Children can be taught their name, address, and phone number. Teaching good touch/bad touch is also initiated at this stage of development. Nutritional needs are changing, and children need an adequate calorie intake of low-fat nutritious food. Cognitive and psychological growth can be fostered by providing a safe environment and new places and toys for preschoolers to explore, limiting TV, and discouraging aggressive behavior. Talking with and reading to children enhances their language skills. Social interaction with other children is facilitated by visiting friends or attending preschool. Consistent rules and praise for positive behavior will make this a happy and fulfilling period for the family.

The Head Start health promotion case was chosen for this chapter because health supervision of infants and children is the sixth most common visit in primary care settings. Head lice is a common health problem that children may encounter when they first attend school. Dermatitis is a recurrent disease that can be controlled with appropriate intervention and health education. Flu, cold, and allergic rhinitis represent a set of the most common problems seen in ambulatory care settings. It is important to recognize the differences and commonalities of presenting signs and symptoms to determine the appropriate diagnosis and treatment.

## REFERENCES

Burns C., Barber N., Brady, M., Dunn, A. (eds.). (1996). *Pediatric Primary Care: A Handbook for Nurse Practitioners.* Philadelphia: W. B. Saunders.

Centers for Disease Control and Prevention. (1996). Immunization of Adolescents: Recommendations of the Advisory Committee on Immunization Practices, the American Medical Association. *Morbidity Mortality Weekly Report 45,* No. RR-13, pp. 3–9.

Committee on Practice and Ambulatory Medicine. (1995). Recommendations for preventive pediatric health care. *Pediatrics 92*(6), 751.

Erikson, E. (1963). *Childhood and Society.* New York: Norton.

Murray, R., Zentner, J. (1997). *Health Assessment and Promotion Strategies Through the Life Span,* 6th ed. Stamford, CT: Appleton & Lange.

Pulaski, M. A. (1971). *Understanding Piaget: An Introduction to Children's Cognitive Development.* New York: Harper & Row.

U.S. Preventive Services Task Force. (1996). *Guide To Clinical Preventive Services,* 2d ed. Baltimore: Williams & Wilkins.

Woolf, S., Jonas, S., Lawrence, R. (eds.). (1996). *Health Promotion and Disease Prevention in Clinical Practice.* Baltimore: Williams & Wilkins.

# 5

# Health Promotion

*Marie L. Talashek*
*Dorothy Kent*

Dejon B., a 36-month-old African American boy, was brought to the inner-city clinic by his grandmother for a Head Start physical. Since his birth, Dejon has received all health care at the clinic. He was last seen in the clinic 6 months ago with a low-grade fever and diarrhea, which resolved after 3 days, and prior to that at 18 months of age for well-child care. Dejon continues to live with his 20-year-old mother, who is a college student, and his grandmother, who also cares for his 24-month-old cousin during the day. Dejon plays with blocks as the history is taken from Mrs. B.

## CHIEF COMPLAINT

"I have the school form that needs to be filled out. Does Dejon need any shots for preschool?" (See Fig. 5-1 for a sample child health examination form.)

## HISTORY OF PRESENT ILLNESS

Despite his otherwise normal history, Dejon's grandmother is concerned that Dejon has been wetting the bed about once a week. He has been bowel- and bladder-trained during the day for the past 5 months. She also wonders if he is eating enough, as he seems less interested in food than he was at the last visit.

## PAST MEDICAL HISTORY

Dejon's immunization record and blood lead levels are reviewed:

Hepatitis B (Hep B)                    (Birth, 1 month, and 6 months)
Diphtheria-pertussis-tetanus (DTP)     (2 months, 4 months,
                                        6 months, and 18 months)

H. Serv. 101 — (Rev. 9-81)
Com. No. 291

# CERTIFICATE OF CHILD HEALTH EXAMINATION

**CHICAGO PUBLIC SCHOOLS**
Bureau of Medical and
School Health Services

*(Information on this form may be shared with appropriate personnel for health and educational purposes)*

| PUPIL'S NAME | | | | | |
|---|---|---|---|---|---|
| (Please Print or Type) | LAST | FIRST | MIDDLE | I.D. NO. | BIRTHDATE _____ MO. DAY YR. |

SEX ☐ M ☐ F

ADDRESS _____ STREET - CITY - ZIP CODE _____ SCHOOL _____ GRADE LEVEL _____

PARENT OR GUARDIAN _____ PHONE NO. _____ HOME / WORK _____ ADDRESS _____

**IMMUNIZATION:** Please provide the month, day and year for every dose administered. The day and month is required if you cannot determine if the vaccine was given prior to the minimum interval or age.

| Dose | Mo. Day Yr. | Mo. Day Yr. | Mo. Day Yr. | Mo. Day Yr. | Mo. Day Yr. |
|---|---|---|---|---|---|
| | | 1 | 2 | 3 | 4 |
| DIPHTHERIA, PERTUSSIS AND TETANUS (DPT) . . . . . | | | | | |
| DIPHTHERIA AND TETANUS (Td) OR (TD) . . . . . | | | | | |
| ORAL POLIO . . . . . . | | | | | |
| COMBINED MEASLES/MUMPS/ RUBELLA (MMR) . . . . | | | | | |
| COMBINED MEASLES AND RUBELLA (MR) . . . . . | | | | | |
| RUBEOLA (RED MEASLES) LIVE VIRUS VACCINE . . . . | | | | | |
| RUBELLA (3 DAY OR GERMAN MEASLES) . . . . . | | | | | |
| MUMPS . . . . . . . | | | | | |
| *TB SKIN TEST . . . . | RESULTS | | | | |

*Mandated for Child Care Facilities.

1. CLINICAL DIAGNOSIS IS ACCEPTABLE IF VERIFIED BY PHYSICIAN.

MEASLES _____ MONTH _____ DAY _____ YEAR

MUMPS _____ MONTH _____ DAY _____ YEAR

2. LABORATORY CONFIRMATION OF ANY DISEASE IS ACCEPTABLE.

DISEASE _____ MONTH _____ DAY _____ YEAR

LAB RESULT _____

PHYSICIAN'S SIGNATURE _____

**HEALTH PROVIDER SIGNATURE (PHYSICIAN, SCHOOL HEALTH PROFESSIONAL OR HEALTH OFFICIAL) (VERIFYING THAT IMMUNIZATIONS WERE GIVEN)**

SIGNATURE _____ DATE _____

SIGNATURE _____ DATE _____

SIGNATURE _____ DATE _____

## MEDICAL HISTORY

(To be Completed by Parent)

| | |
|---|---|
| CHICKEN POX . . . . . . . | YEAR: |
| SCARLET FEVER/STREP . . . | YEAR: |
| T.B./T.B. CONTACT . . . . | YEAR: |
| CONGENITAL DEFECTS . . . . | |
| DIABETES . . . . . . . | |
| EPILEPSY . . . . . . . | |
| HEART DISEASES . . . . . | |
| FREQUENT EAR INFECTION . . | |
| INJURIES/ACCIDENTS . . . . | YEAR: |
| RESULTS | |
| PERMANENT DISABILITY . . . | YEAR: |
| TYPE | |
| RESULTS | |
| SURGERY (OPERATIONS) . . . | YEAR: |
| TYPE | |
| RESULTS | |
| ALLERGIES (LIST) | |

ROUTINE MEDICATIONS (LIST) _____

OTHER _____

PARENT'S SIGNATURE _____ DATE _____

(To be Completed by Physician)

## PHYSICAL EXAMINATION

| EVALUATION: | (REQUIRED) | | | | (STRONGLY RECOMMENDED) | | |
|---|---|---|---|---|---|---|---|
| | Normal | Abnormal | Follow-Up — Comment | | Date | Normal | Abnormal Results |
| HEIGHT ____ WEIGHT ____ | | | | HEMOGLOBIN . . . . . | | | |
| SKIN . . . . . . . | | | | HEMATOCRIT . . . . . | | | |
| EYES . . . . . . . | | | | URINALYSIS . . . . . | | | |
| EARS . . . . . . . | | | | LEAD SCREENING . . . | | | |
| NOSE . . . . . . . | | | | SICKLE CELL . . . . . | | | |
| THROAT . . . . . . | | | | MEDICATIONS ____ | | | |
| THROAT/DENTAL . . . | | | | DIET RESTRICTION/NEEDS ____ | | | |
| CARDIOVASCULAR B/P . | | | | SPECIAL EQUIPMENT NEEDED ____ | | | |
| RESPIRATORY . . . . | | | | ALLERGIES ____ | | | |
| GASTROINTESTINAL . . | | | | OTHER ____ | | | |
| GENITO-URINARY . . . | | | | GENERAL COMMENTS ____ | | | |
| NEUROLOGICAL . . . . | | | | | | | |
| MUSCULAR SKELETAL . . | | | | | | | |
| SCOLIOSIS SCREENING . | | | | | | | |
| NUTRITIONAL STATUS . | | | | | | | |
| OTHER | | | | | | | |

ON THE BASIS OF THIS EXAMINATION ON THIS DAY I APPROVE THIS CHILD'S PARTICIPATION IN:

INTERSCHOLASTIC SPORTS ☐ YES ☐ NO
(FOR 1 YEAR)
PHYSICAL EDUCATION ☐ YES ☐ NO

IF NO, PLEASE ATTACH EXPLANATION.

PHYSICIAN'S SIGNATURE ____    DATE ____

ADDRESS ____    TELEPHONE ____

| | PRE-SCHOOL — DURING FIRST YEAR OF ENROLLMENT | | | | | | | | | SCHOOL AGE — DURING SCHOOL YEAR AT REQUIRED GRADE LEVEL | | | | | | | |
|---|---|---|---|---|---|---|---|---|---|---|---|---|---|---|---|---|---|
| DATE | | | | | | | | | | | | | | | | | |
| GRADE | | | | | | | | | | | | | | | | | |
| | R | L | R | L | R | L | R | L | R | L | R | L | R | L | R | L | |
| VISION | | | | | | | | | | | | | | | | | |
| HEARING | | | | | | | | | | | | | | | | | |

CODE
P — Pass
F — Fail
R — Referred

FIGURE 5-1. Certificate of child health examination.

| | |
|---|---|
| *Haemophilus influenzae* type b | (2 months, 4 months, 6 months, and 12 months) |
| Poliovirus (OPV) | (2 months, 4 months, and 18 months) |
| Measles-mumps-rubella (MMR) | (12 months) |
| Blood lead | 6 µg/dL at 12 months and 7 µg/dL at 24 months |

QUESTION 1. What additional historical information is required? (Select all that apply.)
   A. Diet history
   B. Sleep patterns
   C. Play behavior
   D. Language development

## PHYSICAL FINDINGS

All findings in the physical exam are normal. Dejon's height and weight are both in the 50th percentile.

QUESTION 2. Which of the following screening tests should be completed at this visit? (Select all that apply.)
   A. Tuberculin test
   B. Hematocrit or hemoglobin
   C. Blood lead level
   D. Urinalysis (dipstick)
   E. Complete blood count

QUESTION 3. Which of the following immunizations is recommended at this time?
   A. DTP
   B. OPV
   C. MMR
   D. Varicella virus

QUESTION 4. All of the following are reported by Dejon's grandmother. Which one is potentially related to preschool adjustment problems?
   A. Sleeps 10 h a night with one nap during the day.
   B. Separates from mother or grandmother with some apprehension.
   C. Distorts reality with make-believe.
   D. Unable to pronounce some consonants.
   E. Often becomes angry and hits his cousin.

QUESTION 5. What is the management for the enuresis?
   A. Explain that bed wetting is usually not considered a problem until the age of 6.
   B. Initiate pharmacologic therapy.
   C. Initiate a Sleep Dry Program.
   D. Rule out urinary tract infection and diabetes.

QUESTION **6.** What nutritional guidance should be provided to the grand-mother? (Select all that apply.)
A. A copy of the Food Guide Pyramid.
B. Caloric needs are less because Dejon is growing less at this time than he was as an infant.
C. Appetites do not remain constant during the preschool years.
D. Eating should not become a "battle of wills" between Dejon and his mother and grandmother.

## ANSWERS

QUESTION **1.** What additional historical information is required?
A. *YES.* The diet history is an integral part of well-child care. A 24-h diet recall should be done, along with questions about vitamins, fluoride, and iron supplements. The recall should include amount and type of solids and liquids. The food preferences of the child should also be considered. Additionally, it is important to assess family eating patterns. Some families eat together at the table, whereas others watch television or individuals may eat alone when they are hungry. Some social atmospheres are more conducive to eating than others.
B. *YES.* Number of hours of sleep, including night and naps, and whether the child sleeps through the night is important information for evaluating adequacy of sleep. It is also helpful to know if the child can return to sleep alone after awakening during the night.
C. *YES.* Play is assessed because it is the way children practice developmental skills. Play is the work of childhood. Knowledge of the child's ability to sit and pay attention for short periods of time and patterns of interactions with peers will help with the assessment of school readiness.
D. *YES.* Language development is an important developmental parameter. Oral-motor development, the auditory ability to perceive sentences and words, the cognitive ability to understand the meaning and context of the words, and the motivation to use language are prerequisite to language development.

QUESTION **2.** Which of the following screening tests should be completed at this visit?
A. *YES.* A tuberculin test is usually required for entry into school, including preschool and Head Start programs. Antigen skin testing using the standardized dose of purified protein derivative (PPD) is recommended. The Mantoux intracutaneous injection is recommended because it has 99 percent specificity for detecting active tuberculosis cases. The multiple puncture preparations are not recommended, as they have as low as 90 percent specificity.
B. *YES.* Either hematocrit or hemoglobin screening for anemia is recommended.
C. *YES.* Children at risk should have initial screening for blood lead between 9 and 12 months of age. Screening should also include questions to identify environmental risk. Children who live near highways and in

older neighborhoods with lead paint are at risk. If the blood lead level is less than 10 μg/dL and high-risk exposures are not identified, further screening is not required. Dejon lives in the inner city, where the potential for lead exposure is high; therefore he should be rescreened annually.

D. *YES*. A dipstick urinalysis is recommended during the early childhood period. This is often done during health screening for school admission. A dipstick urinalysis is a quick and relatively inexpensive test to measure pH, sugar, protein, ketones, and hemoglobin. Abnormal findings need to be further investigated.

E. *NO*. A complete blood count is not needed unless the hematocrit or hemoglobin is abnormal.

QUESTION 3. Which one of the following immunizations is recommended at this time?

A. *NO*. The fifth dose of DTP is not needed until between 4 and 6 years of age. Either DTP or DTaP vaccine can be used at that time. DTaP is diphtheria and tetanus toxoid with acellular pertussis vaccine and is licensed for the fifth and sixth dose if the child is more than 15 months of age.

B. *NO*. The fourth dose of OPV is not due until between 4 and 6 years of age.

C. *NO*. The second dose of MMR can be given between 4 and 6 years of age or at age 11 or 12 years.

D. *YES*. It is recommended that varicella virus vaccine be given any time after 12 months of age. Dejon should be immunized because he will be attending preschool and will likely be exposed to varicella (chicken pox). Chicken pox is usually a self-limiting illness. However, one in 1000 children experiences encephalitis, and children who scratch the lesions may become infected with staphylococci or group A ß-hemolytic streptococci. There are other, less common problems associated with varicella. Thus, this is a recommended vaccination (see Table 5-1 for the CDC Immunization Guidelines).

QUESTION 4. Which one of the following is potentially related to preschool adjustment problems?

A. *NO*. Dejon is like most 3-year-olds, who require 10 to 12 h of sleep a night and one nap during the day.

B. *NO*. Dejon is like most 3-year-olds, who may still be hesitant to separate from significant others. Attending the Head Start program will allow Dejon to be away from home in a place where he can feel safe. One of the strengths of this type of program is that it socializes children into the routine of school.

C. *NO*. Dejon's distortion of reality with make-believe is common. Children of this age enjoy pretending and learn through trying numerous activities. Because they have limited experience, their explanations of events are often incorrect. Magical thinking is rare after 5 years of age because previous experiences allow for a frame of reference based in reality.

D. *NO*. Dejon's problem with *r* and *l* sounds is common in 3-year-olds. Sentence structure is not perfect in this age group, but 90 percent of speech is usually intelligible. School will provide an opportunity for Dejon to reinforce correct sentence structure by hearing stories and conversing with teachers.

**E.** *YES.* Anger and hitting may be related to school adjustment problems. These behaviors are unacceptable in the school setting, and a child may be removed from preschool until he has gained the social skills required for playing with other children. Dejon needs consistent limit setting and should never be allowed to hit or bite. Physical punishment will aggravate the behavior. Appropriate time out and play time alone can be effective. It is also important for him to be successful in his play activities. He should get lots of approval from his mother and grandmother when he behaves appropriately.

**QUESTION 5.** What is the management for the enuresis?

**A.** *YES.* Bed wetting (nocturnal enuresis) is not considered a problem until after the age of 6 years. Dejon is progressing very well with toilet training, as he has only occasional nocturnal enuresis. His mother and grandmother may want to use a diaper at night; however, children often refuse to be diapered, as they no longer consider themselves to be "babies."

**B.** *NO.* Imipramine (Tofranil) should not be used in children under the age of 6 years because it interferes with sleep patterns and has an antidepressant effect. However, it may be used to treat older children because of its anticholinergic effects of urinary retention and delayed micturation. Desmopressin acetate (DDAVP) may be effective used alone or adjunctive to nonpharmacological interventions for nocturnal enuresis in children over 6 years of age. Approximately 50 percent of children have a remission. It is administered as a nasal spray, and patients should be monitored for fluid and electrolyte balance. Nasal burning, rhinitis, and gastric irritation may also occur from using nasal sprays.

**C.** *NO.* Sleep Dry Programs are based on behavior modification. A buzzer or bell goes off, waking the child, when urination begins; wetness sets off the alarm. Research has shown that bed-wetting alarm systems demonstrate longer-term effectiveness than does drug therapy. There is no reason to initiate this program in children less than 5 or 6 years of age.

**D.** *NO.* The history and dipstick urinalysis do not indicate the need for a workup of diabetes mellitus, diabetes insipidus, or urinary tract infection at this time.

**QUESTION 6.** What nutritional guidance should be provided to the grandmother?

**A.** *YES.* The Food Guide Pyramid designed by the Department of Agriculture provides a guide to daily food choices (see Fig. 5-2 for the Food Guide Pyramid). These recommendations provide a diet that is low in fat and high in fiber and nutrients. This pattern of eating should be followed throughout life. A serving for a preschooler is approximately 1 tablespoon for each year of age or about one-fourth to one-third of an adult serving.

TABLE 5-1  Recommended Childhood Immunization Schedule. United States, January–December 1997

*Vaccines^a are listed under the routinely recommended ages. ⃞Bars⃞ indicate range of acceptable ages for vaccination. ▨Shaded bars▨ indicate catch-up vaccination: at 11-12 years of age, Hepatitis B vaccine should be administered to children not previously vaccinated, and Varicella Virus vaccine should be administered to unvaccinated children who lack a reliable history of chickenpox.*

| Age ▶ / Vaccine ▼ | Birth | 1 month | 2 months | 4 months | 6 months | 12 months | 15 months | 18 months | 4-6 years | 11-12 years | 14-16 years |
|---|---|---|---|---|---|---|---|---|---|---|---|
| Hepatitis B^{b,c} | Hep B-1 | | Hep B-2 | | Hep B-3 | | | | | Hep B^c | |
| Diphtheria, Tetanus, Pertussis^d | | | DTaP or DTP | DTaP or DTP | DTaP or DTP | | DTaP or DTP^d | | DTaP or DTP | Td | |
| H. influenzae type b^e | | | Hib | Hib | Hib^e | Hib^e | | | | | |
| Polio^f | | | Polio^f | Polio | Polio^f | | Polio^f | | Polio | | |
| Measles, Mumps, Rubella^g | | | | | | MMR | | | MMR^g | or MMR^g | |
| Varicella^h | | | | | | Var | | | | Var^h | |

^a This schedule indicates the recommended age for routine administration of currently licensed childhood vaccines. Some combination vaccines are available and may be used whenever administration of all components of the vaccine is indicated. Providers should consult the manufacturers' package inserts for detailed recommendations.

b_Infants born to **HBsAg-negative mothers**_ should receive 2.5 µg of Merck vaccine (Recombivax HB®) or 10 µg of SmithKline Beecham (SB) vaccine (Engerix-B®). The 2nd dose should be administered ≥1 mo after the 1st dose.
_Infants born to **HBsAg-positive mothers**_ should receive 0.5 mL hepatitis B immune globulin (HBIG) within 12 hrs of birth, and either 5 µg of Merck vaccine (Recombivax HB®) or 10 µg of SB vaccine (Engerix-B®) at a separate site. The 2nd dose is recommended at 1-2 mos of age and the 3rd dose at 6 mos of age.
_Infants born to mothers whose **HBsAg status is unknown**_ should receive either 5 µg of Merck vaccine (Recombivax HB®) or 10 µg of SB vaccine (Engerix-B®) within 12 hrs of birth. The 2nd dose of vaccine is recommended at 1 mo of age and the 3rd dose at 6 mos of age. Blood should be drawn at the time of delivery to determine the mother's HBsAg status; if it is positive, the infant should receive HBIG as soon as possible (no later than 1 wk of age). The dosage and timing of subsequent vaccine doses should be based upon the mother's HBsAg status.

cChildren and adolescents who have not been vaccinated against hepatitis B in infancy may begin the series during any childhood visit. Those who have not previously received 3 doses of hepatitis B vaccine should initiate or complete the series during the 11-12 year-old visit. The 2nd dose should be administered at least 1 mo after the 1st dose, and the 3rd dose should be administered at least 4 mos after the 1st dose, and at least 2 mos after the 2nd dose.

dDTaP (diphtheria and tetanus toxoids and acellular pertussis vaccine) is the preferred vaccine for all doses in the vaccination series, including completion of the series in children who have received ≥1 dose of whole-cell DTP vaccine. Whole-cell DTP is an acceptable alternative to DTaP. The 4th dose of DTaP may be administered as early as 12 mos of age, provided 6 mos have elapsed since the 3rd dose, and if the child is considered unlikely to return at 15-18 mos of age. Td (tetanus and diphtheria toxoids, adsorbed, for adult use) is recommended at 11-12 yrs of age if at least 5 yrs have elapsed since the last dose of DTP, DTaP, or DT. Subsequent _routine_ Td boosters are recommended every 10 yrs.

eThree _H. influenzae_ type b (Hib) conjugate vaccines are licensed for infant use. If PRP-OMP (PedvaxHIB® [Merck]) is administered at 2 and 4 mos of age, a dose at 6 mos is not required. After completing the primary series, any Hib conjugate vaccine may be used as a booster.

fTwo poliovirus vaccines are currently licensed in the US: inactivated poliovirus vaccine (IPV) and oral poliovirus vaccine (OPV). The following schedules are all acceptable by the ACIP, the AAP, and the AAFP, and parents and providers may choose among them:
  1. IPV at 2 and 4 mos; OPV at 12-18 mos and 4-6 yrs
  2. IPV at 2, 4, 12-18 mos, and 4-6 yrs
  3. OPV at 2, 4, 6-18 mos, and 4-6 yrs

The ACIP routinely recommends schedule 1. IPV is the only poliovirus vaccine recommended for immunocompromised persons and their household contacts.

gThe 2nd dose of MMR is routinely recommended at 4-6 yrs of age or at 11-12 yrs of age, but may be administered during any visit, provided at least 1 mo has elapsed since receipt of the 1st dose, and that both doses are administered at or after 12 mos of age.

hSusceptible children may receive Varicella vaccine (Var) during any visit after the 1st birthday, and unvaccinated persons who lack a reliable history of chickenpox should be vaccinated during the 11-12 year-old visit. Susceptible persons ≥13 yrs of age should receive 2 doses, at least 1 mo apart.

_Note:_ Approved by the Advisory Committee on Immunization Practices (ACIP), the American Academy of Pediatrics (AAP), and the American Academy of Family Physicians (AAFP).

SOURCE: American Academy of Pediatrics, Committee on Infectious Diseases. (1997). Recommended childhood immunization schedule—United States. _Pediatrics 99_, 136-138.

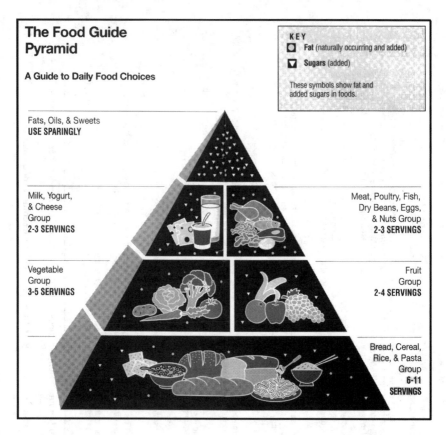

**FIGURE 5-2.**    The Food Guide Pyramid. [U.S. Department of Agriculture. (1992). *The Food Guide Pyramid*, Home and Garden Bulletin No. 252. Washington, D.C.]

B.  *NO.* Dejon's growth has slowed. However, his body mass is larger, and thus increased calories are required to meet body mass needs and energy expenditure. A 3-year-old requires 102 kcal/kg per day.

C.  *YES.* Appetites vary in this age group; small amounts of food should be offered during the day. Children may not want to sit down, so finger foods may be more acceptable. Good choices include a variety of fresh fruits and vegetables. It is important that children not fill up on juice or milk. After age 2, milk should be changed to 1 percent to assure a low fat intake, and bottles should no longer be used. This practice will also prevent tooth decay.

D.  *YES.* Eating should be a pleasurable event, and forcing a child to eat just does not work. Children should be allowed some say in what they eat, and parents should provide a variety of foods so that nutritional requirements are met. The child can be included in food preparation; children love to be helpful, and involvement can also encourage an interest in trying new foods. The TV may need to be turned off, as preschoolers are easily distracted.

# REFERENCES

Boynton, R., Dunn, E., Stephens, G. (1994). *Manual of Ambulatory Pediatrics*, 3d ed. Philadelphia: J. B. Lippincott.

Burns, C., Barber, N., Brady, M., Dunn, A. (eds.). (1996). *Pediatric Primary Care: A Handbook for Nurse Practitioners.* Philadelphia: W. B. Saunders.

Centers for Disease Control and Prevention. (1996). Immunization of adolescents: Recommendations of the Advisory Committee on Immunization Practices. *Morbidity Mortality Weekly Report 45*, No. RR-13, pp. 3–9.

Monda, J., Husmann, D. (1995). Primary nocturnal enuresis: A comparison among observation, imipramine, desmopressin acetate and bed-wetting alarm systems. *J Urol 154*(2), 745–748.

Overview of well child care. (1989). In M. Avery, L. First (eds.), *Pediatric Medicine*, 1–29. Baltimore: Williams & Wilkins.

Smellie, J., McGrigor, V., Rose, S., Douglas, M. (1996). Nocturnal enuresis: A placebo controlled trial for two antidepressant drugs. *Arch Dis Child 75*(1), 62–66.

U.S. Department of Agriculture. *The Food Guide Pyramid.* Home and Garden Bull. No. 252. Hyattsville, MD: Human Nutrition Information Service, 1992. Order from Food and Drug Administration (product FDA93-2259), Information and Outreach Staff, HFE-88, Room 16-63, 5600 Fisher Lane, Rockville, MD 29857, 301-443-3170.

# 6

# Dermatitis

*Marlene G. Smith*
*Arlene Miller*

Nicole W., aged 4, is brought to the office by her mother for a recurring rash. She has received all her health care at this clinic since birth, and was last seen 3 months ago at her annual 4-year-old well-child visit. At that time there were no concerns or complaints. Nicole is cooperative during the exam. Although she appears to be in some general discomfort, she is in no acute distress.

## CHIEF COMPLAINT

"Her rash came back 3 weeks ago and is getting worse, even though we are using ointment."

## HISTORY OF PRESENT ILLNESS

Three weeks ago the antecubital fossae of Nicole's arms became increasingly red and itchy. In addition, the rash was present on the dorsal aspect of her lower legs near her ankles. There was no pus or oozing, but scabs have formed where Nicole has scratched herself repeatedly. Her mother has been applying hydrocortisone 1% ointment to the area twice a day with some, but not complete, improvement.

QUESTION 1. What additional information is needed to complete the history? (Select all that apply.)
   A. Similar symptoms in family members and/or friends
   B. Changes in detergents, lotions, or soaps
   C. Travel outside of her usual community
   D. Vomiting and diarrhea
   E. Symptoms of upper and lower respiratory involvement

## PAST MEDICAL HISTORY

The rash was first noted when, at 2 months of age, Nicole experienced an episode of oozing crusts on an erythematous base on her forehead and cheeks

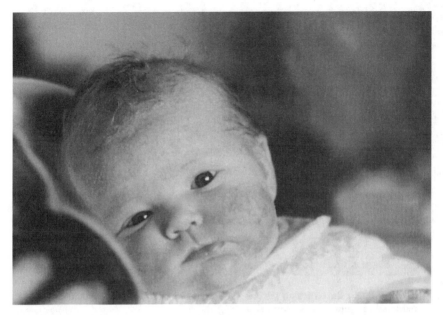

FIGURE 6-1.   Infantile eczema (see Color Plate 2). (M. L. Talashek, personal photograph, January 1997.)

(Fig. 6-1). This was diagnosed as infantile eczema and resolved within 2 weeks after treatment with topical corticosteroids. Since then she has had occasional recurrences once or twice a year. By 2 years of age the rash developed in the antecubital fossae of both arms, but it did not recur on the face. Allergy skin testing done 1 year ago revealed sensitivity to wool, cats, and dust mites. Currently, Nicole is developmentally on schedule and is up to date with her immunizations. Nicole eats a well-balanced diet, selecting foods from all food groups. She lives with her parents and 6-year-old brother in a moderate-sized suburb of a large, Midwest city and attends preschool twice a week.

## PHYSICAL FINDINGS

General:   A well-developed child in moderate discomfort who is trying hard not to scratch her arms and legs.

Skin:   Erythematous, papular rash in early stage of healing, in bilateral antecubital fossae and on dorsal aspect of her lower legs near ankles (Fig. 6-2).

Head, eyes, ears, nose, throat:   External and internal ears are clear; conjunctiva are clear; nasal turbinates are pale and boggy with some clear discharge; throat is clear, without redness or exudate; no lymphadenopathy present.

Lungs:   Clear bilaterally.

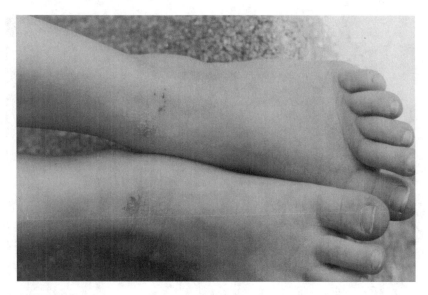

FIGURE 6-2.  Current skin lesions (see Color Plate 3). (M. L. Talashek, personal photograph, September 1997.)

QUESTION 2. Which one of the following best describes the lesions on the lower legs in Fig. 6-2?
A. Erythema, lichenification, and scabs
B. Oozing crusts
C. Pustules and open comedones
D. Hypopigmented patches
E. Delicate scaling areas with skin-colored linear ridges

## ASSESSMENT

Nicole has an exacerbation of atopic dermatitis.

QUESTION 3. Which of the following data are necessary to make the diagnosis of atopic dermatitis?
A. Family history of diabetes mellitus
B. Fine, flesh-colored papular rash on the trunk
C. Itchy skin within the past 12 months
D. Episodes of insomnia

## MANAGEMENT

Nicole is treated with both topical and oral medications.

QUESTION 4. What pharmacologic interventions are used in the management of atopic dermatitis? (Select all that apply.)
A. Oral antibiotics
B. Oral antipruritics

   **C.** Topical antipruritics

   **D.** Topical anti-inflammatories

**QUESTION 5.** Recommended nonpharmacologic interventions include which of the following?

   **A.** Keeping skin well hydrated

   **B.** Eliminating all grain foods from diet

   **C.** Frequent bathing

   **D.** Restrict clothing to synthetic materials

**QUESTION 6.** What is the long-term outlook for those affected with atopic dermatitis?

   **A.** Quick, permanent resolution once treatment is started

   **B.** Slow but permanent resolution after first occurrence

   **C.** Infrequent recurrences, typically after long periods of remission

   **D.** Chronic, frequent exacerbations that may continue until adulthood

## ANSWERS

**QUESTION 1.** What additional information is needed to complete the history?

   **A.** *YES.* The exact pathogenesis of atopic dermatitis is not completely known, but there appears to be a significant genetic predisposition. Two-thirds of patients have family members with hay fever, asthma, food and environmental allergies, or atopic dermatitis. Other nonallergic familial disorders have no bearing on the predisposition for atopic dermatitis. Acute problems that present in a manner similar to the chronic illness may be missed if a complete history is not obtained. Scabies, for example, can mimic the itchy, red rash of atopic dermatitis, but since scabies is contagious, it is likely to be found in family members or playmates also.

   **B.** *YES.* "Allergic skin" is sensitive to irritating substances, such as lotions, soaps, or detergents, which can cause a flare-up in atopic dermatitis or can represent a localized contact dermatitis from new substances. Other irritants that can be triggers for atopic dermatitis in susceptible individuals include hot baths, warm temperatures, wool, animal contact, perfumes, feathers, plants, smoke, dust, cosmetics, and stress.

   **C.** *YES.* A travel history is important, as it can give a clue to whether the cause of the rash may be a regionally occurring agent. Exposure to new or different elements can also cause an exacerbation in atopic dermatitis.

   **D.** *NO.* Vomiting and diarrhea are not associated with atopic dermatitis. If they are present, further assessment for a causative agent is necessary.

   **E.** *YES.* Asthma, allergic rhinitis (itchy, watery eyes and sneezing), and atopic dermatitis make up the triad of "atopic" disorders that are genetically based and have a hypersensitive or allergic component.

**QUESTION 2.** Which one of the following best describes the lesions on the lower legs in Fig. 6-2?

   **A.** *YES.* Atopic dermatitis often presents with the skin changes of erythema, lichenification, and scabs as a result of prolonged scratching from chronic itching.

B. *NO*. Oozing crusts may be present, but this usually represents a secondary infection such as impetigo.
C. *NO*. Pustules and open comedones are manifestations of acne vulgaris.
D. *NO*. Hypopigmentation can occur as a postinflammatory response, but it is not present here.
E. *NO*. Scaling skin with linear ridges can be found in psoriasis.

QUESTION 3. Which of the following data are necessary to make the diagnosis of atopic dermatitis?
A. *NO*. Atopic dermatitis is an allergic familial disorder, and there is a genetic link between atopic dermatitis, asthma, and other allergic disorders. Other genetically based disorders have no relationship to atopic dermatitis.
B. *NO*. Fine, flesh-colored papules often represent the scarlatina rash of group A beta-hemolytic *streptococci* pharyngitis.
C. *YES*. See Table 6-1, a list of diagnostic minimal criteria for atopic dermatitis.
D. *NO*. Though itching skin may keep the patient awake, atopic dermatitis is not related to true insomnia or early wakening.

QUESTION 4. What pharmacologic interventions are used in the management of atopic dermatitis?
A. *NO*. Unless there is a secondary skin infection, oral or topical antibiotics are not beneficial for the management of atopic dermatitis.
B. *YES*. Because of the pruritic and allergic components of atopic dermatitis, antipruritics can be helpful. Diphenhydramine hydrochloride (Benadryl) can be given at a dose of 1.25 mg/kg P.O. every 4 to 6 h as needed. Hydroxyzine hydrochloride (Atarax, Vistaril), 50 mg daily p.r.n. in divided doses q.i.d. can be given to children under 6 years old, and for adults and children over 6 years 50 to 100 mg daily divided q.i.d. p.r.n. are commonly used. Both act as antihistamines by competing with histamine for cell receptor sites on effector cells. This prevents histamine access, which then restricts histamine-induced allergic symptoms. Both drugs have anticholinergic properties that lead to the common side effects of sedation and dry mouth.

**Table 6-1   Minimal Criteria for Diagnosis of Atopic Dermatitis**[a]

Itchy skin must be present within the past 12 months, plus three or more of the following:
  Rash involvement of skin creases
  Personal history of asthma or allergic rhinitis[b]
  History of generalized skin dryness in the past year
  Flexural dermatitis on exam
  Onset before the age of 2[c]

[a]Developed by H. Williams (1996), based on Hanifin and Rajka criteria. With permission.
[b]In children less than 4 years old, history of atopic disease in a first-degree relative.
[c]Not used in children less than 4 years old.

**Table 6-2  Commonly Used Topical Corticosteroid Preparations Based on Vasoconstrictive Activity (not an exhaustive list)**

| |
|---|
| Low Potency |
|   Hydrocortisone 0.5%, 1%, and 2.5% cream, lotion, ointment (Hytone, Cortaid, Nutracort) |
|   Dexamethasone 0.1% gel, ointment (Decadron) |
| Moderate Potency |
|   Triamcinolone acetonide 0.1% cream, ointment, lotion (Kenalog, Aristocort) |
|   Betamethasone valerate 0.1% cream (Valisone) |
| High Potency |
|   Desoximetasone 0.25% cream, ointment (Topicort) |
|   Fluocinonide 0.05% cream, gel, lotion, solution (Lidex) |
| Very High Potency |
|   Betamethasone dipropionate 0.05% cream, ointment, solution (Diprolene) |

C. *NO.* Topical antipruritics have not been shown to be helpful in reducing the pruritic effects of atopic dermatitis. Since these medications are often drying (e.g., calamine, Burow's solution), they can exacerbate the dry skin component of atopic dermatitis.

D. *YES.* Topical anti-inflammatories are the mainstay of atopic dermatitis management. Pharmacologically classified as glucocorticoids, these agents increase enzyme synthesis needed to decrease the inflammatory response. Inflammation is reduced by the steroids' action of vasoconstriction, stabilizing lysosomal membranes, and decreasing the amount of polymorphonuclear leukocytes and monocytes in the inflammatory infiltrate. Hydrocortisone, a corticosteroid secreted by the adrenal cortex, is most commonly used. Drug choice is based on using the lowest level of potency that provides a therapeutic effect. Low-potency drugs (e.g., hydrocortisone ½ to 1%) should be used on delicate skin such as the face, eyelids, axilla, diaper area, and groin, as these areas have greater penetration and absorption rates. Thicker, lichenificated skin may need a higher-potency, fluorinated corticosteroid such as triamcinolone. Cortisone in an ointment base is absorbed more effectively and is generally recommended for areas of thicker skin. Creams and lotions are indicated for hairy areas such as the scalp. All preparations should be applied in a thin film b.i.d. for no more than 2 weeks at a time (see Table 6-2).

**QUESTION 5.** Recommended nonpharmacologic interventions include which of the following?

A. *YES.* Because atopic dermatitis is essentially a superdry skin condition, well-hydrated skin will be less symptomatic. The goal of skin hydration is to replace the moisture in the stratum corneum and decrease loss of transdermal water. Baths of 15 to 20 min are necessary to hydrate the skin. After bathing, skin should be patted dry, not rubbed, as this can be irritating. An emollient cream should be applied over the damp skin within 3 min of the bath to trap in moisture. A thick cream, without perfume or coloring, holds moisture better than a lotion. Emollients that contain lanolin should be avoided because of the frequency of wool allergy or sensitivity with atopic dermatitis. An inexpensive cream that is readily available is solid vegetable shortening. Apply cream at least b.i.d. In humid or tropical climates, less frequent use may be necessary. Cream can be applied over cortisone to increase absorption of the medication. Increasing room humidity may also aid in skin hydration.

**B.** *NO.* Eliminating food needs to be done only if a specific allergy is found. Wheat is the most common grain allergy for the atopic dermatitis patient.

**C.** *NO.* Frequent bathing (more than once a day) is not recommended because of its drying effect. Water should be lukewarm, as hot water has a greater drying effect. Soaps can also be drying. Superfatted or nondrying soaps such as Dove are the best. Prolonged exposure to chemically treated water, such as in a swimming pool, may also exacerbate the skin condition.

**D.** *NO.* Natural fibers, with the exception of wool, are less irritating to atopic dermatitis skin. Soft cotton and linen clothes are best.

**QUESTION 6.** What is the long-term outlook for those affected with atopic dermatitis?

**A.** *NO.* Though some respond quickly to treatment, it is more common for resolution to take several weeks.

**B.** *NO.* Atopic dermatitis is a disorder with frequent recurrences. Complete resolution may not occur for years.

**C.** *NO.* Periods between recurrences can be short, and recurrences frequent.

**D.** *YES.* Atopic dermatitis is a chronic disorder for which there is no cure. It is characterized by periods of exacerbation and remission. In severe cases, skin may never be totally symptom free. Spontaneous resolution occurs in 40 percent of infants by age 5. Overall, a 40 to 50 percent recovery rate by 15 years of age has been reported. Those who do not experience a total resolution often have a decrease in severity by that age. Though less common, the onset of atopic dermatitis has been noted during adolescence and adulthood.

## REFERENCES

Krowchuk, D. (1987). Practical aspects of the diagnosis and management of atopic dermatitis. *Pediatric Ann 16*(1), 57–66.

Priff, N. (ed.). (1996). *Nurse practitioner's drug handbook.* Springhouse, PA: Springhouse Corporation.

Romeo, S. (1995). Atopic dermatitis: The itch that rashes. *Pediatric Nursing 21*, 157–163.

Williams, H. (1996). Diagnostic criteria for atopic dermatitis. *Lancet 348*, 1391–1392.

# 7

# Head Lice

*Lorrita Verhey*
*Arlene Miller*

Patti S. was brought to the health center by her mother. Her immunization record is up to date, with no history of adverse reactions reported. Patti was last seen 6 months ago for a preschool physical exam. At that time, her exam revealed a heathy 4-year-old with normal growth and development and good hygiene.

## CHIEF COMPLAINT

"For the past week and a half, Patti has been scratching the back of her head."

## HISTORY OF PRESENT ILLNESS

Patti had a haircut approximately 1 month ago, at which time no abnormal scalp problems were noted. She has no personal or family history of eczema or allergies. She takes no routine p.r.n. medications. Patti attends preschool in a suburban setting and plays well with her classmates. Approximately 10 days ago, her mother noticed her vigorously scratching the back of her head, sometimes leaving redness that lasted several hours. She has not had similar episodes in the past.

QUESTION 1. Important additional information might include which of the following? (Select all that apply.)
   A. Fitful sleep
   B. Similar problems in any of Patti's playmates at home or at school
   C. Relief measures that have been tried, and their degree of success
   D. Similar itching at other sites on the body

## PHYSICAL FINDINGS

Patti is a well-nourished 4½-year-old girl who is enthusiastic, very active, cooperative, and friendly.

Vital signs:    Temperature 98°F, pulse 88, respirations 22, blood pressure 82/60.

Head:    Symmetric; skin is soft with good turgor; scalp examination reveals no areas of erythema, crusting, papules, pustules, or flaking. On close examination, small grey-white oval spots are seen that seem to be attached to the hair shafts. Along the nape of her neck and behind her left ear, small black specks and excoriations are noted. There are some slightly tender and enlarged superficial nodes along the occipital border of her scalp. No rash is noted on the upper trunk, arms, or face.

QUESTION 2. Which of the following should be considered as a likely diagnosis?
   A. Scabies
   B. Tinea capitis
   C. Pediculosis capitis
   D. Eczema

## ASSESSMENT

Pediculosis capitis.

## PLAN

A plan that includes application of a pediculicide, removing the nits, and cleaning the environment is instituted (see Fig. 7-1).

QUESTION 3. Which of the following is effective for pediculosis capitis? (Select as many as apply.)
   A. Pyrethrins with piperonyl butoxide (RID)
   B. Lindane (Kwell) shampoo
   C. Malathion lotion 0.5%
   D. Hydrocortisone 1%
   E. Permethrin 1% (Nix)

QUESTION 4. Which of the following are appropriate treatment plans regarding the application of shampoo for head lice? (Select all that apply.)
   A. Apply lindane (Kwell) shampoo to dry hair and work in well. After 4 min, rinse hair thoroughly.
   B. After applying permethrin shampoo, comb wet hair with a fine-tooth comb.
   C. Reapply the shampoo within 24 h.
   D. The shampoo should be used also as a body wash to eliminate the likelihood of spread of head lice to the pubic area.

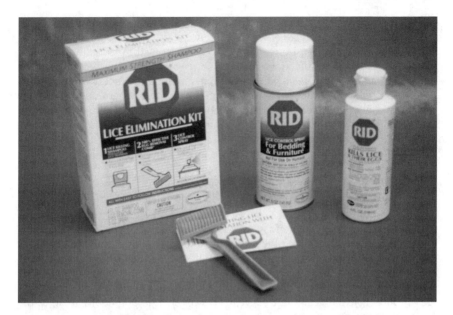

**FIGURE 7-1.** Pediculicide. (RID is a registered trademark of Pfizer Inc.)

**QUESTION 5.** What additional instructions should be given to Mrs. S.? (Select all that apply.)
  A. Instruct Patti *not* to share articles like hats, combs, or hair ornaments.
  B. Rinse combs and brushes in warm water and air-dry.
  C. Wash bed linen and headgear.
  D. Encourage frequent hand washing to remove lice or nits from under her fingernails.
  E. Patti may return to school after one week.

## ANSWERS

**QUESTION 1.** Important additional information might include which of the following?
  A. *YES.* Fitful sleep associated with increased itching during the night would be indicative of scabies.
  B. *YES.* Similar problems in any of Patti's playmates at home or at school would suggest that the condition is contagious. Both pediculosis and scabies are extremely contagious, and are spread through close contact and shared clothing or linen.
  C. *YES.* Relief measures such as dandruff shampoo or medications and their degree of success would be important to establish, to help narrow the differential diagnosis.
  D. *YES.* Similar itching at other sites on the body would be unlikely in pediculosis capitis, and pediculosis corpus is not seen in conjunction with head lice. Scabies lesions are more commonly found on the webs of fingers, folds of wrists, elbows, armpits, or genitalia.

**Question 2.** Which of the following is the most likely diagnosis?
- **A.** *NO.* Scabies lesions are more likely to be found on the body and appear as curving burrows or itchy papules with excoriation, possibly with secondary infection.
- **B.** *NO.* The lesions seen with tinea capitis include red, scaly round lesions and hair loss. Thickened, broken-off hairs with erythema and scaling of the underlying scalp are distinguishing features.
- **C.** *YES.* The mites may be seen as small black specks and may move. Nits (eggs) appear as gray-white oval cases that are attached to the hair shafts when laid by the female louse. Unlike dandruff, they are not flakes and are not be easily shaken out.
- **D.** *NO.* Atopic dermatitis may be present on the face of infants. This would not be the usual finding in children after infancy.

**Question 3.** Which of the following is effective for pediculosis capitis?
- **A.** *YES.* Pyrethrins with piperonyl butoxide (RID) is currently a treatment of choice because of its safety and efficacy. It can be purchased without a prescription (see Fig. 7-1).
- **B.** *YES.* Lindane (Kwell) shampoo kills mites, nits, and ova effectively (85 percent) with a single treatment. However, it is potentially toxic to the nervous system and is contraindicated in infants and during pregnancy. It requires a prescription.
- **C.** *YES.* Although its potential toxicity is still being investigated, malathion lotion 0.5% may be a newer alternative treatment. However, it is flammable and must be used cautiously.
- **D.** *NO.* Hydrocortisone 1% is not a treatment for pediculosis and is not necessary for the excoriations, which will clear up as the infestation and itching are eliminated.
- **E.** *YES.* Permethrin 1% (Nix) is currently a treatment of choice because of its safety and efficacy. It is 99 percent effective with a single treatment in most cases and has a 10-day residual effect. It is available without a prescription.

**Question 4.** Which of the following are appropriate treatment plans regarding the application of shampoo for head lice?
- **A.** *YES.* Apply lindane (Kwell) shampoo to dry hair and work in well. After 4 min, rinse hair thoroughly. A second treatment is usually not necessary for head or body lice, but it should be reapplied in 2 weeks for pubic lice.
- **B.** *YES.* Permethrin is a pediculicide but not an ovacide. Therefore, it is especially important to comb them out.
- **C.** *NO.* A second treatment may be advisable in 2 weeks with permethrin, since it is not an ovacide and nits that are not removed may mature in 7 to 10 days. An alternative second therapy is to apply olive oil to the scalp and hair, because lice may be resistant to a pediculicide. The olive oil will smother remaining lice and facilitate the removal of nits and eggs.
- **D.** *NO.* Pediculosis capitis does not spread to the body or pubic area.

**QUESTION 5.** What additional instructions should be given to Mrs. S.?

**A.** *YES.* The most likely mode of transmission for pediculosis capitis is through sharing articles like hats, combs, or hair ornaments. Lice do not jump from one person to another.

**B.** *NO.* Combs and brushes should be soaked in alcohol (or a pediculicide) for 1 h and rinsed in hot water.

**C.** *YES.* Wash bed linen and headgear and dry in a dryer for at least 20 min, or dry clean. Articles that cannot be cleaned should be stored in a closed plastic bag for 1 month.

**D.** *NO.* Lice and nits are not harbored under fingernails.

**E.** *NO.* Patti may return to school after the initial treatment. A follow-up visit in 10 to 14 days may be helpful to ensure complete resolution of the infestation.

## REFERENCES

Burns, C. E., Barber, N., Brady, M. A., Ardys, M. S. (1996). *Pediatric primary care: A handbook for nurse practitioners.* Philadelphia: W. B. Saunders.

Hay, W. W., Groothuis, J. R., Hayward, A. R., Levin, M. J. (eds.). (1995). *Current pediatric diagnosis and treatment,* 12th ed. Norwalk, CT: Appleton & Lange.

# 8

# Allergic Rhinitis, Common Cold, and Influenza

*Patricia A. Furnace*
*Arlene Miller*

Ramona P., a 4-year-old Latina, is accompanied to a rural health clinic by her mother. Ramona was last seen in the clinic 4 months ago for conjunctivitis, which resolved without sequelae. Her immunizations have been administered at the health department and are up to date. Her height and weight have consistently followed the growth curve at the 75th percentile.

## CHIEF COMPLAINT

"Ramona just doesn't feel good. She hasn't gotten better with Tylenol."

## HISTORY OF PRESENT ILLNESS

Ramona has a 3-day history of rhinorrhea, nasal congestion, sneezing, scratchy throat, and generalized malaise.

QUESTION 1. What information is important to obtain at this time? (Select all that apply.)
A. Similar problem in her family or playmates
B. Frequent upward rubbing of her nose
C. Fever in the past few days
D. Previous history of similar symptoms
E. Color of nasal discharge

## PAST MEDICAL HISTORY

Ramona's past medical history is unremarkable.

QUESTION 2. Which of the following information would help differentiate among allergic rhinitis, common cold, and influenza? (Select all that apply.)
A. Age of the child
B. Family history of allergic problems such as asthma, atopic dermatitis, or seasonal allergies

C. Season of the year, i.e., spring, summer, fall, winter
D. Sex of the child
E. Denver II

## PHYSICAL FINDINGS

Appears ill, sitting quietly in mother's lap

| | |
|---|---|
| Vital signs: | Temperature 99°F, pulse 90, respirations 20. |
| Head: | Normocephalic without tenderness. |
| Eyes: | Pupils equal, round, react to light and accommodate. |
| | Conjunctiva without erythema or exudate. |
| Ears: | Tympanic membranes are pearly gray. Canals are patent without exudate. |
| Nose: | Erythematous, clear rhinorrhea is present. |
| Face: | No discolorations or sinus tenderness. |
| Throat: | Tonsils are 1+, without exudate, erythema, or lesions. |
| Neck: | Supple, nontender. |
| Lungs: | Clear to auscultation and percussion. |
| Cardiovascular: | Regular rate and rhythm without murmur. |
| Abdomen: | Bowel sounds are present. Soft with no masses or areas of tenderness. |

QUESTION 3. What history or physical examination findings would be expected with allergic rhinitis? (Select all that apply.)
A. Dark circles under the eyes
B. Clear rhinorrhea
C. Pale, boggy mucous membranes
D. Edema and erythema of nasal mucus membranes
E. Erythematous, bulging tympanic membranes

QUESTION 4. What history or physical examination findings would be expected with the common cold? (Select all that apply.)
A. Nasal mucosa edema
B. Inspiratory wheezing
C. Sneezing
D. Sudden onset of symptoms
E. Clear nasal discharge

QUESTION 5. What history or physical examination findings would be expected with influenza? (Select all that apply.)
A. Systemic symptoms (myalgia, malaise) overshadow respiratory symptoms (rhinorrhea)
B. Sudden onset of symptoms
C. Erythematous tympanic membranes
D. Cervical lymphadenopathy
E. Dark circles under the eyes

## ASSESSMENT

QUESTION 6. Which of the following would be the most likely diagnosis for this patient?
A. Allergic rhinitis
B. Common cold
C. Influenza
D. Acute otitis media

## PLAN

QUESTION 7. Management of influenza would include which of the following? (Select all that apply.)
A. Education on prevention of influenza
B. Amoxicillin
C. Antipyretics
D. Amantadine
E. Symptomatic treatment (saline gargles, saline nasal spray)

QUESTION 8. Management of the common cold would include which of the following? (Select all that apply.)
A. Topical or oral decongestant
B. Expectorant
C. Antibiotic
D. Education about the transmission of colds
E. Consumption of additional fluids

QUESTION 9. Management of allergic rhinitis would include which of the following? (Select all that apply.)
A. Education regarding allergen avoidance
B. Oral antihistamines/decongestants
C. Cromolyn nasal spray
D. Steroid nasal spray
E. Skin testing/immunotherapy

## ANSWERS

QUESTION 1. What information is important to obtain at this time?
A. *YES.* Acute viral and bacterial infections occur more frequently in close, confined groups.
B. *YES.* Rubbing the nose upward or "allergic salute" is commonly seen in allergic rhinitis.
C. *YES.* Sudden onset of a high fever occurs with influenza. A mild increase in temperature may be seen with the common cold. Usually no fever accompanies allergic rhinitis.
D. *YES.* Recurrence of symptoms is seen with allergic rhinitis, since it is a chronic health problem.
E. *YES.* Nasal discharge is clear with allergic rhinitis and influenza. The common cold produces clear, thin nasal discharge. Bacterial infections or presence of a foreign body produces purulent discharge.

QUESTION 2. Which of the following information would help differentiate among influenza, common cold, and allergic rhinitis?
A. *YES.* The age of the child can help you determine which problem is most likely to occur. The average age of onset of allergic rhinitis in children is 10 years. The common cold is most prevalent in kindergarten children, followed by those of preschool years. School-age children will have approximately seven colds per year. The incidence of the common cold decreases with age. Sequelae from influenza occur most often in the very young and the elderly, especially if they have any coexisting health problems.
B. *YES.* Allergic rhinitis has a strong genetic predisposition. It can be seen in families with a history of other allergic health problems.
C. *YES.* Influenza will usually occur during the winter. The common cold can occur throughout the year. Allergic rhinitis may be either seasonal or perennial. Seasonal allergic rhinitis is associated with trees, grasses, and pollen, which usually cause more symptoms in the spring and fall. Perennial allergic rhinitis is associated with dust mites and mold antigens.
D. *NO.* Allergic rhinitis, common cold, and influenza affect both sexes equally.
E. *NO.* The Denver II is helpful in assessing gross motor, language, fine motor-adaptive, and personal-social development. It will not help in differentiating among allergic rhinitis, common cold, and influenza.

QUESTION 3. What history or physical examination findings would be expected with allergic rhinitis?
A. *YES.* Dark circles under the eyes or "allergic shiners" are associated with allergic rhinitis.
B. *YES.* Clear rhinorrhea is part of the constellation of symptoms occurring with allergic rhinitis.
C. *YES.* Pale, boggy mucous membranes occur in allergic rhinitis as a result of exposure to an allergen. The allergen binds to IgE antibodies, precipitating the release of histamine, leukotrienes, and prostaglandins, causing the allergic response.
D. *NO.* Erythema and edema of the nasal mucous membranes occur with the common cold. Erythema of the nasal mucous membranes occurs with influenza.
E. *NO.* Acute otitis media will have erythematous, bulging tympanic membranes on physical examination.

QUESTION 4. What history or physical examination findings would be expected with the common cold?
A. *YES.* Edema of the nasal mucosa occurs as a result of infection by one of the approximately 200 different viral strains that have been identified as causing the common cold.
B. *NO.* Inspiratory wheezing is heard in lower respiratory tract illnesses. The common cold affects the upper respiratory tract, especially the nasal passages.
C. *YES.* Sneezing occurs in 50 to 70 percent of patients with the common cold. The patient will frequently sneeze during the history and/or physical examination.

   D. *NO.* Sudden onset of symptoms occurs with influenza. The common cold presents with a more gradual onset of symptoms.
   E. *YES.* Clear nasal discharge will be seen on physical examination of a patient with the common cold.

**QUESTION 5.** What history or physical examination findings would be expected with influenza?
   A. *YES.* The individual will appear acutely ill, usually more so than an individual with either the common cold or allergic rhinitis. The discomfort is generalized on physical examination.
   B. *YES.* The sudden onset of symptoms is a hallmark of influenza infections. This, along with the systemic symptoms of myalgia and malaise, contributes to the acutely ill appearance of the individual.
   C. *NO.* Erythematous tympanic membranes are seen in acute otitis media. However, otitis media is a possible sequela of an influenza infection.
   D. *YES.* Cervical lymphadenopathy is frequently found in influenza infections.
   E. *NO.* "Allergic shiners" or dark circles under the eyes are seen in allergic rhinitis. The individual with influenza may appear tired.

**QUESTION 6.** Which of the following would be the most likely assessment for this patient?
   A. *NO.* If she had allergic rhinitis, pale, boggy mucous membranes would have been seen on physical examination. Itchy eyes, nose, ears, or palate would have been a predominant complaint. A transverse crease across the nose from rubbing the nose (allergic salute) might also be present on physical examination.
   B. *YES.* Ramona is presenting with the classic symptoms of the common cold. The positive physical findings of a slight fever and erythema with clear rhinorrhea on nasal examination along with the negative findings on examination of the head, eyes, ears, face, mouth and throat, neck, and lungs aids in this assessment.
   C. *NO.* Influenza presents with a sudden onset of symptoms. On physical examination, cervical lymphadenopathy should have been present. Usually children with influenza appear acutely ill.
   D. *NO.* Examination of her ears revealed pearly gray tympanic membranes. This finding is inconsistent with acute otitis media. Otitis media can be a complication of influenza.

**QUESTION 7.** Management of influenza would include which of the following?
   A. *YES.* Since acute viral and bacterial infections occur more frequently in close, confined groups, education about the transmission of influenza is important. It is transmitted person to person, usually through aerosolization. An individual is most contagious during the peak of the symptoms. Incubation of influenza is 1 to 4 days.
   B. *NO.* Use of antibiotics for viral infections is ineffective.
   C. *YES.* Antipyretics are helpful in lowering fever and alleviating myalgia. Aspirin should be avoided in children less than 16 years of age because of the risk of Reye's syndrome.

**D.** *NO.* For amantadine to be effective, it must be administered within 48 h of onset of symptoms. It is recommended for individuals at high risk for complications of influenza.

**E.** *YES.* Symptomatic treatment such as saline gargles and saline nasal spray may increase the comfort level of the individual for the duration of the illness. It will not shorten the course of the illness.

**QUESTION 8.** Management of the common cold would include which of the following?

**A.** *YES.* Topical (nasal) or oral decongestants may promote drainage and relieve congestion by decreasing the edema of the nasal mucosa, but their use is somewhat controversial, since they do not shorten the course of the disease. Also, although topical decongestants have fewer systemic effects, they can cause rebound rhinorrhea if used for more than 3 to 5 days. Oral decongestants do not cause rebound rhinorrhea and can be used for a longer period of time.

**B.** *NO.* The efficacy of expectorants has not been proven. Water is the best expectorant and is less expensive.

**C.** *NO.* Antibiotics are not effective for viral infections and may promote antibiotic-resistant organisms.

**D.** *YES.* The viruses causing the common cold are spread from person to person via contaminated nasal secretions. Rhinoviruses will survive for hours on the hands. Careful hand washing and avoidance of touching the eyes or nose will help to minimize exposure to viruses associated with the common cold. Symptoms usually last 6 to 10 days.

**E.** *YES.* Consumption of additional fluids helps to liquefy secretions and increases the comfort level of the individual.

**QUESTION 9.** Management of allergic rhinitis would include which of the following?

**A.** *YES.* Initial management of allergic rhinitis would include client education about avoiding or minimizing exposure to allergens and irritants to which the patient is sensitive. For persons sensitive to animal dander, pets should be kept outside or, at a minimum, out of the patient's bedroom. Dust or dust mite sensitivity requires controlling house dust, especially in the bedroom; covering the mattress and pillow in an allergen-impermeable cover; and washing sheets and blankets weekly in hot water. Carpets should be vacuumed weekly or, if possible, removed from the bedroom. Feather pillows should be replaced with polyester pillows. Patients should avoid damp basements; moldy surfaces should be cleaned. Persons with seasonal pollen allergies should keep windows and doors closed to decrease pollen influx; air conditioning may be helpful. The patient should be advised not to smoke, and there should be no smoking in the home.

**B.** *YES.* Oral antihistamines are primary sources of symptomatic relief from itching, sneezing, and rhinorrhea. It may be necessary to try several products before an effective agent is found; over time, the patient may develop a tolerance that requires switching to another agent. The newer generation of H1-receptor antagonists, such as loratadine (Claritin) and fexofenadine (Allegra), are less sedating and are the agents of choice. Decongestants help to decrease nasal obstruction and can be used alone or in conjunction with antihistamines. Topical decongestants can be used in cases of severe nasal congestion, but for no longer than 3 to 4 days because of rebound effects.

C. *YES.* Cromolyn nasal spray (Nasalcrom) is used prophylactically to prevent mast cell release of histamine and other chemical mediators of the allergic response. Cromolyn requires consistent, regular use, has minimal side effects, and is now available over the counter. It may take 2 to 4 weeks to see an effect.

D. *YES.* Steroid nasal sprays, such as beclomethasone (Vancenase, Beconase) and fluticasone (Flonase), are very effective in reducing inflammation of the nasal mucosa. Onset of activity takes about 2 weeks. These agents are often used in conjunction with antihistamines/decongestants for persons with significant symptoms.

E. *YES.* Referral for skin testing or serologic testing for specific allergens, and desensitization via immunotherapy, should be considered for persons whose symptoms are unable to be controlled with traditional management and for persons with significant year-round symptoms.

## REFERENCES

Bernstein, B. M. (1996). Common cold. In J. Noble (ed.), *Textbook of Primary Care Medicine*, 2d ed., 1517–1522. St. Louis: Mosby.

Burns, C. E., Barber, N., Brady, M. A., Ardys, M. S. (1996). *Pediatric Primary Care: A Handbook for Nurse Practitioners.* Philadelphia: W. B. Saunders.

Effros, R. M., Kaufman, J. (1996). Asthma and other allergic disorders. In J. Noble (ed.), *Textbook of Primary Care Medicine*, 2d ed. 1522–1531. St. Louis: Mosby.

Frankenurg, W. K. (1988). *Denver II Screening Manual.* Denver: University of Colorado Health Sciences Center.

Graft, D. F. (1996). Allergic and nonallergic rhinitis. *Postgrad Med* 100(2), 64–74.

Griffith, H. W. (1997). *5-Minute Clinical Consult—1997.* Philadelphia: Lea & Febiger.

Herzon, F. S. (1996). Rhinorrhea and nasal stuffiness. In R. H. Rubin et al. (eds.), *Medicine: A Primary Care Approach*, 96–99. Philadelphia: W. B. Saunders.

Noble, J. E. (1996). Allergic disease. In C. D. Berkowitz (ed.), *Pediatrics: A Primary Care Approach*, 216–221. Philadelphia: W. B. Saunders.

Shaw, J. C., Robertson, M. H., Parker, F. (1996). Common skin disorders. In J. Noble (Ed.), *Textbook of Primary Care Medicine*, 2d ed., 345–347. St. Louis: Mosby.

Small, B. E. (1996). Common pediatric infections. In R. H. Rubin et al. (eds.), *Medicine: A Primary Care Approach*, 454–459. Philadelphia: W. B. Saunders.

Uphold, C. R., Graham, M. V. (1994). *Clinical Guidelines in Family Practice*, 2d ed. Gainsville, FL: Barmarrae Books.

# III

## SCHOOL AGE

# Introduction

## Marie L. Talashek

Primary care providers recognize the need for school-age children to become more independent. As children near adolescence, they will gradually assume the role of historian, with parents providing less information. Some clinicians choose to interview parents while the child is being weighed and measured. They then interview and examine the child alone so that sensitive matters can be discussed privately. However, if joint interviews are conducted, children should be included in the discussion. Fostering independence is important, because children must assume grater responsibility for lifestyle choices as they age. If it appears that a private conversation with the parent is necessary, it should be conducted prior to the examination. Private conversations held after the examination may frighten the child and/or the parent.

The American Academy of Pediatrics recommends visits at ages 6, 8, 10, and 12 years. Each visit should include the following:

1. History of health and wellness since the last visit should be taken.
2. A complete physical examination should be given.
3. Height, weight, and blood pressure should be graphed.
4. Vision and hearing screening should be done.
5. A developmental/behavioral assessment should be made.
6. Immunization status should be assessed and brought into compliance with Centers for Disease Control and Prevention (CDC) recommendations.
7. Hematocrit or hemoglobin and urinalysis should be done once during this time period.
8. Biennial screening for tuberculosis is recommended by the Committee on Infectious Diseases. (Longer intervals may be appropriate for children living in areas of very low occurrence.)
9. Anticipatory guidance should be given.

According to Erikson, during the school years children progress through the stage of industry vs. inferiority. Industry rather than inferiority is fostered by guarding against placing children in situations for which they are not ready. School-age children are in the Piagetian stage of concrete operations. Their pattern of thinking is logical and reversible, and they are able to think about part–whole relationships. Children are enthusiastic and anxious to learn, but failures result in feelings of inferiority. Parents should be encouraged to identify areas where children can be successful and facilitate participation in these activities. For some parents, recognizing their children's need for increased independence and responsibility as they move through childhood is a difficult task.

The Preventive Service Task Force recommends that primary care include promoting healthy eating, regular physical exercise, and antitobacco messages. Counseling pertinent to injury prevention for this age group includes information on auto, bicycle, and all-terrain vehicle accidents; burns; drownings; poisonings; and youth violence. Parents who understand emerging sexual development are better able to provide age-appropriate information regarding sexual matters.

The cases for this part were chosen to reflect common or important health issues for school-age children. The delayed menses case was included because individuals vary in their rate of pubertal development, causing concern for children and their parents. The reemergence of tuberculosis in all age groups makes it an important topic, and some children, such as recent immigrants or refugees, are at greater risk for the infection. The prevalence of asthma is higher in school-age children (12 to 15 percent) than in the general population (5 percent), and the case provides a vehicle for the discussion of teaching children to take an active role in the management of their illness. Pharyngitis, a common illness among school-age children, is included because practitioners must identify the 10 percent of cases that require antibiotic treatment to prevent serious sequelae. The highly infectious nature of impetigo is relevant because school-age children often touch one another in the process of playing and learning.

## REFERENCES

Committee on Practice and Ambulatory Medicine. (1995). Recommendations for preventive pediatric health care. *Pediatrics 92*(6), 751.

Centers for Disease Control and Prevention. (1996). Immunization of adolescents: Recommendations of the Advisory Committee on Immunization Practices, the American Medical Association. *Morbidity and Mortality Weekly Report 45*, No. RR-13, pp. 3–9.

Erikson, E. (1963). *Childhood and Society*. New York: Norton.

Woolf, S., Jonas, S., Lawrence, R. (eds.). *Health Promotion and Disease Prevention in Clinical Practice*. Baltimore: Williams & Wilkins.

Murray, R., Zentner, J. (1997). *Health Assessment and Promotion Strategies through the Life Span*, 6th ed. Stamford, CT: Appleton & Lange.

Burns, C., Barber, N., Brady, M., Dunn, A. (eds.). *Pediatric Primary Care: A Handbook for Nurse Practitioners*. (1996). Philadelphia: W. B. Saunders.

Pulaski, M. A. (1971). *Understanding Piaget: An Introduction To Children's Cognitive Development*. New York: Harper & Row.

U.S. Preventive Services Task Force. (1996). *Guide To Clinical Preventive Services*, 2d ed. Baltimore: Williams & Wilkins.

# 9

# Growth Delay

*Ricki S. Witz*
*Marie L. Talashek*

Shawna M. is a 14-year-old African American female who lives in a university town. She presents for her required school physical examination. Shawna has a wide circle of friends and a supportive family, and participates in softball and soccer. She has received regular health care since birth. Her major concern today is that she is shorter than her peers, and that she has not reached menarche.

## CHIEF COMPLAINT

"I am a lot shorter than my friends."

## HISTORY OF PRESENT ILLNESS

Shawna is an active adolescent female, accompanied by her mother for this visit. She was last seen at 10 years of age for her required fifth grade physical examination. She has had no health concerns requiring an appointment in the interim. Today, Shawna and her mother express concerns about Shawna's short stature and lack of pubertal maturation. Shawna feels that over the last several years her female friends have surpassed her in height. She feels embarrassed in the gym locker room because of her lack of breast development and her sparse pubic and axillary hair distribution.

## FAMILY HISTORY

There is no family history of gastrointestinal disorders, hepatic disease, pancreatic disease, neurologic disorder, cancer, blood dyscrasias, renal disease, respiratory disorders, cardiovascular disorders, or musculoskeletal disorders. Her mother did not take diethylstilbestrol (DES) during her pregnancy with Shawna.

## PAST MEDICAL HISTORY

Hospitalizations:  Denies previous hospitalizations.

Illnesses:             Two episodes of otitis media prior to 10 years
                       of age without sequelae. She has had varicella,
                       and usually gets 1 to 2 colds each winter.

Menarche:              Denies any episodes of vaginal bleeding or spotting.

Medications:           Denies taking medications, vitamins, or herbal
                       supplements.

Allergies:             Denies medication, food, or seasonal allergies.

Immunizations:         Up to date and without adverse reactions. She will need a
                       tetanus-diphtheria immunization at this encounter.

## SOCIAL HISTORY

Shawna lives with her parents and a sister. Her parents hold professional degrees
and are employed in the community. Her family has few financial concerns,
and has adequate insurance coverage for both acute and health maintenance
visits. Shawna is able to concentrate on her homework without difficulty. She
denies alcohol, tobacco, and recreational drug use. She has not had a boyfriend and denies any type of sexual exposure.

QUESTION 1. What additional subjective information is required to deter-
mine if there is a growth delay? (Select all that apply.)
   A. Parents' heights and ages at the onset of puberty
   B. Nutritional history, habits, and typical 24-h diet recall
   C. Full review of systems
   D. Exposure to electromagnetic fields

## PHYSICAL FINDINGS

Vital signs:   Temperature (oral) 98.2°F, height 152 cm, weight 40 kg,
               respiratory rate 18, blood pressure 104/66.

General:       Pleasant, well-groomed, well-nourished African American
               female, who appears younger than her stated age of 14,
               in no distress.

Head:          Normocephalic. Normal hair distribution.

Eyes:          Pupils equal, round, reactive to light, and accommodation;
               symmetrical corneal light reflex, conjunctiva pink.

Ears:          Canals are clear; tympanic membranes are pearly gray with
               positive light reflex bilaterally.

Nose:          Mucous membranes are pink and moist with a scant amount
               of clear mucus at the turbinates. Septum is midline, nares
               patent bilaterally.

Oropharynx:    Mucosa moist and pink; teeth in good repair; tongue and
               uvula midline with intact gag reflex. Tonsils are not enlarged,
               no exudate noted.

Neck:          Supple without lymphadenopathy. No thyromegaly or masses.

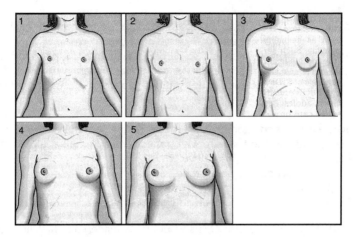

FIGURE 9-1.   Breast development. [Berkowitz, C. D. (ed.). (1996).
*Pediatrics: A Primary Care Approach.* Philadelphia: W. B. Saunders.]
With permission.

| | |
|---|---|
| Lymphatics: | Negative. |
| Lungs: | Clear to auscultation and percussion. |
| Heart: | Rate regular at 72 beats per minute. $S_1$ and $S_2$ audible without $S_3$ or $S_4$, murmurs, heaves, rubs, or clicks. |
| Breasts: | Tanner stage 2. No masses, skin changes, or nipple discharge (see Fig. 9-1). |
| Abdomen: | Active bowel sounds in all four quadrants; normal tympany noted; no organomegaly or masses; no pain to palpation. |
| Genitalia: | Normal female genitalia. Pubic hair Tanner stage 2 (see Fig. 9-2). |

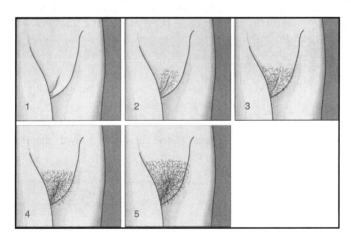

FIGURE 9-2.   Pubic hair development. [Berkowitz, C. D. (ed.). (1996).
*Pediatrics: A Primary Care Approach.* Philadelphia: W. B. Saunders.]
With permission.

Musculoskeletal:  No scoliosis, muscle weakness, or asymmetry bilaterally.
Skin:  Without lesions.
Neurologic:  Cranial nerves II to XII are grossly intact. Upper and lower extremity reflexes 2+ and equal bilaterally.
Extremities:  All extremities are without cyanosis, edema, or clubbing. Pulses are intact.

QUESTION 2. What additional objective information is required to determine if there is constitutional short stature with pubertal delay? (Select all that apply.)
  A. Past and current height and weight
  B. Upper/lower body segment ratio
  C. Vaginal and bimanual pelvic examination
  D. Denver Development Screening Tool (Denver II)

QUESTION 3. What laboratory tests would be considered in first-line testing? (Select all that apply.)
  A. Complete blood count (CBC) with differential
  B. Monospot
  C. Chemistry profile
  D. Thyroid function tests

QUESTION 4. What radiologic studies might be considered? (Select all that apply.)
  A. Hand/wrist x-rays
  B. Bilateral hip x-rays
  C. Lateral skull x-ray
  D. Chest x-ray

QUESTION 5. Which of the following relationships among bone age (BA), height age (HA), and chronological age (CA) are most consistent with constitutional short stature?
  A. BA < HA < CA
  B. HA ≤ BA < CA
  C. HA < BA = CA
  D. HA = BA < CA
  E. BA ≤ HA < CA

QUESTION 6. Which of the following are causes of growth disturbances in the adolescent? (Select all that apply.)
  A. Osgood-Schlatter disease
  B. Endocrine disorders
  C. Systemic illness
  D. Exercise-induced asthma

## ASSESSMENT

The diagnosis is constitutional short stature with pubertal delay.

QUESTION 7. Which of the following are characteristics of constitutional short stature? (Select all that apply.)
   A. Normal laboratory studies
   B. Normal physical examination
   C. Linear growth of 2.0 cm per year
   D. Bone age delay of 1.5 to 4.0 years, compared with chronological age

## PLAN

QUESTION 8. What are the plans for follow-up? (Select all that apply.)
   A. Annual monitoring of growth.
   B. Growth hormone (GH) is indicated and should be administered.
   C. Refer to a consulting physician.
   D. Discuss causes for constitutional growth delay.

## ANSWERS

QUESTION 1. What additional subjective information is required to determine if there is a growth delay?
   A. *YES.* Parents' heights and ages at onset of puberty are important in identifying familial trends in pubertal and growth delay. More than 60 percent of individuals with growth delay have a positive family history of constitutional short stature. Shawna's mother reports a history of menarche at age 15 and an adult height of 157 cm.
   B. *YES.* An individual's overall nutritional state is a significant factor in physical growth and development. Malnutrition can be responsible for growth delay related to a lack of sufficient calories, protein, carbohydrates, and vitamins to support cellular growth and physical maturation.
   C. *YES.* Growth delay may have pathological causes. In order to perform a reliable physical examination, a full and comprehensive review of systems must be conducted. A thorough review of systems helps the examiner to rule out systemic illness and will provide a basis for a systematic, focused physical examination.
   D. *NO.* There is no evidence to suggest that exposure to electromagnetic fields (high-intensity power lines, video computer terminals, etc.) will cause growth delay.

QUESTION 2. What additional objective information is required to determine if there is constitutional short stature with pubertal delay?
   A. *YES.* Information regarding historical growth trends is used to assess for deviations from normal growth and to predict growth trends over time.
   B. *YES.* The upper/lower body segment ratio (U/L) is defined as

$$\frac{\text{Height from top of head to symphysis pubis}}{\text{Height from symphysis pubis to the floor}}$$

The U/L is used in the assessment of pathologic growth delay. By 10 years of age the U/L should be 1.0, and in adulthood it should be 0.9 to 1.0. In African Americans, the U/L is usually 0.85 to 0.9; this is related to longer limb lengths. A U/L of greater than 1.0 may indicate hypothyroidism or chondrodysplasia, and a U/L of less than 1.0 may indicate hypogonadism. A normal U/L is found in constitutional short stature and delay of puberty.

C. *YES.* An external vaginal and bimanual pelvic examination is indicated in an amenorrheic adolescent female with constitutional short stature and pubertal delay to assess for abnormalities in the external genitalia or for an imperforate hymen. A bimanual pelvic examination is used to assess for the presence or absence of the uterus and ovaries.

D. *NO.* The Denver Developmental Screening Tool is used to assess social, gross motor, fine motor, and language development in infants and preschoolers.

**QUESTION 3.** What laboratory tests would be considered in first-line testing?

A. *YES.* A CBC is useful to diagnose anemias, leukocytosis, nutritional status, and possibility of infection, all of which may contribute to pathological growth disturbances.

B. *NO.* A monospot is useful in diagnosing infectious mononucleosis, which would not contribute to growth delay.

C. *YES.* A chemistry profile should be done to assess glucose, renal function, hepatic function, serum calcium, phosphorus, albumin, and protein. Abnormalities in these parameters may indicate chronic disease, which can cause growth delay.

D. *YES.* Primary or secondary hypothyroidism can cause growth delay and delay of sexual maturity and pubescence.

**QUESTION 4.** What radiologic studies might be considered?

A. *YES.* Hand/wrist x-rays are used to assess bone age.

B. *NO.* Bilateral hip x-rays are unnecessary in the determination of causes of growth delay.

C. *YES.* A lateral skull x-ray will give information regarding sella turcica changes that may affect growth. This test would be done only after bone age evaluation.

D. *NO.* There are no indications for a chest x-ray, and it would not contribute to formulating a diagnosis.

**QUESTION 5.** Which of the following relationships among bone age (BA), height age (HA), and chronological age (CA) are most consistent with constitutional short stature?

A. *NO.* BA < HA < CA reflects hypothyroidism.

B. *NO.* HA ≤ BA < CA indicates skeletal dysplasia.

C. *NO.* HA < BA = CA signifies a relationship consistent with a genetic growth delay.

**D.** *YES.* HA = BA < CA shows the proper relationship for constitutional short stature.

**E.** *NO.* BA ≤ HA < CA symbolizes a growth pattern consistent with hypogonadism.

**QUESTION 6.** Which of the following are causes of growth disturbances in the adolescent?

**A.** *NO.* Osgood-Schlatter disease is a localized disorder characterized by inflammation of the tibial tuberosity.

**B.** *YES.* Various endocrine disorders, such as primary hypothyroidism and insulin-dependent diabetes mellitus, can result in delayed growth and pubescence.

**C.** *YES.* Systemic illnesses that can produce growth delay include, but are not limited to, anorexia nervosa, inflammatory bowel disease, sickle cell anemia, chronic heart disease, and systemic lupus erythematosus.

**D.** *NO.* Although uncontrolled chronic asthma may be responsible for growth delay, exercise-induced bronchospasm does not play a role in overall growth patterns.

**QUESTION 7.** Which of the following are characteristics of constitutional short stature?

**A.** *YES.* Normal laboratory values support a diagnosis of constitutional short stature. Abnormal laboratory values would suggest a pathological cause for growth delay.

**B.** *YES.* Normal physical examination findings are required to consider a diagnosis of constitutional short stature.

**C.** *NO.* Linear growth should be at least 3.7 cm/year to support a diagnosis of constitutional short stature. Linear growth of less than 3.7 cm/year is indicative of a pathologic cause for growth delay.

**D.** *YES.* A bone age delay of 1.5 to 4.0 years as compared with the client's chronological age should be apparent.

**QUESTION 8.** What are the plans for follow-up?

**A.** *NO.* Linear growth and weight should be monitored every 4 to 6 months. Development of secondary sex characteristics and growth catch-up may occur. If an acceleration of growth and maturation does not occur, then further intervention may be considered.

**B.** *NO.* Growth hormone is not indicated in all situations. In view of this client's age and family history of delayed sexual maturity, hormonal treatment is not indicated. However, the time of puberty may be quickened in boys treated with low doses of testosterone, but their final height is not affected by treatment.

**C.** *NO.* However, referral to a consulting physician and/or pediatric endocrinologist is indicated in cases where pathologic growth delay is demonstrated.

**D.** *YES.* Educating the family and client is essential for the adequate understanding of constitutional short stature with pubertal delay. It is important for the clinician to realize the impact of short stature and delayed puberty on the adolescent's self-esteem and self-concept. Discussing predicted growth and sexual maturation as well as providing reassurance may help to allay the adolescent's feelings and fears about her body image.

## REFERENCES

Cheffer, N. D., Brady, A. M. (1996). Endocrine and metabolic diseases. In C. Burns, N. Barber, M. Brady, A. Dunn (eds.), *Pediatric Primary Care: A Handbook for Nurse Practitioners*, 513–528. Philadelphia: W. B. Saunders.

Gotlin, R. W., Kappy, M. S., Slover, R. H. (1997). Endocrine disorders. In W. Hay, J. Groothuis, A. Hayward, M. Levin (eds.), *Current Pediatric Diagnosis and Treatment*, 820. Stamford, CT: Appleton & Lange.

Neinstein, L., Kaufman, F. (1996). Abnormal growth and development. In L. S. Neinstein (ed.), *Adolescent Health Care: A Practical Guide*, 3d ed., 165–193. Baltimore: Williams & Wilkins.

# 10

# Asthma

*Linda Farrand*
*Jeanne M. Ondyak*

Beth H., a 7-year-old, lives on a farm with her parents and three siblings. At age 4 she was diagnosed as having asthma. At that time she also had skin tests done, which showed her to be allergic to several pollens, dust mites, cats, and dogs. Her father smokes one pack of cigarettes a day. Beth receives care at a Midwest rural health clinic.

## CHIEF COMPLAINT

"Beth has been wheezing more, both during the day and at night, for the past month."

## HISTORY OF PRESENT ILLNESS

Beth's episodes of wheezing have increased from less than once weekly to two to three times a week during the past month. In addition, her nighttime symptoms, cough and occasional wheezing, have increased from about twice a month to four times a month. She is now using her current medication, albuterol (Proventil, Ventolin), 1–2 puffs as needed, about three times per week. She last used her albuterol early this morning, about 6 h ago. Her mother states that she has not had an upper respiratory infection recently.

## PAST MEDICAL HISTORY

As an infant, Beth had three episodes of otitis media that resolved with amoxicillin. During her preschool years, she had only one further episode of otitis media, but before her diagnosis of asthma at age 4, she had several episodes of bronchiolitis and persistent nonproductive cough, especially at night. She was seen in the emergency room once about this time last year for an acute wheezing episode that occurred at night and was not controllable with albuterol. She did not require admission. Her past history is positive for allergic rhinitis, for which she takes intranasal cromolyn (Nasalcrom) and occasional antihistamines, but negative for eczema and pneumonia.

**QUESTION 1.** What additional historical information is necessary? (Select all that apply.)
A. Symptom history
B. Family history
C. Nutritional history
D. Social history

**QUESTION 2.** For the asthmatic individual with seasonal allergies, worsening symptoms in early spring are most likely due to which of the following?
A. Tree pollen
B. Grass pollen
C. Weed pollen
D. Dust mite
E. Fungi (molds)

## PHYSICAL FINDINGS

| | |
|---|---|
| General: | Slender, Caucasian girl with pleasant affect and an easy smile; able to speak in sentences; alert, with intermittent cough but no audible wheezing. |
| Vital signs: | Temperature 98.6° F, pulse 90, respirations 24, blood pressure 100/64, height 49 in, weight: 55 lb. |
| Skin: | Pink. |
| Head: | No sinus tenderness. |
| Eyes: | Conjunctivae clear without discharge. |
| Ears: | Canals clear, tympanic membranes pearly grey with positive light reflex bilaterally, landmarks visualized, movable bilaterally. |
| Nose: | Horizontal crease on bridge of nose, mucosa pale, thin clear discharge present, turbinates slightly swollen, no polyps or lesions. |
| Throat: | Mucosa pink, tonsils 2+, no exudate, no postnasal drainage. |
| Neck: | No lymphadenopathy. |
| Chest: | Chest expansion symmetric, no retractions or accessory muscle use, tactile fremitus equal bilaterally; resonant to percussion throughout. |
| Lungs: | Few mild end-expiratory wheezes at bases. |
| Heart: | Normal $S_1$-$S_2$, no murmur. |

**QUESTION 3.** Which additional test is necessary to evaluate Beth's current status?
A. Complete blood count (CBC)
B. Erythrocyte sedimentation rate (ESR)
C. Peak expiratory flow (PEF)
D. Oxygen saturation (pulse oximetry)

## ASSESSMENT

Beth's peak flow is 79 percent of her average predicted value; this increases to 90 percent 20 min after taking 1 puff of albuterol.

**QUESTION 4.** Based on the National Institutes of Health 1997 guidelines, how would the severity of Beth's asthma be classified?
A. Mild intermittent
B. Mild persistent
C. Moderate persistent
D. Severe persistent

## PLAN

**QUESTION 5.** Which of the following medications would be the first choice to add to Beth's regimen for long-term control of her asthma symptoms?
A. Cromolyn sodium (Intal)
B. Theophylline (Theo-Dur)
C. Salmeterol (Serevent)
D. Flunisolide (Aerobid)
E. Zafirlukast (Accolate)

**QUESTION 6.** What are the key points on which to educate Mrs. H. and Beth about the use of inhaled cromolyn sodium? (Select all that apply.)
A. Mechanism of action
B. Dosage
C. Onset of action
D. Inhaler technique
E. Side effects

**QUESTION 7.** How could Beth's environment be altered to decrease exposure to allergens and other triggers? (Select all that apply.)
A. Encase mattress and pillow in allergen-impermeable covers.
B. Keep pets outside.
C. Use a chemical agent on carpeting to denature the dust mite antigen.
D. Do not allow smoking in the home.
E. Use a humidifier.

**QUESTION 8.** It is important to teach Mrs. H. and Beth to recognize symptoms that indicate inadequate control. Which of the following is an *early* sign/symptom of worsening asthma severity?
A. Increased use of accessory muscles
B. Speaking in short phrases
C. Frequent coughing, decreased exercise tolerance
D. Overly sleepy—not easily roused

Beth and her mother have agreed to use an asthma diary to monitor symptoms, medication use, and peak expiratory flow, to be reviewed at her next visit.

QUESTION 9. What are the critical points to cover in teaching the use of a peak flow meter? (Select all that apply.)
A. How to get an accurate reading
B. How often to use the meter
C. How to interpret the result
D. How to clean the meter

## ANSWERS

QUESTION 1. What additional historical information is necessary?
A. *YES.* Important information to obtain as part of the symptom history includes (1) the typical presenting symptoms (cough, wheeze, chest tightness, shortness of breath, sputum production); (2) the pattern of symptoms (perennial, seasonal, continuous, episodic, onset, duration, frequency, diurnal variation, nocturnal awakening); (3) precipitating or aggravating factors (environmental allergens, such as pollen, mold, dust mites, cockroaches, and animal dander; irritants, such as smoke, cold air, strong odors, chemicals, and aerosols; exercise; upper respiratory infections or sinusitis; strong emotional expressions; drugs; food or food additives); and (4) a profile of a typical exacerbation (usual prodromal signs and symptoms, usual patterns of management).
B. *NO.* At an initial work-up, it would be important to assess for a positive family history of allergy or asthma, as this would contribute to making the diagnosis. At this point in time, however, Beth has already been diagnosed with asthma, and thus exploring family history would not add information necessary to manage her condition.
C. *NO.* A complete nutritional history would not be indicated for this focused visit; however, as noted above, it would be important to question Mrs. H. regarding whether she has noticed that any foods have precipitated asthma symptoms in Beth. Possible offenders are milk, eggs, peanuts, shellfish, soy, wheat, and chocolate.
D. *YES.* Important information to obtain regarding the social history includes (1) the characteristics of the home, especially the rooms where the patient spends the most time (i.e., bedroom, living room), including heating and air conditioning systems, carpeting, humidifier, stuffed furniture, stuffed toys, fireplace, and presence of mold, mildew, or cockroaches; (2) smokers in the home or day care; (3) support for asthma management in the school and day care setting (presence of a school nurse, access to inhaler medication, the classroom teacher's and physical education teacher's awareness of the condition); (4) the impact of asthma on the child and the family (number of days missed from school, limitation of activity, economic impact, effect on behavior and school performance); and (5) the child's and family's perceptions of the disease (belief in the chronicity of asthma, ability to cope with illness).

QUESTION 2. For the asthmatic individual with seasonal allergies, worsening symptoms in early spring are most likely due to which of the following?
A. *YES.* Trees pollinate in early spring. Troublesome offenders include alder, birch, oak, cottonwood, and elm, although species vary according to locale.
B. *NO.* Grass pollinates in late spring.

C. *NO.* Weeds pollinate in late summer through fall. Ragweed is the most notorious culprit causing seasonal allergy symptoms, with pollen counts peaking from mid-August through mid-September and lasting until the first frost.
D. *NO.* Dust mite allergy causes perennial symptoms that are typically worse in the winter. While the medical history is usually sufficient to determine sensitivity to seasonal allergens, allergy testing (skin testing or in vitro testing) is the only reliable way to determine sensitivity to perennial indoor allergens. The clinical significance of positive allergy tests must be assessed in relation to the patient's history.
E. *NO.* Indoor molds cause perennial symptoms, and outdoor molds such as *Alternaria* and *Cladosporium* are present in summer and fall.

**QUESTION 3.** Which additional test is necessary to evaluate Beth's current status?
A. *NO.* A CBC would not be indicated except to rule out infection, anemia, or some other acute process; Beth's history and physical findings do not suggest the presence of these conditions.
B. *NO.* An ESR is a nonspecific indicator of an infectious disease and is not indicated in this case.
C. *YES.* Peak expiratory flow is a measure of lung function that is obtained using a peak flow meter. Peak expiratory flow indicates the maximum rate of flow attained during forced expiration starting with fully inflated lungs. Peak flow meters are small, portable, and inexpensive and can be easily used in the office or at home to help assess the severity of asthma and evaluate response to therapy. While predicted values corrected for height, sex, race, and age are available (see Fig. 10-1), the patient's values may be consistently higher or lower. Thus, objectives for therapy need to be based on the patient's personal best PEF value and typical daily variability. Peak flow meters are tools for ongoing monitoring, not diagnosis. Spirometry is recommended at the time of initial diagnosis, after treatment has stabilized symptoms and PEF in order to document "normal" airway function, and every 1 to 2 years thereafter.
D. *NO.* Measurement of oxygen saturation by pulse oximetry is indicated in moderate to severe respiratory distress or with a PEF <50 percent of the predicted personal best value; Beth's physical findings do not reflect significant respiratory distress. Pulse oximetry is a noninvasive procedure that measures the arterial oxygen saturation of hemoglobin using a small cliplike sensor placed on a finger. In mild asthma, the oxygen saturation will be normal, with values >95 percent; values in asthma of moderate severity will range from 90 to 95 percent, and values in severe attacks will be <90 percent.

**QUESTION 4.** Based on the National Institutes of Health 1997 guidelines (Fig. 10-2), how would the severity of Beth's asthma be classified?
A. *NO.* Prior to her recent increase in symptoms, the severity of Beth's asthma fit the mild intermittent classification; however, her current daytime and nighttime symptoms have increased, placing her in a higher category.
B. *YES.* Beth's current symptoms fit most closely with the category of mild persistent asthma.

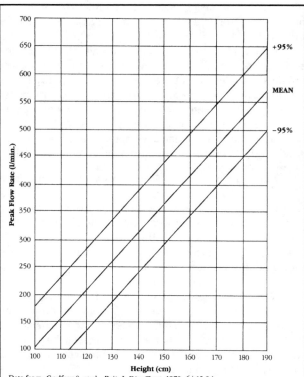

Data from: Godfrey S. et al., *Brit. J. Dis. Chest*, 1970; 64:15-24.

**Predicted Average Peak Expiratory Flow for Normal Children and Adolescents**

**(liters per minute)**

| Height (inches) | Males & Females | Height (inches) | Males & Females |
|---|---|---|---|
| 43 | 147 | 56 | 320 |
| 44 | 160 | 57 | 334 |
| 45 | 173 | 58 | 347 |
| 46 | 187 | 59 | 360 |
| 47 | 200 | 60 | 373 |
| 48 | 214 | 61 | 387 |
| 49 | 227 | 62 | 400 |
| 50 | 240 | 63 | 413 |
| 51 | 254 | 64 | 427 |
| 52 | 267 | 65 | 440 |
| 53 | 280 | 66 | 454 |
| 54 | 293 | 67 | 467 |
| 55 | 307 | | |

Data from: Polger, G, Promedhat V: *Pulmonary function testing in children: Techniques and standards.* Philadelphia, W.B. Saunders, 1971.

**FIGURE 10-1.** Peak expiratory flow rate nomogram. National Institutes of Health, National Heart, Lung, and Blood Institute. (1991). *Guidelines for the Diagnosis and Management of Asthma.* NIH Publication No. 91-3042. Bethesda, MD: Author.

# Clinical Features Before Treatment*

| | Symptoms** | Nighttime Symptoms | Lung Function |
|---|---|---|---|
| STEP 4<br>Severe Persistent | ■ Continual symptoms<br>■ Limited physical activity<br>■ Frequent exacerbations | Frequent | ■ $FEV_1$ or PEF ≤60% predicted<br>■ PEF variability >30% |
| STEP 3<br>Moderate Persistent | ■ Daily symptoms<br>■ Daily use of inhaled short-acting $beta_2$-agonist<br>■ Exacerbations affect activity<br>■ Exacerbations ≥2 times a week, may last days | >1 time a week | ■ $FEV_1$ or PEF >60%–<80% predicted<br>■ $PEF^1$ variability >30% |
| STEP 2<br>Mild Persistent | ■ Symptoms >2 times a week but <1 time a day<br>■ Exacerbations may affect activity | >2 times a month | ■ $FEV_1$ or PEF ≥80% predicted<br>■ PEF variability 20–30% |
| STEP 1<br>Mild Intermittent | ■ Symptoms ≤2 times a week<br>■ Asymptomatic and normal PEF between exacerbations<br>■ Exacerbations brief (from a few hours to a few days); intensity may vary | ≤2 times a month | ■ $FEV_1$ or PEF ≥80% predicted<br>■ PEF variability <20% |

*The presence of one of the features of severity is sufficient to place a patient in that category. An individual should be assigned to the most severe grade in which any feature occurs. The characteristics noted in this figure are general and may overlap because asthma is highly variable. Furthermore, an individual's classification may change over time.

**Patients at any level of severity can have mild, moderate, or severe exacerbations. Some patients with intermittent asthma experience severe and life-threatening exacerbations separated by long periods of normal lung function and no symptoms.

FIGURE 10-2. Classification of asthma severity. National Institutes of Health, National Heart, Lung, and Blood Institute. (1997). *Guidelines for the diagnosis and Management of Asthma.* NIH Publication No. 97-4051. Bethesda, MD: Author.

C. *NO*. Beth's symptoms are not severe enough to be characterized as moderate persistent asthma.

D. *NO*. Beth's symptoms are not this severe.

**QUESTION 5.** Which of the following medications would be the first choice to add to Beth's regimen for long-term control of her asthma symptoms?

A. *YES*. The use of inhaled cromolyn sodium (Intal), a nonsteroidal anti-inflammatory medication, is a good first choice for children for long-term control of asthma because of its strong safety profile. Nedocromil (Tilade) is a similar nonsteroidal anti-inflammatory drug, also without any known long-term side effects, and is another possible choice for initial daily long-term therapy. Nedocromil is especially useful when cough is a prominent feature and may be more potent than cromolyn in inhibiting exercise-induced bronchospasm (see Figs. 10-3 and 10-4).

B. *NO*. Sustained-release theophylline, a mild to moderate bronchodilator, is an alternative, but not preferred, long-term control medication because of its modest clinical efficacy and potential for toxicity. Its principal use now is as adjuvant therapy to inhaled corticosteroids for the prevention of nocturnal asthma symptoms. It may also be considered when there are issues of cost or com-pliance; however, monitoring of serum concentration levels is required.

C. *NO*. Salmeterol (Serevent) is a long-acting inhaled $\beta_2$ agonist with a duration of at least 12 h after a single dose. This drug is used as an adjunct to inhaled corticosteroids for long-term control, especially for control of nocturnal symptoms and prevention of exercise-induced bronchospasm. It does not provide quick relief and should not be used for exacerbations.

D. *NO*. While inhaled corticosteroids, such as flunisolide (Aerobid), beclomethasone (Beclovent), and triamcinolone (Azmacort), are considered to be the most effective therapy for long-term control of persistent asthma, a trial of cromolyn or nedocromil is the first choice of treatment for children with mild persistent asthma because of the relative safety of these medications. However, if these do not provide adequate control, an inhaled corticosteroid will be necessary for long-term therapy. To reduce the potential for adverse effects, the lowest possible dose should be used. Children's growth should be monitored as some studies have identified growth delay in children treated with inhaled corticosteroids; this appears to be dose-related, with the majority of studies showing that dosages of 400 to 800 µg a day do not have a negative effect on growth. Also, inhaled steroids should be administered with a spacer device and patients should be instructed to rinse their mouths afterwards (rinse and spit) to minimize the risk of oral candidiasis (thrush).

E. *NO*. Zafirlukast (Accolate) and zileuton (Zyflo) belong to a new class of drugs called *leukotriene modifiers*, which may be used as alternative therapy to cromolyn, nedocromil, or low doses of inhaled steroids in persons with mild persistent asthma; however, their use has not been approved in patients ≤12 years of age, and further study is needed to clarify their role in therapy.

**QUESTION 6.** What are the key points at which to educate Mrs. H. and Beth about the use of inhaled cromolyn sodium?

   **A.** *YES.* Cromolyn is an anti-inflammatory drug that works by preventing mast cell release of inflammatory mediators. A simple explanation regarding the mechanism of action and purpose of the medication is appropriate. Beth and her mother should know that this medication helps to prevent symptoms and is for long-term control, not for quick relief. It is important to stress that Beth should continue to use her albuterol for immediate relief of acute symptoms.

   **B.** *YES.* To be effective, Beth needs to take her cromolyn 1 to 2 puffs, three to four times a day. Inadequate dosage is a factor that can contribute to treatment failure.

   **C.** *YES.* An adequate duration of therapy is necessary, as it can take up to 4 weeks for cromolyn to be effective; at that time, a decrease in the frequency of wheezing and night symptoms should be noticed.

   **D.** *YES.* According to a 1994 study, three-quarters of asthma patients use their inhalers incorrectly. Even though Beth has been using an inhaler, it is important to review technique and have her do a return demonstration (see Fig. 10-5). Use of a spacer device allows for easier coordination of inhalation and generally increases lung delivery of the medication.

   **E.** *YES.* Cromolyn is a safe and effective drug. Side effects are uncommon and primarily include unpleasant taste, hoarseness, and coughing, which can be minimized by the use of a spacer.

**QUESTION 7.** How could Beth's environment be altered to decrease exposure to allergens and other triggers?

   **A.** *YES.* Essential actions to control dust mites include encasing Beth's mattress and pillow in allergen-impermeable covers and washing the sheets and blankets weekly at a temperature ≥130°F. Other desirable interventions include reducing indoor humidity to less than 50 percent, removing the carpet from the bedroom, and minimizing the number of stuffed toys in the child's bedroom.

   **B.** *YES.* Ideally, any dogs or cats should be given away to a good home, since Beth is sensitive to these pets; if this is not acceptable, the animals should be kept outside if the climate permits. At a minimum, the pets should be kept out of her bedroom and her bedroom door kept closed. Atopic persons can become sensitized to any warm-blooded animal, including rodents and birds. Contrary to popular belief, the length of the animal's hair does not determine allergenicity; the sources of animal allergen are dander, saliva, and urine (rodents). Animals excrete differing amounts of allergenic protein, thus individuals may report being more or less sensitive to different animals of the same species. Beth should avoid any farm animals that trigger her symptoms. Also, her pillow should be made of hypoallergenic material, not feathers or down. In the future, Beth may be able to minimize her allergy symptoms to cats by receiving Allervax cat vaccine. Potentially available as early as 1998, this vaccine will require a series of four injections over 2 to 4 weeks, and a possible booster shot every 6 to 12 months.

*(text continues on page 93)*

| | Treatment | | Preferred treatments in bold print. |
| --- | --- | --- | --- |
| | Long-Term Control | Quick Relief | Education |
| **STEP 4**<br>**Severe**<br>**Persistent** | Daily medications:<br>■ **Anti-inflammatory: inhaled corticosteroid (high dose)**<br>AND<br>■ **Long-acting bronchodilator: either inhaled long-acting beta$_2$-agonist,** sustained release theophylline, or long-acting beta$_2$-agonist tables<br>AND<br>■ Corticosteroid tablets or syrup long term (2 mg/kg/day, generally do not exceed 60 mg per day). | ■ Short-acting bronchodilator: **inhaled beta$_2$-agonists** as needed for symptoms.<br>■ Intensity of treatment will depend on severity of exacerbation; see component 3–Managing Exacerbations.<br>■ Use of short-acting inhaled beta$_2$-agonists on a daily basis, or increasing use, indicates the need for additional long-term-control therapy. | Steps 2 and 3 actions plus:<br>■ Refer to individual education/counseling |
| **STEP 3**<br>**Moderate**<br>**Persistent** | Daily medication<br>■ Either<br>**Anti-inflammatory: inhaled corticosteroid (medium dose)**<br>OR<br>**Inhaled corticosteroid (low-medium dose)** and add a long-acting bronchodilator, especially for nighttime symptoms: either **long-acting inhaled beta$_2$-agonist,** sustained-release theophylline, or long-acting beta$_2$-agonist tablets.<br>■ If needed<br>**Anti-inflammatory: inhaled corticosteroids (medium high dose)**<br>AND<br>**Long-acting bronchodilator,** especially for nighttime symptoms; either **long-acting inhaled beta$_2$-agonist,** sustained release theophylline, or long-acting beta$_2$-agonist tablets. | ■ Short-acting bronchodilator: **inhaled beta$_2$-agonists** as needed for symptoms.<br>■ Intensity of treatment will depend on severity of exacerbation; see component 3–Managing Exacerbations.<br>■ Use of short-acting inhaled beta$_2$-agonists on a daily basis, or increasing use, indicates the need for additional long-term-controlled therapy. | |
| **STEP 2**<br>**Mild**<br>**Persistent** | One daily medication:<br>■ **Anti-inflammatory: either inhaled corticosteroid** (low doses) or cromolyn or nedocromil (children usually begin with a trial of cromolyn or nedocromil). | ■ Short-acting bronchodilator: **inhaled beta$_2$-agonists** as needed for symptoms.<br>■ Intensity of treatment will depend on severity of exacerbation; see component 3–Managing Exacerbations. | Step 1 actions plus:<br>■ Teach self-monitoring<br>■ Refer to group education if available<br>■ Review and update self-management plan |

Step 1 actions plus:
■ Teach self-monitoring
■ Refer to group education if available
■ Review and update self-management plan.

| | | |
|---|---|---|
| ■ Sustained release theophylline, to serum concentration of 5-15 mcg/mL is an alternative, but not preferred, therapy. Zafirlukast or zileuton may also be considered for patients ≥12 years of age, although their position in therapy is not fully established. | ■ Use of short-acting inhaled $beta_2$-agonists on a daily basis, or increasing use, indicates the need for additional long-term-control therapy. | |
| **STEP 1**<br><br>**Mild**<br>**Intermittent** | ■ No daily medication needed. | ■ Short-acting bronchodilator: **inhaled** $beta_2$**-agonists** as needed for symptoms.<br>■ Intensity of treatment will depend on severity of exacerbation; see component 3–Managing Exacerbations.<br>■ Use of short-acting inhaled $beta_2$-agonists more than 2 times a week may indicate the need to initiate long-term-control therapy. | ■ Teach basic facts about asthma<br>■ Teach inhaler/spacer/holding chamber technique<br>■ Discuss roles of medications<br>■ Develop self-management plan<br>■ Develop action plan for when and how to take rescue actions, especially for patients with a history of severe exacerbations<br>■ Discuss appropriate environmental control measures to avoid exposure to known allergens and irritants<br><br>(See component 4) |

↑ **Step up**
If control is not achieved, consider step up. First, review patient medication technique, adherence, and environmental control (avoidance of allergens or other factors that contribute to asthma severity).

**Step down**
Review treatment every 1 to 6 month; a gradual stepwise reduction in treatment may be possible.

**NOTES:**
■ The stepwise approach presents guidelines to assist clinical decisionmaking; it is not intended to be a specific prescription. Asthma is highly variable; clinicians should tailor specific medication plans to the needs and circumstances of individual patients.
■ Gain control as quickly as possible; then decrease treatment to the least medication necessary to maintain control. Gaining control may be accomplished by either starting treatment at the step most appropriate to the initial severity of their condition or by starting at a higher level of therapy (e.g., a course of systemic corticosteroids or higher dose of inhaled corticosteroids).
■ A rescue course of systemic corticosteroids may be needed at any time and at any step.
■ Some patients with intermittent asthma experience severe and life-threatening exacerbations separated by long periods of normal lung function and no symptoms. This may be especially common with exacerbations provoked by respiratory infections. A short course of systemic corticosteroids is recommended.
■ At each step, patients should control their environment to avoid or control factors that make their asthma worse (e.g., allergens, irritants), this requires specific diagnosis and education. Referral to an asthma specialist for consultation or comanagement is *recommended* if there are difficulties achieving or maintaining control of asthma or if the patient requires step 4 care. Referral may be *considered* if the patient requires step 3 care (see also component 1–Initial Assessment and Diagnosis).

**FIGURE 10-3.** **Stepwise approach for managing asthma in adults and children older than 5 years of age. National Institutes of Health, National Heart, Lung, and Blood Institute. (1997). *Guidelines for the Diagnosis and Management of Asthma*. NIH Publication No. 97-4051. Bethesda, MD: Author.**

| | Long-Term Control | Quick Relief |
|---|---|---|
| **STEP 4**<br>**Severe**<br>**Persistent** | ■ Daily anti-inflammatory medicine—<br>High-dose inhaled corticosteroid with spacer/<br>holding chamber and face mask<br>If needed, add systemic corticosteroids 2 mg/kg/day<br>and reduce to lowest daily or alternate-day dose<br>that stabilizes symptoms | ■ Bronchodilator as needed for symptoms (see step 1)<br>up to 3 times a day |
| **STEP 3**<br>**Moderate**<br>**Persistent** | ■ Daily anti-inflammatory medication. Either:<br>Medium-dose inhaled corticosteroid with spacer/<br>holding chamber and face mask<br>OR, once control is established:<br>Medium-dose inhaled corticosteroid and nedocromil<br>OR<br>Medium-dose inhaled corticosteroid and long-acting<br>bronchodilator (theophylline) | ■ Bronchodilator as needed for symptoms (see step 1)<br>up to 3 times a day |
| **STEP 2**<br>**Mild**<br>**Persistent** | ■ Daily anti-inflammatory medication. Either:<br>Cromolyn (nebulizer is preferred; or MDI) or nedocromil<br>(MDI only) tid–qid<br>Infants and young children usually begin with a trial of<br>cromolyn or nedocromil<br>OR<br>Low-dose inhaled corticosteroid with spacer/holding<br>chamber and face mask | ■ Bronchodilator as needed for symptoms (see step 1) |
| **STEP 1**<br>**Mild**<br>**Intermittent** | ■ No daily medication needed. | ■ Bronchodilator as needed for symptoms <2 times a week.<br>Intensity of treatment will depend upon severity of<br>exacerbation (see component 3-Managing Exacerbations).<br>Either:<br>Inhaled short-acting beta$_2$-agonist by nebulizer or face<br>mask and spacer/holding chamber<br>OR<br>Oral beta$_2$-agonist for symptoms |

■ With viral respiratory infection:
  Bronchodilator q 4–6 hours up to 24 hours (longer with physician consult) but, in general, repeat no more than once every 6 weeks
  Consider systematic corticosteroid if
    Current exacerbation is severe
    OR
    Patient has history of previous severe exacerbations

**Step down**
Review treatment every 1 to 6 months. If control is sustained for at least 3 months, a gradual stepwise reduction in treatment may be possible.

**Step up**
If control is not achieved, consider step up. But first, review patient medication technique, adherence, and environmental control (avoidance of allergens or other precipitant factors).

NOTES:
■ **The stepwise approach presents guidelines to assist clinical decisionmaking. Asthma is highly variable; clinicians should tailor specific medication plans to the needs and circumstances of individual patients.**
■ Gain control as quickly as possible; then decrease treatment to the least medication necessary to maintain control. Gaining control may be accomplished by either starting treatment at the step most appropriate to the initial severity of their condition or by starting at a higher level of therapy (e.g., a course of systemic corticosteroids or higher dose of inhaled corticosteroids).
■ A rescue course of systemic corticosteroid (prednisolone) may be needed at any time and step.
■ In general, use of short-acting beta$_2$-agonist on a daily basis indicates the need for additional long-term-control therapy.
■ It is important to remember that there are very few studies on asthma therapy for infants.
■ Consultation with an asthma specialist is *recommended* for patients with moderate or severe persistent asthma in this age group. Consultation should be *considered* for all patients with mild persistent asthma.

FIGURE 10-4.   Stepwise approach for managing asthma in infants and young children (5 years of age and younger). National Institutes of Health, National Heart, Lung, and Blood Institute. (1997) *Guidelines for the Diagnosis and Management of Asthma.* NIH Publication No. 97-4051. Bethesda, MD: Author.

*Please demonstrate your inhaler technique at every visit*

1. Remove the cap and hold inhaler upright.
2. Shake the inhaler.
3. Tilt your head back slightly and breathe out slowly.
4. Position the inhaler in one of the following ways (A or B is optimal, but C is acceptable for those who have difficulty with A or B. C is required for breath-activated inhalers):

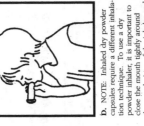

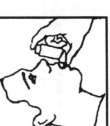

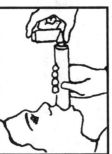

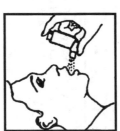

**A.** Open mouth with inhaler 1 to 2 inches away.

**B.** Use spacer/holding chamber (that is recommended especially for young children and for people using corticosteroids).

**C.** In the mouth. Do not use for corticosteroids.

**D.** NOTE: Inhaled dry powder capsules require a different inhalation technique. To use a dry powder inhaler, it is important to close the mouth tightly around the mouthpiece of the inhaler and to inhale rapidly.

5. Press down on the inhaler to release medication as you start to breathe in slowly.
6. Breathe in slowly (3 to 5 seconds).
7. Hold your breath for 10 seconds to allow the medicine to reach deeply into your lungs.
8. Repeat puff as directed. Waiting 1 minute between puffs may permit second puff to penetrate your lungs better.
9. Spacers/holding chambers are useful for all patients. They are particularly recommended for young children and older adults and for use with inhaled corticosteroids.

*Avoid common inhaler mistakes. Follow these inhaler tips:*
- Breathe out *before* pressing your inhaler.
- Inhale *slowly*.
- Breathe in through your mouth, not your nose.
- Press down on your inhaler at the *start* of inhalation (or within the first second of inhalation).
- Keep inhaling as you press down on inhaler.
- Press your inhaler only *once* while you are inhaling (one breath for each puff).
- Make sure you breathe in evenly and deeply.

NOTE: Other inhalers are becoming available in addition to those illustrated above. Different types of inhalers may require different techniques

**FIGURE 10-5.** Steps for using your inhaler. National Institutes of Health, National Heart, Lung, and Blood Institute. (1997). *Guidelines for the Diagnosis and Management of Asthma.* NIH Publication No. 97-4051. Bethesda, MD: Author.

C. *NO.* Routine use of chemicals on carpeting or upholstered furniture to kill dust mites or to denature the antigen is no longer recommended because of their minimal and short-lived effects.

D. *YES.* Smoke is a significant respiratory irritant, and persons with asthma should not be exposed. Beth's father should be counseled to quit smoking; at least, there should be no smoking in the home. Wood-burning stoves and fireplaces that do not draw well may also trigger symptoms.

E. *NO.* Humidifiers should not be used in the homes of persons sensitive to dust mites or mold, as increased humidity encourages the growth of both. Use of air conditioning during warm weather is recommended, as this reduces humidity and limits dust mite growth. Air conditioning is also helpful for persons sensitive to outdoor allergens such as pollens and seasonal molds.

**QUESTION 8:** It is important to teach Mrs. H. and Beth to recognize symptoms that indicate inadequate control. Which of the following is an *early* sign/symptom of worsening asthma severity?

A. *NO.* The increased use of accessory muscles to breathe is a sign of moderate to severe asthma; the patient may also have difficulty breathing lying down and prefer to sit.

B. *NO.* Speaking in short phrases is a sign of breathlessness that occurs with moderate asthma severity; with a severe asthma attack, the patient is usually only able to speak in single words.

C. *YES.* Increased coughing, especially at night, is a cardinal early sign, as is decreased exercise tolerance. The patient may prefer not to exert herself and to stay quiet.

D. *NO.* Drowsiness or confusion, concomitant with other symptoms of respiratory distress in the patient with asthma, is a late and ominous sign indicating impending respiratory arrest. Bradycardia and absense of wheezing also indicate that respiratory arrest is imminent.

**QUESTION 9.** What are the critical points to cover in teaching the use of a peak flow meter?

A. *YES.* Peak flow readings are dependent on patient effort and technique. To obtain an accurate reading, the user must stand up, inhale deeply, seal lips around the mouthpiece, and exhale into the meter as fast and hard as possible. Note the value to which the indicator moves. This manuever should be repeated twice more, and the best value of the three efforts should be recorded. Because of the variability of readings between meters, patients should use the same meter consistently and bring their own meter to return visits.

B. *YES.* Recommendations for frequency of PEF monitoring vary depending on the purpose. (1) To establish an individual's personal best PEF, measurements should be recorded once a day in the early afternoon over a 2- to 3-week period when the patient's asthma is under good control. Early afternoon is the recommended time of day for measurement, as this time generally reflects optimal lung function. A reading should also be taken after each use of a short-acting ß agonist. The highest PEF reading achieved is considered to be the personal best value. A child's personal best should be reassessed periodically to reflect changes in PEF due to growth. (2) To determine the severity of a patient's asthma and to evaluate the response to a change in chronic maintenance therapy, short-term daily monitoring over a 2- to 3-week period is recommended. This measurement should be performed daily upon awakening, before taking a bronchodilator. If the reading is below 80 percent of the patient's personal best PEF, additional readings should be taken during the day to determine if the asthma is worsening or improving after medication. (3) Long-term daily peak flow monitoring is recommended for patients with moderate to severe persistent asthma or unstable asthma.

C. *YES*. When the peak flow is more than 80 percent of the personal best measurement, asthma is considered to be under good control; this is a "green light," and medicines should be taken as usual. A reading between 50 and 80 percent signals caution; this is a "yellow light" and indicates the need to take quick relief medicine (short-acting β agonist) and to contact the health care provider and have medications adjusted. A reading below 50 percent signifies a "red light." This indicates a need for prompt medical attention: The patient should contact the office immediately or go straight to the closest emergency room. Ranges based on the personal best PEF should be calculated by the provider, and the patient should be given a written action plan along with verbal instructions. If PEF values consistently increase 20 percent or more when measured before and after short-acting bronchodilators, this may indicate the need for a step-up in pharmacotherapy.

D. *YES*. Cleaning the meter is best done following the manufacturer's directions.

## REFERENCES

Berlow, B. A. (1997). Eight key questions to ask when your patient with asthma doesn't get better. *American Family Physician 55*(1), 183–189.

Larsen, J. S., Hahn, M., Ekholm, B., Wick, K. A. (1994). Evaluation of conventional press-and-breathe metered-dose inhaler technique in 501 patients. *J Asthma 31*, 193–199.

National Institutes of Health, National Heart, Lung, and Blood Institute. (1991). *National Asthma Education and Prevention Program Expert Panel Report: Guidelines for the Diagnosis and Management of Asthma.* NIH Publication No. 91-3042. Bethesda, MD: Author.

National Institutes of Health, National Heart, Lung, and Blood Institute. (1997). *National Asthma Education and Prevention Program Expert Panel Report 2: Guidelines for the Diagnosis and Management of Asthma.* NIH Publication No. 97-4051. Bethesda, MD: Author.

National Jewish Center for Immunology and Respiratory Medicine. (1997). Cat lovers take heart. *New Directions and Lung Line Letter 25*(3), 6.

Pearlman, D. S., Greos, L. S., Vitanza, J. M. (1997). Allergic disorders. In W. W. Hay, J. R. Groothuis, A. R. Hayward, M. J. Levin (eds.), *Current Pediatric Diagnosis and Treatment*, 922–943. Stamford, CT: Appleton & Lange.

# 11

# Positive Mantoux Test

*Bernard P. Tadda*
*Marie Lindsey*

Hang D. is a 12-year-old Vietnamese girl who comes with her family for the standard physical examination required of all refugees arriving in the United States. It is common for immigrants and refugees in this rural area to come to this clinic for their initial assessment, as well as for follow-up care. An interpreter assists in conducting the history and physical examination.

## CHIEF COMPLAINT

"Our daughter needs to be examined so that she can start school."

## PRESENT HEALTH STATUS

Hang has no significant complaints other than occasional "bloody noses," which occur once every month or two and seem to be related to "weather changes" by the mother's report. The girl has also just gotten over a "cold," which seems to be gone today.

## PAST MEDICAL HISTORY

The mother reports that Hang has had no significant health problems or hospitalizations. Hang had a couple of ear infections when she was between 10 months and 2 years old, which resolved without sequelae. At the age of 11 months she had a rash for about a week that was treated with some "Chinese medicine." The interpreter cannot offer any better translation of what the medicine was.

## REVIEW OF SYSTEMS

Hang denies any cough, fever, chills, night sweats, or weight loss. Parents deny a family history of tuberculosis (TB) or any contact with TB-positive individuals. The rest of the review of systems was also negative.

## PHYSICAL FINDINGS

| | |
|---|---|
| Vital signs: | Temperature 98.6°F, pulse 84, respirations 20, blood pressure 94/60. |
| General: | Alert, cooperative Vietnamese girl in no acute distress. |
| Skin: | Soft, warm, good turgor, without edema. Seven faint erythematous surface abrasions across upper back and lower neck. Abrasions are 4 to 5 cm long, ½ cm wide, with a linear distribution on the neck and back. |
| Eyes: | Sclera clear; pupils equal, round, reactive to light, and accommodation; red reflex noted. |
| Nose: | Patent; nasal mucosa pink, moist. |
| Throat: | No tonsillar enlargement, erythema, or exudate. |
| Ears: | Tympanic membranes pearly grey, mobile, with landmarks and light reflex noted. |
| Neck: | Few small anterior cervical nodes palpable. Thyroid palpable but not enlarged. |
| Lungs: | Clear in all fields. |
| Heart: | Regular rate and rhythm; $S_1 > S_2$ at apex; no $S_3$, $S_4$, or murmurs. |
| Abdomen: | Soft, nontender, no masses or organomegaly. |
| Musculoskeletal: | Full range of motion and good strength of upper and lower extremities. Spine straight. |
| Neurologic: | Grossly within normal limits. |
| Genitalia: | Normal external female genitalia, Tanner stage 2. Breast: No masses, Tanner stage 2. |

The results of the following diagnostic tests were as follows:

| | |
|---|---|
| Complete blood count: | Hemoglobin, hematocrit, white blood count within normal limits |
| Blood chemistry panel: | All lab values normal except alkaline phosphatase mildly elevated |
| Urinalysis: | Within normal limits |
| Rapid plasma reagin (RPR): | Negative |
| Human immuno-deficiency virus: | Negative |
| Hepatitis B surface antigen (HbsAg): | Negative |
| Mantoux test, left forearm: | 22 mm induration |

## ASSESSMENT

QUESTION 1. Hang's Mantoux test and history suggest which of the following?
   A. She probably has active TB and should be isolated.
   B. She should have a repeat TB skin test in 2 weeks to check for a "booster effect."
   C. She probably has inactive TB and will need preventive medication.
   D. She needs a bacille Calmette-Guérin (BCG) vaccine to prevent her TB from becoming active.

QUESTION 2. Which of the following additional tests are needed? (Select all that apply.)
  A. Urine culture and sensitivity
  B. Chest x-ray
  C. Erythrocyte sedimentation rate (ESR)
  D. Sputum for acid-fast bacilli
  E. Electrocardiogram (ECG)

QUESTION 3. Hang's alkaline phosphatase was slightly elevated. This is probably related to which of the following?
  A. Her age and normal bone growth
  B. Gallbladder disease
  C. Her TB status
  D. Underlying bone disease

QUESTION 4. The abrasions on Hang's back are most likely related to which of the following?
  A. Rubbing the back with a coin based on the belief that this will help to relieve any infirmity
  B. Child abuse on the part of the parents
  C. A skin reaction caused by TB
  D. Scabies

QUESTION 5. In working with an interpreter and non-English-speaking patients, the provider should be aware of which of the following?
  A. Using a family member is preferable because he or she can interpret a patient's medical history in a more personal way than a medical interpreter.
  B. A good bilingual translator makes the best medical interpreter.
  C. Having the interpreter put the instructions in writing will ensure that the right message is conveyed.
  D. Having the interpreter repeat the provider's question in English before translating will help clarify whether he or she understands what is being asked.

## PLAN

QUESTION 6. Treatment of inactive TB (with a normal chest x-ray and no symptoms) is called preventive therapy and usually involves which of the following medications? (Select all that apply.)
  A. Rifampin
  B. Ethambutol
  C. Isoniazid (INH)
  D. Azithromycin

QUESTION 7. Watching for adverse effects of the medication for inactive TB includes close monitoring of which of the following laboratory indices? (Select all that apply.)
  A. Urinalysis to check for ketonuria
  B. Aspartate transaminase (AST) and alanine transaminase (ALT) to check for liver enzyme elevation
  C. Creatine phosphakinase (CPK) to check for muscle disease
  D. Electrocardiogram to check for QRS widening

## ANSWERS

QUESTION 1. Hang's Mantoux test and history suggest which of the following?
  A. NO. A positive TB skin test does not give information about the activity or inactivity of the disease. It indicates that a person has been exposed to the disease and has developed antibodies. Hang probably does not have an *active* case of TB, since she has no signs or symptoms of the disease. Classic symptoms of pulmonary TB include productive cough, fever, night sweats, chills, and weight loss. For nonimmuno-compromised patients, a Mantoux reading of 10 mm or more of induration at the injection site is considered positive for TB infection.
  B. NO. The 22-mm induration of the TB skin test indicates that Hang has been infected with the tuberculosis bacterium. Since her result is already significant (greater than 10 mm induration), a repeat test would produce similar results and offer no new information.
  C. YES. The size of the induration of Hang's skin test indicates that she has been infected with the tuberculosis bacterium. As she does not have any symptoms at this point, it appears that she has no signs of active TB and so will need medication to treat the infection in its *inactive* state. This is also known as preventive therapy.
  D. NO. As a prophylactic agent, the BCG vaccine is of questionable value. Its use is far more widespread in countries other than the United States. If it is to be effective, it must be administered *prior* to TB exposure. It may be indicated in a tuberculin-negative infant who resides in a household where repeated TB exposure is likely. Individuals who have received BCG vaccine should not be excluded from skin testing. The protection provided by the vaccination wanes and its effectiveness is weak; therefore, any reaction ≥ 10 mm should be considered positive for TB infection.

QUESTION 2. Which of the following additional tests are needed?
  A. NO. Although TB can affect the kidneys, Hang has no signs or symptoms to suggest this presentation. If there were symptoms, a urine culture and sensitivity would not be appropriate because a special urine culture for acid-fast bacilli would be required to diagnose urinary TB.
  B. YES. A chest x-ray is needed to look for any pulmonary lesions, as TB is a disease that primarily affects the lungs.
  C. NO. The ESR is a nonspecific test for inflammation and would yield no valuable information in what appears to be inactive TB.

D. *NO*. While examining sputum for acid-fast bacilli is an excellent confirmatory test for active TB, it is unwarranted for someone like Hang who has no respiratory symptoms.

E. *NO*. An ECG would yield no valuable information in this case, given Hang's young age and the absence of active infection.

**QUESTION 3.** Hang's alkaline phosphatase was slightly elevated. This is probably related to which of the following?

A. *YES*. The alkaline phosphatase is often elevated in children, as their bones are growing.

B. *NO*. While an elevated alkaline phosphatase can indicate gallbladder disease, this is unlikely given Hang's age and lack of symptoms.

C. *NO*. Elevated alkaline phosphatase is not related to a positive TB skin test with inactive disease.

D. *NO*. While an elevated alkaline phosphatase can indicate bone disease, this is unlikely given Hang's age and lack of symptoms.

**QUESTION 4.** The abrasions on Hang's back are most likely related to which of the following?

A. *YES*. This is a technique called "coin rubbing" that is employed by the Vietnamese in an attempt to relieve infirmities. Often this appears like a "hickey" or surface abrasion and has been mistaken for child abuse (see Fig. 11-1).

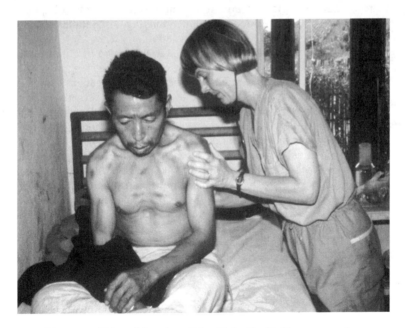

**FIGURE 11-1.** Skin coining (see Color Plate 4). (P. Fox, personal photograph, January 1990.) With permission.

   B.  *NO*. Although child abuse needs to be considered in the presence of
       any unusual skin presentations, knowledge of the Vietnamese culture
       and a complete history taking would eliminate this possibility.
   C.  *NO*. TB does not cause a localized skin rash of this type.
   D.  *NO*. The skin lesion from scabies is papular and does not usually affect
       this area of the back.

**QUESTION 5.** In working with an interpreter and non-English-speaking
patients, the provider should be aware of which of the following?
   A.  *NO*. Untrained family members may not understand the importance of
       certain questions, and may be more concerned with maintaining their
       relationship with the patient than with providing accurate information
       for the health care provider. Using a family member may interfere with
       collecting sensitive information, particularly when the family member
       is the patient's child. In addition, untrained interpreters are more likely
       to take shortcuts or use their own discretion. There are five common errors
       made by untrained interpreters. *Omission* occurs when the interpreter
       chooses to completely or partially delete a part of the speaker's mes-
       sage. *Addition* is the interpreter's tendency to include new information.
       *Condensation* is the tendency to simplify and explain, and *substitution*
       is the tendency to replace concepts. *Role exchange* occurs when an
       interpreter replaces the health care provider's questions with his or her
       own, in effect taking over the role of interviewer.
   B.  *NO*. The translation process refers only to communicating information
       from one language into another, usually written, form. Adequate oral
       interpretation requires accurate understanding of the intent of the mes-
       sage, and is more than a literal translation.
   C.  *NO*. There is no guarantee that an interpreter who is able to speak a
       language is equally skilled in reading or writing that language. In addi-
       tion, before providing written instructions in the patient's native lan-
       guage, the provider must ensure that the patient is literate in his or her
       own language. Providing simple instructions in English may be useful
       only if patients have access to others in their community who can pro-
       vide adequate translation if necessary.
   D.  *YES*. A practical way to clarify whether the interpreter understands the
       health care provider's question is to ask him or her to reiterate or para-
       phrase it in English before translating it into the patient's language.
       Unfortunately, this does not ensure that the question will be accurately
       interpreted in the second language, or that the patient will understand
       the intent of the message.

**QUESTION 6.** Treatment of inactive TB (with a normal chest x-ray and no
symptoms) is called preventive therapy and usually involves which of the following medications?
   A.  *NO*. Rifampin is not indicated unless there is suspicion of an active
       case of TB.
   B.  *NO*. Ethambutol is not indicated unless there is suspicion of an active
       case of TB.

C. *YES.* The recommended treatment for inactive TB (preventive therapy) is to give INH for at least 6 months. Other medications are indicated only if there appears to be an active case of TB.

D. *NO.* Azithromycin is not indicated in the treatment of TB, active or inactive.

**QUESTION 7.** Watching for adverse effects of the medication for inactive TB includes close monitoring of which of the following laboratory indices?

A. *NO.* Unless there is coexisting diabetes, there is no need to monitor urine ketones.

B. *YES.* With INH therapy, it is necessary to monitor for any INH-induced hepatotoxicity by checking the liver function tests and monitoring for any symptoms.

C. *NO.* There is no need to monitor the CPK, as muscle disease is not a common side effect of TB medications.

D. *NO.* There is no need to monitor the ECG, as heart disease is not a common side effect of TB medications.

## REFERENCES

Centers for Disease Control and Prevention. (1994). *Core Curriculum on Tuberculosis: What the Clinician Should Know,* 3d ed. Washington, DC: U.S. Department of Health & Human Services, Public Health Service.

Centers for Disease Control and Prevention. (1996). The role of BCG vaccine in the prevention and control of tuberculosis in the United States. *Morbidity and Mortality Weekly Report 5,* No. RR-4, pp. 1–14.

Fischbach, F. (1996). *A Manual of Laboratory and Diagnostic Tests.* Philadelphia: J. B. Lippincott.

Purnell, L. D., Paulanka, B. J. (1998). Purnell's model for cultural competence. In L. D. Purnell, B. J. Paulanka (eds.), *Transcultural Health Care: A Culturally Competent Approach,* 7–15. Philadelphia: F. A. Davis.

Stauffer, R. Y. (1995). Vietnamese Americans. In J. N. Giger, R. E. Davidhizar (eds.), *Transcultural Nursing: Assessment and Intervention,* 2d ed., 441–472. St. Louis: Mosby.

Vasquez, C., Javier, R. (1991). The problem with interpreters: Communicating with Spanish-speaking patients. *Hospital and Community Psychiatry 42*(2), 163–165.

Walsh, K. (1994). Guidelines for the prevention and control of tuberculosis in the elderly. *Nurse Pract 19*(11), 79–84.

# 12

# Pharyngitis with Impetigo

*Patricia A. Furnace*
*Arlene Miller*

Tommy W. is an 11-year-old African American male living in the suburban area of a major Midwestern city. He presents to the office, accompanied by his mother, with a 4-day history of a sore throat. Tommy has been followed regularly for his well-child examinations since he was born. His height and weight have followed the growth curve at the 90th percentile. His last office visit was 1 year ago for his fifth-grade physical examination. All of his immunizations are current.

## CHIEF COMPLAINT

"Bad sore throat all the time for 4 days that doesn't go away with Tylenol."

## HISTORY OF PRESENT ILLNESS

He has had malaise, anorexia, and intermittent, generalized headaches. He had a fever between 101° and 102°F yesterday. The fever went down after taking acetaminophen, but returned about 4 to 6 h later. Tommy denies any pain or pressure in his ears, rhinorrhea, postnasal drainage, cough, or hoarseness. He has no known allergies. The only medication he has been taking is acetaminophen 4 times a day.

QUESTION 1. What additional information would be important to obtain? (Select all that apply.)
A. Difficulty swallowing
B. Presence of a rash
C. Similar problem in anyone else in his family or at school
D. History of environmental allergies

## PHYSICAL FINDINGS

Vital signs: Temperature 101.8°F, pulse 88, respirations 18.
Ears: Tympanic membranes are pearly gray. Canals are without obstruction.

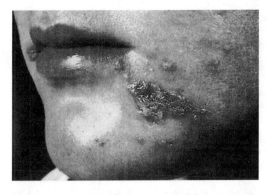

FIGURE 12-1.   Skin findings
(see Color Plate 5).
[Lookingbills, D. P., Marks, J. G.
(eds.). (1986). *Principles of
Dermatology.* Philadelphia:
W. B. Saunders.]
With permission.

Nose:  Patent without exudate or lesions.
Face:  No sinus tenderness. Several small vesicles, a few of which have
       ruptured, with moist, honey-colored crusts on chin (see Fig. 12-1).
Throat: 2+ tonsils, erythematous without exudate or lesions.
Neck:  Supple. Bilateral cervical lymphadenopathy.
Lungs: Clear to auscultation and percussion.

QUESTION 2. Grading tonsillar enlargement aids in the description of find-
ings. Which description is the best for describing 2+ enlargement of the tonsils?
  A. Just visible beyond the tonsillar pillar
  B. Touching each other
  C. Midway between the tonsillar pillar and the uvula
  D. Touching the uvula

QUESTION 3. Common bacterial and viral causes of pharyngitis would include
which of the following? (Select all that apply.)
  A. Adenoviruses
  B. Staphylococcus
  C. Streptococci
  D. Epstein-Barr virus (EBV)
  E. Histoplasma

QUESTION 4. Laboratory testing may be done to confirm a diagnosis. Which
of the following tests would be appropriate to order for this patient? (Select all
that apply.)
  A. Rapid screen for group A β-hemolytic streptococci (GABHS)
  B. Monospot
  C. Complete blood count (CBC)
  D. Random blood sugar

QUESTION 5. When obtaining a throat culture, contact should be made with
which anatomical areas? (Select all that apply.)
  A. Soft palate
  B. Uvula
  C. Both tonsillar regions

D. Posterior wall of oropharynx
E. Papillae on posterior tongue

## ASSESSMENT

QUESTION 6. Which of the following would be an appropriate assessment of this patient?
A. Influenza
B. Infectious mononucleosis
C. Pharyngitis (rule out GABHS)
D. Upper respiratory tract infection

QUESTION 7. The rash on Tommy's face is most likely associated with which of the following?
A. Scarlet fever
B. Cellulitis
C. Impetigo
D. Herpes simplex

## PLAN

QUESTION 8. What medication would be the first choice for treatment if the rapid screen for GABHS is positive?
A. Cefaclor
B. Trimethoprin/sulfamethoxazole
C. Tetracycline
D. Penicillin V

QUESTION 9. Which of the following would be appropriate additional treatment measures for this patient? (Select all that apply.)
A. Increase fluid intake.
B. Soak and soften crusts on face.
C. Follow-up throat culture in 10 days.
D. Analgesics.
E. Antibiotic therapy for facial lesions.

## ANSWERS

QUESTION 1. What additional information would be important to obtain?
A. *YES.* Knowledge of the presence of pain or difficulty with swallowing may help differentiate among the etiologies of a sore throat. Common viral and bacterial infections are accompanied by pain with swallowing, whereas peritonsillar and pharyngeal abscesses are accompanied by more significant dysphagia or difficulty swallowing. A pharyngeal abscess should be suspected if fever persists after 4 days of antibiotic treatment for GABHS.
B. *YES.* The presence of a rash can help narrow the differential diagnosis. An erythematous macular rash with erythematous flexor creases is fre-

quently seen with streptococcal pharyngitis. GABHS pharyngitis may also present with fine, discrete petechiae on the upper abdomen or trunk.
C. *YES.* Acute viral and bacterial pharyngeal infections are more frequent in close, confined groups.
D. *YES.* A sore throat can be caused by postnasal discharge secondary to allergic rhinitis.

QUESTION 2. Grading tonsillar enlargement aids in the description of findings. Which description is best for describing 2+ enlargement of the tonsils?
A. *NO.* Tonsils that are just visible beyond the tonsillar pillar is the description for 1+ or normal tonsils.
B. *NO.* Tonsils that are touching each other describes 4+ enlargement.
C. *YES.* Tonsils that are midway between the tonsillar pillar and the uvula is the best description for 2+ tonsillar enlargement.
D. *NO.* Tonsils that are touching the uvula describes 3+ tonsillar enlargement.

QUESTION 3. Common bacterial and viral causes of pharyngitis would include which of the following?
A. *YES.* Exudative pharyngitis in young children is frequently caused by adenoviruses. The child will usually have a high fever, exudative tonsillitis, and conjunctivitis.
B. *NO.* Staphylococci are not a frequent cause of pharyngitis.
C. *YES.* Groups A, B, C, and G streptococci may be associated with pharyngitis, but only pharyngitis caused by GABHS must be treated with antibiotics. Treatment is necessary primarily because of the potential sequelae of rheumatic fever and glomerulonephritis.
D. *YES.* Epstein-Barr virus causes infectious mononucleosis. Pharyngitis is part of its symptom complex.
E. *NO.* Histoplasma is a fungus that is the causative agent for histoplasmosis. A sore throat is not a symptom in this disease.

QUESTION 4. Laboratory testing may be done to confirm a diagnosis. Which of the following tests would be appropriate to order for this patient?
A. *YES.* A rapid screen for GABHS will provide an answer within 5 to 10 min, whereas routine throat culture results may take 24 to 48 hours. Sources differ regarding treatment in the absence of a positive rapid screen, which may have a 5 to 10 percent false negative rate. Waiting for results of routine throat culture delays prompt treatment, which may increase symptom duration.
B. *NO.* A monospot is helpful in diagnosing infectious mononucleosis. In infectious mononucleosis, the sore throat is usually present 1 week before a positive result will be obtained.
C. *NO.* A CBC will not be helpful at this time. It can indicate the presence of an infection, but it cannot identify the type of infection.
D. *NO.* A blood sugar would be important to consider in an individual with frequent infections. Tommy has no history of other infections.

QUESTION 5. When obtaining a throat culture, contact should be made with which anatomical areas?
A. *NO.* Culture of the soft palate may miss the presence of pathogens.
B. *NO.* The uvula does not readily harbor pathogens.
C. *YES.* Both of the tonsillar regions should be swabbed. GABHS may be retained in the tonsillar crypts.
D. *YES.* The posterior pharyngeal wall should be swabbed in addition to the tonsillar areas to ensure the most accurate results.
E. *NO.* Culture of the papillae on the posterior tongue may miss the presence of pathogens.

QUESTION 6. Which of the following would be an appropriate assessment of this patient?
A. *NO.* Influenza may present with a sore throat and high fever, but sudden onset of myalgia, nonproductive cough, chills, rhinorrhea, sneezing, and high fever are typically part of the symptom complex.
B. *NO.* It is too early to test for infectious mononucleosis for this patient. A negative monospot at this time would not rule out the disease.
C. *YES.* The patient presents with classic symptoms of pharyngitis (see Table 12-1). A rapid screen for GABHS or a throat culture at this time would help make a more specific diagnosis of the type of pharyngitis.
D. *NO.* An upper respiratory tract infection usually presents with sneezing, nasal congestion, cough, and slightly elevated or normal temperature.

QUESTION 7. The rash on Tommy's face is most likely associated with which of the following?
A. *NO.* The rash associated with scarlet fever is most intense in the axilla and groin areas, and the skin appears diffusely erythematous. It usually appears within 24 h of the onset of fever and spreads rapidly during the next 1 to 2 days. Scarlet fever, caused by GABHS, also affects the surface of the tongue, which appears white with enlarged, red papillae ("white strawberry tongue") early in the disease and later red ("red strawberry tongue").
B. *NO.* Cellulitis may be caused by streptococci, *Hemophylis influenzae*, or *Staphylococcus aureus*. Cellulitis is a rapidly spreading infection of the subcutaneous tissues, usually preceded by disruption of a skin lesion such as an insect bite or penetrating wound. Cellulitis is characterized by warm, tender, erythematous areas of skin with irregular borders.
C. *YES.* Impetigo is a superficial bacterial infection caused by GABHS, *S. aureus*, and *Streptococcus pyogenes*. Lesions are most commonly found on the face, extremities, or perineum and are accompanied by lymphadenopathy. The rash begins as a papule that becomes a vesicle. The vesicles rupture, leaving denuded areas covered by classic, honey-colored crusts. Impetigo may be seen in conjunction with pharyngitis caused by GABHS.
D. *NO.* Although the lesions of herpes simplex may include clusters of small vesicles with an erythematous base that progress to yellowish crusts, they are usually limited to the anterior portion of the mouth and

TABLE 12-1  Differential Diagnosis of the Three Most Commonly Seen Causes of Pediatric Pharyngitis

| Condition | History | Fever | Exudate | Lymphadenopathy | Other Findings | Diagnostic Studies |
|---|---|---|---|---|---|---|
| Group A beta-hemolytic streptococcal | Rapid onset Few systemic symptoms Seasonal Infection in family | ≥100°F | Yellow Marked erythema | Anterior cervical | Scarlatiniform rash Tachycardia | + Rapid strep test + Throat culture |
| Viral | Rapid onset Systemic symptoms | ≥100°F | Less likely Swollen, pale pharynx | — | Cough Congestion Rhinitis Malaise Conjunctivitis | − Rapid strep test − Throat culture |
| Infectious mononucleosis | Gradual onset Fatigue and malaise | ≥102°F | White or gray-green Palatine petechiae | Posterior cervical | Hepatosplenomegaly Headache | + Monospot Lymphocytosis |

*Source:* Used with permission from Ruppert, S.D. (1966). Differential diagnosis of common causes of pediatric pharyngitis. *Nurse Pract* 21(4): 38–48. Copyright © Springhouse Corporation. With permission.

lips and are accompanied by burning and pain. In children, primary herpes simplex infection may present with high fever, sore throat, malaise, and decreased fluid intake; secondary infections are less severe and are marked by burning, tingling, and itching at the involved site. Herpes simplex is a viral infection that is not particularly associated with GABHS.

**QUESTION 8.** What medication would be the first choice for treatment if the rapid screen for GABHS is positive?

   **A.** *NO.* Cefaclor is not a first-line antibiotic for GABHS infections. However, treatment with a ß-lactamase–resistant antibiotic would be considered if the patient remains symptomatic after initial treatment.
   **B.** *NO.* Trimethoprin/sulfamethoxazole is not indicated in the treatment of GABHS infections.
   **C.** *NO.* Tetracycline will not eradicate GABHS infections.
   **D.** *YES.* Penicillin is the antibiotic of choice in the treatment of GABHS infections. It can be given either orally or intramuscularly. A 10-day course of the antibiotic is needed to treat this infection and prevent serious sequelae, including rheumatic fever and poststreptococcal glomerulonephritis. Penicillin can prevent rheumatic fever if given within 9 days of the onset of a sore throat caused by GABHS. GABHS is the only causative agent of pharyngitis for which an antibiotic is necessary. Children can return to school after they have been on antibiotics for at least 24 h if they are afebrile.

**QUESTION 9.** Which of the following would be appropriate additional treatment measures for this patient?

   **A.** *YES.* Adequate fluid intake will prevent dehydration and will help the patient feel more comfortable.
   **B.** *YES.* Applying compresses with warm water or Burow's solution to the lesions will soften and remove the crusts on his face. Education regarding cleanliness, hand washing, and spread of the disease should be included.
   **C.** *NO.* A culture following treatment is not necessary in the asymptomatic patient.
   **D.** *YES.* Analgesics will help the patient feel more comfortable. Use of aspirin-containing products should be avoided in children up to the age of 16 because of the risk of Reye's syndrome.
   **E.** *YES.* Treatment of very mild lesions includes topical antibiotics such as mupirocin t.i.d. for 5 to 14 days. If there is no improvement within 3 days, oral antibiotic treatment, preferably penicillin, is recommended if the infection is caused by GABHS.

## REFERENCES

Berkowitz, C. D. (1996). *Pediatrics: A Primary Care Approach*, 216–221. Philadelphia: W. B. Saunders.

Griffith, H. W. (1997). *5 Minute Clinical Consult.* Philadelphia: Lea & Febiger.

Inkelis, S. H. (1996). In C. D. Berkowitz (ed.), *Pediatrics: A Primary Care Approach*, 186–191. Philadelphia: W. B. Saunders.

Jarvis, C. (1992). *Physical Examination and Health Assessment.* Philadelphia: W. B. Saunders.

Noble, J., Green, H. L., Levinson, W., Modest, G. A., Young, M. (eds.), (1996). *Textbook of Primary Care Medicine,* 2d ed. St. Louis: Mosby-Yearbook.

Ruppert, S. D. (1996). Differential diagnosis of common causes of pediatric pharyngitis. *Nurse Pract 21*(4), 39–48.

Stein, P. G. (1996). Sore throat. In R. H. Rubin, C. Voss, D. J. Derksen, A. Gateley, R. W. Quenzer (eds.), *Medicine: A Primary Care Approach,* 103–106. Philadelphia: W. B. Saunders.

# IV

# ADOLESCENT

# Introduction

## Marie L. Talashek

Effective primary care providers for adolescents understand the psychosocial developmental issues of this age group and enjoy the challenge of guiding each adolescent to attain his or her optimal level of health. Adolescents assume the role of primary historian, with parents supplementing the information. Adolescents must be prepared to assume responsibility for lifestyle choices. During this developmental period, decisions are made that alter the course of one's life, including those involving school activities and employment, as well as initiating sexual relations or substance use.

The American Academy of Pediatrics recommends visits at ages 14, 16, 18, and 20 years. Each visit should include the following:

1. A history of health and wellness since the last visit should be taken.
2. A complete physical examination should be given.
3. Height, weight, and blood pressure should be graphed.
4. Vision and hearing screening should be done.
5. Developmental/behavioral assessment should be done.
6. Immunization status should be assessed and brought into compliance with Centers For Disease Control and Prevention (CDC) recommendations.
7. Hematocrit or hemoglobin and urinalysis should be done at least once during this time period.
8. Screening for tuberculosis should be done at least once during this time period.
9. Anticipatory guidance should be given.
10. Sexually active females should have an annual Pap smear and be screened for sexually transmitted diseases (STDs).

According to Erikson, the developmental task of adolescence is to develop ego identity rather than role diffusion; an adolescent links the past, present, and future for an understanding of self. Adolescents are in the Piagetian stage of formal operational thought, which is characterized by abstract reasoning. Formal operational thought also includes future orientation, reasoning about chance and probability, and generating and evaluating alternatives.

Anticipatory guidance, according to the U.S. Preventive Task Force, includes promoting healthy eating by limiting fat and cholesterol, maintaining caloric balance and adequate calcium intake, and engaging in regular physical activity. Injury prevention counseling includes use of lap/shoulder belts; helmet use with bicycles, motorcycles, and ATVs; smoke detectors; and safe storage of firearms. Substance use is an area of great importance for this age group. The avoidance of smoking, underage drinking, illicit drug use, and substance use while driving, swimming, and boating must be stressed. Sexual behavior, including prevention of STDs and unintended pregnancy, is to be addressed. Although the effectiveness of this has not been proven, advising abstinence should be part of clinical counseling about high-risk behaviors. Contraception for pregnancy prevention and consistent use of condoms with spermicide for STD prevention should be encouraged for all sexually active teens. Counseling also includes regular visits to dental care providers, flossing, and brushing with fluoride toothpaste.

The cases for this part were chosen to reflect common issues/conditions occurring during adolescence. Emerging sexual behaviors and lack of planning for intercourse may result in sexually transmitted diseases, urinary tract infections, and adjustment disorders. Suicide is the third leading cause of mortality for males aged 15 to 24 years. The National Adolescent Student Health Survey found that 12 percent of eighth and tenth graders reported that someone had raped or tried to rape them, and 54 percent of females surveyed in a national sample of college students reported some sort of sexual victimization. Eating disorders are also common during adolescence, with approximately 20 percent being overweight and more than 3 percent having anorexia nervosa or bulimia. Exercise-induced asthma can be managed to allow for exercise, resulting in a healthier lifestyle that can continue through adulthood.

## REFERENCES

Burns, C., Barber, N., Brady, M., Dunn, A. (eds). (1996). *Pediatric Primary Care: A Handbook for Nurse Practitioners*. Philadelphia: W. B. Saunders.

Centers for Disease Control and Prevention. (1996). Immunization of Adolescents: Recommendations of the Advisory Committee on Immunization Practices. *Morbidity and Mortality Weekly Report* 45, No. RR-13, pp. 3–9.

Committee on Practice and Ambulatory Medicine. (1995). Recommendations for preventive pediatric health care. *Pediatrics 92*(6), 751.

DeKeseredy, W. S. (1988). *Woman Abuse in Dating Relationships: The Role of Support*. Toronto: Canadian Scholars Press.

Erikson, E. (1963). *Childhood and Society*. New York: Norton.

Inhelder, B., Piaget, J. (1958). *The Growth of Logical Thinking from Childhood to Adolescence*. New York: Basic Books.

Neinstein, L. S. (1996). *Adolescent Health Care: A Practical Guide*, 3d ed. Baltimore: Williams & Wilkins.

U.S. Preventive Services Task Force. (1996). *Guide To Clinical Preventive Services*, 2d ed. Baltimore: Williams & Wilkins.

Woolf, S., Jonas, S., Lawrence, R. (eds). (1996). *Health Promotion and Disease Prevention in Clinical Practice*. Baltimore: Williams & Wilkins.

# 13

# Adolescent Sexual Activity

*Judith McDevitt*
*Marie Lindsey*

Carrie is a 19-year-old Caucasian female who has come to the college health service for a Papanicolaou (Pap) test. She is a sophomore majoring in communications and lives in an apartment nearby with several roommates who are also students. This is her first visit to the college health service.

## CHIEF COMPLAINT

"I've never had a Pap test, and I just want to make sure everything's okay."

## HISTORY OF PRESENT ILLNESS

Carrie has a new boyfriend with whom she has been having sex several times a week for the past 4 months, most recently 3 days ago. They use condoms most of the time, except during or right after her period. Last week she felt some nontender "bumps" on her vulva when she was washing. Using a mirror, she observed that the lesions resembled small, tan moles. She does not know if they were present before she felt them last week. She denies a past history of a sexually transmitted disease (STD), but is concerned about that possibility.

## PAST HISTORY

Carrie reports a history of good health; the last time she sought health care was for a sore throat one year ago, when she went to her family's health maintenance organization at home. She has never been hospitalized or had surgery, has no allergies, and takes no medications. Carrie feels that she and her boyfriend both are currently monogamous. However, she reports a history of two prior partners, the first of which was when she was 16. Her sexual practices have been limited to vaginal intercourse with males. She does not know much about her boyfriend's sexual history (e.g., how many prior partners, his sexual practices, or history of STDs). She has not noticed any moles, warts, or sores on her boyfriend. Her menstrual periods are on a regular 28-day cycle, have a moderate flow, and last approximately 5 days; her last menstrual period began 12 days ago.

QUESTION 1. Which of the following additional historical information must be obtained from Carrie? (Select all that apply.)
   A. Presence of vaginal discharge, odor, itching
   B. Presence of dark, cloudy, or malodorous urine; urinary frequency, urgency, dysuria, hematuria
   C. Presence of fever, chills, or pelvic pain
   D. Menstrual, obstetric, and contraceptive history

QUESTION 2. What factors in Carrie's history increase the likelihood of an STD?
   A. Onset of sexual activity before age 17
   B. Inconsistent condom use
   C. Multiple sexual partners, or a partner who has had multiple sexual partners
   D. Mutual monogamy

QUESTION 3. Since Carrie has never had a pelvic examination before, how should the examination be conducted? (Select all that apply.)
   A. Explain the examination beforehand.
   B. Show her the speculum you will use.
   C. Teach her how to relax her pelvic muscles.
   D. Raise the head of the examination table.
   E. Offer Carrie a hand mirror so that she can watch the examination and view her own cervix if she so desires.

## PHYSICAL FINDINGS

Vital signs:  Temperature 98.4°F, pulse 74, blood pressure 108/70 (right arm sitting), height 64 in, weight 120 lb.
Skin:  Warm, dry, intact, turgor good. No lesions, birthmarks, or edema. Color uniformly light tan except pale white in a bikini bathing suit distribution.
Hair:  Normal texture, female distribution, no evidence of infestation.
Head:  Normocephalic, no lesions or lumps.
Face:  Expressions symmetrical; no sinus tenderness
Eyes:  Extraocular movements intact, no nystagmus bilaterally
Conjunctivae clear, sclerae white, no lesions or redness
Pupils equal, round, reactive to light, and accommodation.
Ears:  Pinnae without masses or tenderness; canals clear; tympanic membranes pearly gray, landmarks intact.
Nose:  Nares patent, mucosa pink, no lesions.
Mouth:  Oral mucosa pink, no lesions, teeth in good repair. Pharynx pink, no exudate, tonsils 1+.
Neck:  No masses, tenderness, or lymphadenopathy. Trachea midline, thyroid nonpalpable.

Spine/back:   Normal spinal profile, no costovertebral angle tenderness.
Lungs:   Clear to auscultation.
Heart:   Regular rate and rhythm; $S_1 > S_2$ at apex; no $S_3$, $S_4$, clicks, or murmurs.
Breasts:   Symmetric; no dimpling, retractions, or lesions. Contour and consistency firm, homogeneous. No tenderness or masses. Montgomery's tubercles prominent bilaterally. No nipple discharge. No axillary lymphadenopathy.
Abdomen:   Flat, symmetric, soft, nontender, no organomegaly. No inguinal lymphadenopathy.

## PELVIC EXAMINATION

External genitalia:   No evidence of infestation, swelling, or redness. Bartholin's, urethra, and Skene's glands intact. Cluster of three discrete, dry, tan-pink, soft, 3–5 mm papules at fourchette.
Vagina:   Pink with prominent rugae; creamy white secretions without odor, pH 4.1.
Cervix:   Pink, no lesions, copious clear, mucoid discharge. No cervical motion tenderness.
Uterus:   Small, firm, mobile, smooth, nontender, anteverted.
Adnexae:   Right ovary 3 × 2 × 1 cm, nontender; left ovary nonpalpable, nontender.
Rectal:   Rectal wall intact, no masses or tenderness. Brown stool present, guaiac negative.

QUESTION 4. Which of the following findings on Carrie's physical examination are clinical features associated with sexually transmitted infections? (Select all that apply.)
A. Montgomery's tubercles
B. Papules at fourchette
C. Prominent vaginal rugae
D. Vaginal pH of 4.1
E. Copious clear, mucoid cervical discharge

QUESTION 5. Which of the following tests should be done to screen Carrie for STDs? (Select all that apply.)
A. Pap test
B. Screening tests for chlamydia and gonorrhea
C. Rapid plasma reagin (RPR) test or Venereal Disease Research Laboratory (VDRL) test
D. Biopsy of papules
E. Wet prep

QUESTION 6. How should the Pap smear be performed to assure an adequate cytological specimen? (Select all that apply.)
A. Moisten the speculum with water-based lubricant.
B. Gently remove excessive vaginal or cervical discharge with a cotton swab.

C. Collect the Pap smear first, before other specimens.
D. Sample the ectocervix using a spatula, then the endocervical canal using an endocervical brush. Apply both samples to the slide at the same time.
E. Apply fixative within 4 seconds to preserve the specimen.

## ASSESSMENT

Pap test:    Satisfactory sample for evaluation; positive for low-grade squamous intraepithelial lesion (LSIL).
Chlamydia:  Negative.
Gonorrhea:  Negative.
RPR:        Negative.
Wet prep:   Potassium hydroxide (KOH) prep negative for yeast forms. Saline prep negative for clue cells and trichomonads; 0 to 1 white blood cells per high-power field with numerous lactobacilli noted. Whiff test negative.

QUESTION 7. Which of the following can be diagnosed on the basis of Carrie's physical examination and test results? (Select all that apply.)
   A. Genital warts (condyloma acuminata)
   B. Bacterial vaginosis
   C. Cervical cancer

## PLAN

QUESTION 8. What interventions should be planned now? (Select all that apply.)
   A. Removal of visible warts
   B. Refer for colposcopy
   C. STD screening for Carrie's boyfriend
   D. Contraceptive counseling

## ANSWERS

QUESTION 1. Which of the following additional historical information must be obtained from Carrie?
   A. YES. Vaginal discharge, odor, and itching are symptoms of a vaginal infection.
   B. YES. Because of the close anatomical association of the genital and urinary systems, the history should include specific questions to screen for urinary problems.
   C. YES. Fever, chills, or pelvic pain could be symptoms of a more serious infection, such as pelvic inflammatory disease.
   D. YES. Questions about the menstrual, obstetric, and contraceptive history are included in the well-woman visit so that difficulties in these areas can be identified. The menstrual history should cover age at menarche, usual menstrual interval, duration of menses, amount of flow, and

symptoms. Information regarding any pregnancies, their course and outcomes, and future plans regarding childbearing should be obtained. Questions regarding contraceptive history should include current and previously used methods, satisfaction with these methods, and whether the patient would like to change methods.

**QUESTION 2.** What factors in Carrie's history increase the likelihood of an STD?

   **A.** *YES.* Sexually active individuals under the age of 25 are at particularly high risk for STDs and human immunodeficiency virus (HIV) infection. Also, onset of sexual activity at age 17 or younger is a specific risk factor for cervical dysplasia, possibly because this early onset increases the time during which immature metaplastic tissue can be exposed to causative agents.

   **B.** *YES.* Having unprotected sex poses risks for exposure to STDs and HIV. Latex condoms provide some protection, although condoms fail 10 to 15 percent of the time as a result of incorrect use or breakage. Also, condoms do not prevent skin-to-skin contact of the external genitalia, so that STDs affecting these areas can be transmitted.

   **C.** *YES.* Having multiple sexual partners or a partner with multiple sexual partners is associated with particularly high risk for STD and HIV infection.

   **D.** *NO.* Mutual monogamy can prevent STD and HIV infection if both partners are known to be infection-free at the onset of the sexual relationship. However, a series of sexual relationships, even if each relationship is mutually monogamous, means that there have been multiple sexual partners, which is a risk factor for STD and HIV infection.

**QUESTION 3.** Since Carrie has never had a pelvic examination before, how should the examination be conducted?

   **A.** *YES.* Explaining the examination beforehand will help the patient understand what to expect, provide an opportunity for health teaching, and give her an opportunity to ask questions.

   **B.** *YES.* Show the patient which type of speculum will be used, Pederson or Graves. Because of their narrower shape, Pederson specula are recommended for first-time pelvic examinations. The procedure can be demonstrated by curling one's fingers into the palm (to simulate the introitus and vagina) and showing the patient how only the blade of the speculum will be inserted.

   **C.** *YES.* While the patient is still dressed, it is helpful to explain to her how to relax her pelvic muscles by instructing her to tighten and relax her pelvic muscles, as in performing Kegal's exercise. The patient will be more comfortable if she can simulate the relaxed state of this exercise during the examination. Also, the patient should be given an opportunity to empty her bladder prior to the examination.

   **D.** *YES.* With the head of the examination table raised, the patient can see and talk more easily during the examination. Furthermore, the patient can be observed for nonverbal expressions of discomfort. In a semisitting position, the patient will feel more like an active participant in her own health care and less like a passive object being scrutinized.

E.  YES. Allowing a patient to view the procedure and her own cervix promotes education about her own body. In Carrie's case, a mirror will allow her to identify the lesions that are causing her concern.

QUESTION 4. Which of the following findings on Carrie's physical examination are clinical features associated with sexually transmitted infections?

A.  NO. Montgomery's tubercles in the areola are an expected finding on examination. These are small, elevated sebaceous glands that secrete a protective lipid material, especially during lactation.

B.  YES. These growths are most likely genital warts caused by human papillomavirus (HPV), a sexually transmitted infection.

C.  NO. Prominent vaginal rugae are a normal finding in women of childbearing age. Estrogen stimulates the abundant proliferation of the vaginal epithelium, so much so that the uppermost cell layers heap up and fold over on themselves, creating rugae. Without estrogen, the vaginal epithelium thins and atrophies, as is often seen in postmenopausal women.

D.  NO. The normal vaginal pH is 3.8 to 4.2. This low vaginal pH is considered to be a primary mechanism controlling the composition of the vaginal microflora. The acidic environment is thought to inhibit the growth of potentially pathogenic bacteria and protozoa, some of which are sexually transmitted.

E.  NO. Copious clear, mucoid cervical discharge is indicative of impending ovulation, which is likely considering that Carrie is now on day 12 of her cycle. The thin, watery, wet cervical mucus of this phase of the cycle serves to lubricate intercourse and prolongs the life of the sperm cells for up to 3 to 5 days. In contrast, opaque, thick mucus is produced before and after the ovulatory phase and is not associated with fertility, and a purulent cervical discharge is associated with some STDs.

QUESTION 5. Which of the following tests should be done to screen Carrie for STDs?

A.  YES. A Pap test will screen for cervical cancer, now considered to be associated with STDs. Sexually transmitted agents, particularly some forms of HPV, are thought to function as carcinogens.

B.  YES. Screening tests for both chlamydia and gonorrhea are recommended by all major authorities for patients attending STD, family planning, or adolescent health clinics, whether or not they are symptomatic. For gonorrhea testing, a culture is still considered the "gold standard." There are several tests currently available to screen for chlamydia, including culture, enzyme immunoassay, deoxyribonucleic acid (DNA) probe testing, or direct fluorescent antibody testing. Nucleic acid amplification tests are now available that are able to simultaneously detect chlamydial and gonococcal DNA from a single specimen.

C.  YES. Although Carrie most likely has genital warts, the growths observed on the physical examination may also be condylomata lata, a lesion of syphilis. An RPR or VDRL will serve to rule out this possibility and is recommended by the Centers for Disease Control and Prevention (CDC).

**D.** *NO.* Although a biopsy would be required to make a *definitive* diagnosis, it is usually unnecessary for clinical management of genital warts.

**E.** *YES.* On the basis of the physical examination, it is very likely that Carrie has an STD; therefore, a work-up is indicated. A wet prep will screen for vaginal infection, including sexually transmitted vaginal infection.

**QUESTION 6.** How should the Pap smear be performed to assure an adequate cytological specimen?

**A.** *NO.* Moisten the speculum with water only. Lubricants of any kind may contaminate the specimen.

**B.** *YES.* Excessive vaginal or cervical discharge will interfere with effective specimen collection.

**C.** *YES.* Collect the Pap smear first, before other specimens, because there is a risk of bleeding as a result of endocervical sampling. If cultures are taken first and bleeding occurs, blood will be included with the Pap smear and may interfere with its interpretation.

**D.** *YES.* Since both a spatula and a cytobrush are used to collect the Pap specimen, air drying is a problem because of the time needed to transfer material from each to the glass slide. It is now recommended that to avoid air drying of the first specimen, the nurse practitioner should hold on to the spatula while collecting the second specimen, then quickly apply both specimens to the slide.

**E.** *YES.* Applying fixative promptly, ideally within 4 seconds, will minimize air drying and help to properly preserve the specimen. Also, if a spray fixative is being used, it should be applied at a distance of at least 10 in from the slide to avoid distorting the cells.

**QUESTION 7.** Which of the following can be diagnosed on the basis of Carrie's physical examination and test results?

**A.** *YES.* Genital warts (condyloma acuminata) can be diagnosed on the basis of the clinical findings. The only other possibility, condylomata lata, was excluded by the negative RPR. Warts often appear 3 to 6 months after exposure, but the virus can be latent for years. Genital warts are usually benign because the HPV viral types most often associated with them have a low oncogenic potential.

**B.** *NO.* For bacterial vaginosis to be diagnosed, three of the following four signs must be present: a gray, thin, homogeneous discharge that adheres to the vaginal walls, a pH > 4.5, a positive whiff test, or clue cells on microscopic examination. In Carrie's case, the vaginal secretions were creamy white, the pH was 4.1, the whiff test was negative, and there were no clue cells on the wet prep. The lactobacilli seen on the wet prep are the predominant microorganisms found in normal vaginal microflora. They are thought to protect against infection by producing lactic acid, which maintains an acidic pH and inhibits the growth of *Gardnerella vaginalis* and anaerobes such as *Mobiluncus*. It is important to also note that bacterial vaginosis is not considered a sexually transmitted disease.

C. *NO.* While the classification of LSIL indicates histological changes associated with HPV and cervical intraepithelial neoplasia grade I, definitive diagnosis depends on colposcopy and biopsy of abnormal areas for further histological identification. About 60 percent of these lesions will revert to normal on their own, but some may progress to more serious lesions. There are over 60 HPV types, some of which (types 6 and 11) cause generally benign genital warts, and some of which (types 16, 18, 31, and 33) cause subclinical disease and have definite oncogenic potential.

**QUESTION 8.** What interventions should be planned now?

A. *YES.* Visible warts can be removed by applying trichloroacetic acid after first applying xylocaine jelly or petrolatum to the surrounding skin. This nontoxic treatment is simple, cost-effective, and safe to use during pregnancy, and it may be repeated up to 3 times a week. There is a burning sensation lasting about 10 min after the lesions are treated. Other methods include self-treatment by applying podofilox 0.5% at home twice a day for 3 days, but this is contraindicated during pregnancy. More extensive or resistant lesions may be treated by laser therapy, liquid nitrogen, or cryo- or electrocautery. The goal in all cases is to remove visible warts and then wait for the immune system to control viral replication. HPV cannot be eradicated, and genital warts often recur. Also, in 20 to 30 percent of cases the warts will clear spontaneously within 3 months without treatment.

B. *YES.* The presence of vaginal warts and a Pap test positive for LSIL warrants Carrie's being referred for colposcopy, whereby abnormal areas on the cervix will be visualized, biopsied, and sent for histological identification. Although this is costly, the biopsied material would ideally be sent for HPV typing to determine whether Carrie has a high risk for developing cervical cancer. Such information would be helpful in planning subsequent treatment and follow-up. Alternatively, Pap smears can be repeated at 3- to 6-month intervals to monitor the status of identified abnormalities. Excision, ablation, or conization then may be used to manage abnormalities.

C. *NO.* Unlike the situation with gonorrhea and chlamydia, it is not recommended that the partner of an HPV-infected patient receive specific treatment. However, if Carrie's boyfriend had obvious warts that he wanted to have removed, clearly the offer of treatment should be extended to him. As Carrie's tests revealed only an HPV infection, there is no reason for her boyfriend to be screened for other STDs. He is, however, probably already subclinically infected with HPV and should be informed of this probability, as well as of the fact that they both can infect a new partner. They should both be instructed that the use of condoms may reduce transmission, but cannot eliminate the risk altogether.

**D.** *YES.* Carrie is at risk for pregnancy as a result of her reliance on and inconsistent use of condoms. She should receive contraceptive counseling and be offered more reliable methods, such as oral contraceptives, injectable medroxyprogesterone, or spermicides and condoms used together. It must be stressed that as reliable as hormonal methods are for preventing pregnancy, they do not provide protection from STDs.

## REFERENCES

Carson, S. (1997). Human papillomatous virus infection update: Impact on women's health. *Nurse Pract 22*(4), 24–25, 28, 30, 35–37.

Centers for Disease Control and Prevention. (1993). 1993 sexually transmitted diseases treatment guidelines. *Morbidity and Mortality Weekly Report* 42, No. RR-14, 83–91.

Hanson, L. N. (1995). Abnormal cervical cytology. In W. L. Star, L. L. Lommel, M. T. Shannon (eds.), *Women's Primary Health Care: Protocols for Practice,* 12-13–12-17. Washington, D.C.: American Nurses Association.

Mashburn, J., Scharbo-DeHaan, M. (1997). A clinician's guide to Pap smear interpretation. *Nurse Pract 22*(4), 115–118, 124, 126–127, 130, 139.

# 14

# Eating Disorder

*Jill S. Anderson*
*Laina M. Gerace*

Karen J. is a 19-year-old Caucasian college freshman who appears to be of average height and weight. She presents for her first appointment at the College Health Service. Her last physical, to obtain medical clearance for college admission, was 8 months ago, and was performed by a physician in another state. Karen has been taking Ortho-Novum 7/7/7, prescribed by her previous physician, for approximately 7 months. She is requesting a change in her birth control method because of weight gain, which she attributes to the oral contraceptives. She denies any other illnesses, and states that she takes no other medications except occasional over-the-counter diet pills and over-the-counter stimulants (No-Doz) when studying for exams.

## CHIEF COMPLAINT

"I am unhappy with the way I look, and I think 'the pill' has made me gain weight."

## HISTORY OF PRESENT ILLNESS

Karen reports that she was popular and happy in high school. She has had difficulty adjusting to college, both socially and academically. She states that she first began dieting in high school to "maintain her desired weight," and lost 5 lb prior to starting college. She has since regained that weight and an additional 8 lb. She states, "I've been unable to diet successfully since I started taking birth control pills, and I was thinking about changing to the diaphragm." Upon further questioning, Karen also expressed concern about a possible "thyroid problem" because of weight gain. She complains that she is easily fatigued, lacks motivation, and is having trouble keeping up with her course work. She reports a pattern of fasting for a day, followed by episodes of overeating on the weekends. She is reluctant to discuss psychosocial issues, but acknowledges that her relationship with her high school boyfriend is currently strained, and that she is considering dating other men.

QUESTION 1. What are the most likely differential diagnoses to consider at this point? (Select all that apply.)
A. Depression
B. Hypothyroidism
C. Eating disorder
D. Adjustment disorder

## OBJECTIVE DATA

Vital signs: Temperature 98.6°F, blood pressure 102/68 sitting, pulse 70, height 5 ft 4 in, weight 118 lb.

General: A well-developed female of average height and weight who appears younger than her stated age. She appears healthy and in no acute distress.

Skin: Mild acne on face; dry skin on arms; fingernails severely bitten back with scabs on the cuticles. Calluses on the knuckles of the index and middle finger of the right hand.

Head/neck: Mild periorbital edema, nontender mild parotid gland swelling bilaterally. No lymphadenopathy.

Eyes, ears, nose, throat: Mild injection of the conjunctiva bilaterally; ears and nose clear; halitosis present; pharynx reddened and irritated, without exudate. A 7-cm oral ulcer noted on the distal upper palate.

Abdomen: Mild distention with hyperactive bowel sounds. Tenderness noted in the upper right quadrant on palpation.

Lungs: Clear to ausculation.

QUESTION 2. Which of the following areas of inquiry would help to substantiate the diagnosis? (Select all that apply.)
A. History of vomiting
B. Dental sensitivity to temperature changes
C. Laxative use
D. History of sexually transmitted diseases (STDs)

With direct questioning, Karen reluctantly acknowledges the need to "resort to drastic measures" in the past month to control her weight. She minimizes the significance of self-induced vomiting, stating that "everyone in the dorm does it." She admits that she experiences feelings of self-loathing and depression after binges, and that she feels that her eating is out of control. She states that she feels "fat" and "ugly," and begins to cry.

QUESTION 3. Which of the following laboratory tests are needed? (Select all that apply.)
A. Electrocardiogram (ECG)
B. Electrolytes
C. Thyroid function [thyroid-stimulating hormone (TSH) assay]
D. Complete blood count (CBC)
E. Blood urea nitrogen (BUN)

QUESTION 4. What other psychosocial issues might also be problematic for Karen? (Select all that apply.)
   A. Depression with suicidality
   B. Phobias
   C. Substance abuse
   D. Sexual identity disorder

## ASSESSMENT

QUESTION 5. What is the appropriate diagnosis for Karen?
   A. Anorexia nervosa
   B. Bulimia nervosa
   C. Body dysmorphic disorder
   D. Adjustment disorder

## PLAN

QUESTION 6. Apart from psychotherapy, what would be the best community referral option to assist Karen in dealing with this problem?
   A. Overeaters Anonymous
   B. Weight loss clinic
   C. Self-help group for eating disorders
   D. Health club

QUESTION 7. What would be an appropriate medication to consider as part of Karen's treatment?
   A. Selective serotonin reuptake inhibitors (SSRIs) (e.g., Zoloft, Prozac)
   B. Monoamine oxidase (MAO) inhibitor (e.g., Nardil)
   C. Anorexigenic (e.g., Didrex)
   D. Antiemetic (Compazine)

QUESTION 8. The efficacy of medication would be determined by which one of the following?
   A. Weight loss
   B. Satisfaction with appearance
   C. Decrease in binge frequency
   D. Elimination of vomiting behavior

QUESTION 9. Hospitalization should be considered for which of the following? (Select all that apply.)
   A. Cardiac arrhythmias
   B. Suicidality or self-destructive behaviors
   C. Poor response to outpatient treatment
   D. Nonadherence to prescribed medications

## ANSWERS

QUESTION 1. What are the most likely differential diagnoses to consider at this point?

A. *YES.* Karen describes herself as "unhappy" and acknowledges difficulty adjusting to college, along with problems with her boyfriend. Psychosocial stressors can contribute to subjective feelings of depression. She also complains of fatigue, poor motivation, and a sense of being overwhelmed, all of which may be symptoms of a major depression. Further evaluation of depressive symptoms [five or more of the following DSM-IV criteria: depressed mood nearly every day, markedly diminished interest or pleasure in daily activities, significant weight loss (more than 5 percent of body weight), insomnia or hypersomnia nearly every day, psychomotor agitation or retardation observable by others, fatigue or loss of energy, feelings of worthlessness and guilt, inability to think or concentrate, indecisiveness, recurrent thoughts of suicide or death, or suicidal behaviors] is necessary to confirm a diagnosis of depression.

B. *YES.* It is unlikely that Karen's weight gain is due to hypothyroidism, as her symptoms are more consistent with an eating disorder. However, thyroid dysfunction may be a contributing factor to low energy and depression and would need to be ruled out.

C. *YES.* Karen's symptoms are most consistent with bulimia; they include fear of getting fat, uncontrolled binge eating followed by extreme measures to control weight, and a negative self-image attributed to her perception of body weight. Eating disorders are most typically seen in predominantly white upper-middle- and middle-class student groups.

D. *NO.* While Karen does complain about difficulties in adjusting to college life, adjustment disorder is a category used to describe presentations that are in response to an identifiable stressor and that do not meet the criteria for another specific DSM-IV Axis I disorder. In Karen's case, her symptoms point more clearly to an eating disorder.

QUESTION 2. Which of the following areas of inquiry would help to substantiate the diagnosis?

A. *YES.* Self-induced vomiting is a compensatory method frequently used by bulimics to avoid weight gain following binge eating. There is often much shame and/or embarrassment associated with this behavior, and the individual is usually quite secretive about it. A person with bulimia will often not disclose such behavior voluntarily. The noted calluses on the fingers of the right hand are consistent with chronic self-induced vomiting caused by sticking one's fingers down the throat to stimulate the gag reflex.

B. *YES.* The high acidity of vomitus may cause dental caries and dental sensitivity to hot and cold temperatures due to erosion of the dental enamel.

C. *YES.* Laxative abuse occurs frequently in bulimia, and is evidenced by bloating, hyperactive bowel sounds, hemorrhoids, rectal discomfort, and rectal bleeding. Laxative abuse may also cause metabolic acidosis when alkaline intestinal fluids are lost. Severe cases of laxative abuse may result in cardiomyopathy and myocarditis. Other sequelae of laxative abuse include steatorrhea (excess elimination of fats), cathartic colitis, reflex constipation, and edema.

D. *NO.* Bulimia is not correlated with a greater incidence of STDs. Obtaining Karen's sexual history would neither support nor refute a diagnosis of bulimia.

**QUESTION 3.** Which of the following laboratory tests are needed?

A. *YES.* Abnormalities in acid-base balance, particularly $K^+$ and $Ca^+$ levels, may cause cardiac arrhythmias; therefore an ECG is indicated.

B. *YES.* Bulimia may result in metabolic acid-base imbalances due to vomiting and diuretic abuse (metabolic alkalosis) or laxative abuse (metabolic acidosis). The most common electrolyte abnormality seen in bulimics is an elevated bicarbonate level.

C. *YES.* Although thyroid function abnormalities are not usually associated with bulimia, there is a relationship between hypothyroidism and low energy and/or depression. Whereas the prevalence of thyroid disease in depressed females (15 percent) is similar to that in the general population (10.5 percent), there is some evidence of an increased prevalence of thyroid dysfunction in women who have both depression and an eating disorder (24 percent). A TSH assay that tests for both hyperthyroid and hypothyroid states would therefore be useful to rule out thyroid disorder. If the TSH findings are abnormal, then a total serum $T_3$ and a total serum $T_4$ should be ordered. In hypothyroidism the TSH is elevated, and in the later stages the $T_4$ is low, whereas in hyperthyroidism the $T_4$ is elevated and the TSH is low. In some cases the $T_4$ is normal and $T_3$ is elevated in hyperthyroidism.

D. *YES.* A CBC is useful for determining nutritional status, including anemia.

E. *YES.* An elevated BUN is often seen as a result of volume depletion caused by vomiting. Because an elevated BUN causes nausea/vomiting, diarrhea, and headaches, it is important to determine whether the vomiting and diarrhea are due to purging or to an elevated BUN.

**QUESTION 4.** What other psychosocial issues might also be problematic for Karen?

A. *YES.* There is a high comorbidity between depression and bulimia; it has been estimated that over half of persons with bulimia develop major depression. Suicidality, thought to be more common in bulimia than in anorexia, may reflect the high degree of impulsivity, mood swings, and sense of being out of control that is often seen in this disorder.

B. *NO.* Although persons with bulimia have an underlying fear of becoming fat (whereas those with anorexia have a strong desire to be thin), this fear is not regarded as a phobia. Furthermore, a person with bulimia typically does not demonstrate other phobic or anxiety-related symptoms. In individuals with bulimia, a diagnosis of phobia is not given if the avoidance behavior typically seen in specific phobias is limited to avoidance of food and food-related cues.

C. *YES.* There is a high comorbidity between bulimia and other impulse-control disorders, including substance abuse and gambling. About 49

percent of these patients have substance abuse disorders. Bulimia patients may also steal the food that is used for their high-volume binges.
  D.  *NO.* Although Karen has a poor self-image, she does not appear to have issues related to her sexual identity or gender.

**QUESTION 5.** What is the appropriate diagnosis for Karen?
  A.  *NO.* Findings are not consistent with anorexia nervosa. A person with anorexia is typically more than 20 percent below ideal body weight and engages in deliberate self-starvation, continuous dieting, and excessive exercise, as well as denial of hunger. When eating, a person with anorexia is highly controlled (to the point of being ritualistic), and the amount consumed is very restricted. For example, an anorexic person may take over an hour to eat a small salad, meticulously cutting each piece of lettuce, and perhaps eating the different vegetables in a certain order or chewing each mouthful over 100 times. On physical examination, an anorectic usually presents in an emaciated state, with the presence of excessive facial or body hair, possible hair loss on the head, and irregular or absent menses.
  B.  *YES.* Karen's behavior is most consistent with a diagnosis of bulimia nervosa. Symptoms include eating behavior that is out of control in a person of average weight. The added calories are compensated for by extreme methods of weight control. These methods include fasting, self-induced vomiting, diuretic and laxative abuse, abuse of appetite suppressants, and rigorous exercise. Bulimia patients who abuse laxatives develop gastrointestinal symptoms such as eliminating excessive amounts of fats (steatorrhea), bleeding, and bloating.
  C.  *NO.* Body dysmorphic disorder refers to an imagined defect in some aspect of one's appearance that can reach delusional proportions. An example would be someone who is convinced that his or her (normal-appearing) nose is too large, and is the cause of staring and ridicule by others. Such beliefs lead to marked social withdrawal and distress. Overall dissatisfaction with one's body size, with resultant changes in diet, mood, and behavior, is classified as an eating disorder.
  D.  *NO.* Even though Karen reports adjustment problems and relates these to entering college, adjustment disorder is not the appropriate diagnosis. According to the DSM-IV criteria for adjustment disorder, that diagnosis is not given when symptoms meet DSM-IV criteria for another specific Axis I disorder. In addition, having adjustment problems does not necessarily mean that the individual meets the criteria for an actual adjustment disorder. Symptoms of adjustment disorder include marked distress that is in excess of what would be expected from exposure to a specific stressor. In Karen's case, her symptoms point more clearly to bulimia nervosa.

**QUESTION 6.** Apart from psychotherapy, what would be the best community referral option to assist Karen in dealing with this problem?
  A.  *NO.* Overeaters Anonymous addresses overeating in the general population, but does not specifically address the underlying issues that lead to an eating disorder. Treatment of bulimia should not simply focus on eating, but should focus rather on breaking the binge-purge cycle.

   **B.** *NO.* Like Overeaters Anonymous, a weight loss clinic would focus on Karen's weight rather than on the real issues, which are her underlying psychological conflicts or belief systems that are expressed through the development of an eating disorder.

   **C.** *YES.* Self-help groups for eating disorders have been found to be highly effective in providing necessary support, feedback, and confrontation. Patients with bulimia experience a great deal of shame and secrecy in regard to their behavior, and a group approach is an effective means of combating isolation and promoting acceptance and a realistic perspective.

   **D.** *NO.* Although there are health benefits to exercise (including a decrease in depression), enrollment in a health club would address the symptom rather than the problem, and would not be as helpful for Karen as an eating disorders group. Enrolling in a health club is not a specific priority for Karen's problems.

**QUESTION 7.** What would be an appropriate medication to consider as part of Karen's treatment?

   **A.** *YES.* Selective serotonin reuptake inhibitors (SSRIs) have been shown to be effective in treating both the bulimia and the depression seen in this disorder. Antidepressants decrease binging frequencies in both depressed and nondepressed bulimics. Antidepressants should not constitute the sole treatment for bulimia. It is best to combine antidepressant therapy with psychotherapy (either individual or group modality, and either a psychodynamic or a cognitive-behavioral approach). Combining psychotherapy with medications is thought to reduce treatment dropout rates, thereby improving the long-term treatment success rate.

   **B.** *NO.* While MAO inhibitors are effective antidepressants, they require a carefully monitored diet. These medications are rarely a drug of first choice. Patients who take MAO inhibitors must restrict their consumption of tyramine to prevent a hypertensive episode. Tyramine is found in certain foods, such as red wine, beer, aged cheeses, yeasts, avocados, bananas, dairy products, soy sauce, chocolate, and liver. Because of Karen's impulsive and out-of-control eating patterns, this would not be a good choice for her. Furthermore, weight gain is a side effect associated with this antidepressant, and this would preclude it as an acceptable choice for Karen.

   **C.** *NO.* Didrex is an amphetamine drug used in cases of obesity to promote weight loss. It is not an indicated form of treatment for bulimia, and Karen would not be a candidate because of her average-range weight. Appetite suppression is contraindicated in bulimia.

   **D.** *NO.* Compazine is an antiemetic and would not be effective in reducing vomiting, as Karen's vomiting is self-induced and not due to nausea.

**QUESTION 8.** The efficacy of medication would be determined by which one of the following?

   **A.** *NO.* Because her weight is normal, weight loss would not reflect progress for Karen. Depending on how it was attained, weight loss might reflect continuing problems with out-of-control eating patterns.

**B.** *NO.* Medication has not been shown to alter satisfaction with one's appearance. Improved self-image would be an anticipated outcome of pharmacotherapy and psychotherapy, but this would be a later effect, not an early response to treatment.

**C.** *YES.* A decrease in the frequency of binge eating is the most universally reported effect of SSRI medication therapy in the treatment of bulimia. This response may occur whether or not the patient has a concurrent depression. A decrease in weight-regulatory compensatory behaviors (e.g., self-induced vomiting) is also commonly reported.

**D.** *NO.* Self-induced vomiting typically decreases as the patient improves, but it is not usually eliminated until later into treatment. This aspect of the disease is addressed in psychotherapy. Behavioral approaches are very helpful. For example, once the abnormal patterns of eating, binging, and purging have been specifically identified, the patient learns to delay vomiting for longer and longer periods. Learning to delay vomiting helps the patient learn that she has control over the binge-purge cycle.

**QUESTION 9.** Hospitalization should be considered for which of the following?

**A.** *YES.* Cardiac arrhythmias and other medical complications of serious electrolyte imbalance may require hospitalization for specific assessment and close monitoring and treatment.

**B.** *YES.* Suicidal or impulsive, self-destructive behaviors often require hospitalization to protect the patient from self-harm. It has been estimated that suicidal risk is 10 percent in anorexia and 40 percent in bulimia.

**C.** *YES.* Poor response to outpatient treatment may suggest that a more intensive and structured approach, provided by an interdisciplinary team on an inpatient unit, may be necessary to break deeply ingrained patterns of binging and purging.

**D.** *NO.* Failure to comply with prescribed medication needs to be dealt with in an office visit. In fact, most patients with bulimia are best treated as outpatients and should be hospitalized only to manage medical emergencies, or if they are extremely resistant to breaking the binge-purge cycle.

## REFERENCES

American Psychiatric Association. (1994). *Diagnostic and Statistical Manual of Mental Disorders (DSM-IV)*. Washington DC: Author.

Hall, R. C., Dulap, P. K., Hall, R. C., Pachoco, C. A., Blakely, D. K. (1995). Thyroid disease and abnormal thyroid function tests in women with eating disorders and depression. *J Fla Med Assoc 82*(3), 187–192.

Hofland, S. L., Dardis, P. O. (1992). Bulimia nervosa: Associated physical problems. *J Psychosoc Nurs 30*(2), 23–27.

MacKenzie, R., Neinstein, L. S. (1996). Anorexia nervosa and bulimia. In L. S. Neinstein (ed.), *Adolescent Health Care: A Practical Guide*. Baltimore: Williams & Wilkins.

Maxmen, J. S., Ward, N. G. (1995). *Essential Psychopathology and Its Treatment*. New York: Norton.

Townsend, M. C. (1995). *Drug Guide for Psychiatric Nursing*. Philadelphia: F. A. Davis.

Yager, J., Andersen, A., Devlin, M., Mitchell, J., Powers, P., Yates, A. (1993). Practice guidelines for eating disorders: American Psychiatric Association. *Am J Psychiatry 150*(2), 208–228.

# 15

# Sports Physical and Respiratory Symptoms

*Linda Farrand*

*Jeanne M. Ondyak*

Pedro R., a 15-year-old Latino, has an appointment for a sports physical. Pedro was seen last year for his school physical examination which was normal. He denies any illnesses since his examination, last year. He enjoys being in high school and competed on the freshman baseball and soccer teams. Pedro was picked up from track practice by his father, who has accompanied him into the examination room.

## CHIEF COMPLAINT

"I notice that when I run the 400 meters, I become short of breath and wheeze."

## HISTORY OF PRESENT ILLNESS

QUESTION 1. What questions concerning symptoms of shortness of breath and wheezing are critical to ask? (Select all that apply.)
  A. Onset and chronological sequence of symptoms
  B. Associated symptoms
  C. Review of symptoms—abdomen
  D. Aggravating and relieving factors

QUESTION 2. What further historical information is required to explore Pedro's respiratory status? (Select all that apply.)
  A. Past medical history
  B. Family history
  C. Medications
  D. Habits: smoking history/illicit drug use

## PAST MEDICAL HISTORY

Pedro denies taking any medication and has no known allergies. His record shows no history of hospitalizations or injuries.

QUESTION 3. What adolescent issues would you also explore at this visit?
A. Family and peer relationships
B. Diet
C. Contraception
D. Plans after high school
E. Use of seat belts

## PHYSICAL FINDINGS

| | |
|---|---|
| Vital signs: | Temperature 98.6°F, pulse 74, respirations 18, blood pressure 112/68, height 64 in, weight 120 lb. |
| General: | Well-developed, slender male who is able to converse without difficulty. |
| Head: | No sinus tenderness. |
| Eyes: | Conjunctivae clear, no discharge. |
| Ears: | Tympanic membranes within normal limits. |
| Nose: | Nares patent; nasal mucosa pink, turbinates slightly enlarged, no polyps or lesions. |
| Throat: | No tonsillar hypertrophy, no exudate. |
| Neck: | No lymphadenopathy. |
| Lungs: | Mild bilateral expiratory wheezing, no rales, no rhonchi. |
| Heart: | Regular rhythm, normal $S_1$ and $S_2$, no murmurs. |
| Abdomen: | No masses, no tenderness, no bruits heard. |
| Hernia: | None. |
| Back: | No scoliosis; able to touch floor. |
| Neurologic: | Deep tendon reflexes 2+ and equal bilaterally |

QUESTION 4. What additional physical examination data are needed? (Select all that apply.)
A. A "2-min orthopedic exam"
B. Jugular venous pressure (JVP)
C. Peak expiratory flow (PEF)
D. Cranial nerves

## ASSESSMENT

QUESTION 5. Which of the following would be an appropriate assessment of this patient?
A. Aspirated foreign body
B. Exercise-induced bronchospasm (EIB)
C. Acute respiratory infection
D. Vocal cord dysfunction (VCD)

## PLAN

QUESTION 6. Management of EIB for Pedro would include which of the following? (Select all that apply.)
A. Using a short-acting inhaled beta agonist before exercise
B. Including a warm-up period before physical activity
C. Switching to a sport that doesn't require continuous running
D. Prescribing a short burst of an oral steroid

QUESTION 7. Additional issues that would be important to discuss with Pedro and his father include which of the following? (Select all that apply.)
A. School medication policy
B. Notifying the coach of his condition
C. Correct inhaler technique
D. General sports safety issues

QUESTION 8. When should Pedro return for his next appointment?
A. No return appointment is necessary
B. 1 month
C. 6 months
D. Next year for his annual sports physical

## ANSWERS

QUESTION 1. What questions concerning symptoms of shortness of breath and wheezing are critical to ask?
A. *YES.* The onset and chronological sequence of symptoms are important to investigate. It is necessary to explore when the symptoms first occurred, when symptoms occur in relation to exercise (during or after), how long a typical episode lasts, whether symptoms are getting better or worse, and if symptoms occur at other times.
B. *YES.* Information on associated symptoms is necessary. Complaints of chest tightness or a frequent dry cough may indicate ongoing asthma, especially if the cough occurs routinely at night. A productive cough associated with a fever can indicate an infection, either viral or bacterial. Dizziness or syncope with shortness of breath may be an indication of profound air hunger and increased severity of asthma or possible cardiac involvement.
C. *NO.* Review of symptoms for abdominal problems is not related to this chief complaint.
D. *YES.* Ask Pedro if other sports or activities in gym class also precipitate symptoms. Also question Pedro regarding symptoms that occur with exposure to tobacco smoke, cold air, pets, pollens, and other environmental allergens, to determine whether he has triggers other than exercise. Find out what has helped when he is short of breath and whether his breathing improves when he stops running.

QUESTION 2. What further historical information is required to explore Pedro's respiratory status?

A. *YES.* The past medical history should include any history of chronic illnesses and any acute illnesses during the past year. Recent respiratory illnesses must be ruled out. A history of allergic rhinitis or eczema/atopic dermatitis supports the likelihood of asthma or an allergic etiology as the cause of Pedro's symptoms. In addition to exploring respiratory symptoms, the history for a sports physical should focus on the cardiovascular, musculoskeletal, and neurological systems and include questions regarding high blood pressure, heart murmur, palpitations, or syncope; myocardial infarction in any first-degree relative under age 50; previous musculoskeletal trauma; and any central nervous system trauma or condition, including head injury, concussion, or seizure disorders.

B. *YES.* A positive family history for asthma or allergies increases the likelihood that Pedro's symptoms have an allergic basis. The genetic tendency to develop allergies is inherited; however, specific sensitivities are not. If one parent is allergic, there is a 30 to 35 percent chance that the child will develop allergies. If both parents have allergies, the risk increases to 65 percent.

C. *YES.* Prescription medications and over-the-counter drugs can precipitate respiratory symptoms. Aspirin and other nonsteroidal anti-inflammatory drugs can trigger bronchoconstriction in sensitive persons; these patients should be counseled regarding the potential for severe and possibly fatal reactions with continued use. They should be instructed to use acetaminophen instead. The presense of aspirin sensitivity increases with age and asthma severity. ß-blockers can cause asthma symptoms and should be avoided, although patients may be able to tolerate cardioselective β-blockers. Cough may also be precipitated by angiotensin-converting enzyme (ACE) inhibitors. In addition, it is important to determine if Pedro is using over-the-counter antiwheezing medicine, such as Primatene Mist.

D. *YES.* Smoking is on the rise among adolescents; current statistics indicate that 25.4 percent of tenth-graders smoke. Tobacco smoke is a major trigger for asthma symptoms, so it would be important for Pedro to quit if he has started to smoke. Teens respond best to stop smoking messages that appeal to their present situation rather than to distant long-term health concerns. For Pedro, discussing the benefit of improved athletic performance would probably be most influential. Other messages that have meaning for teens include avoiding unpleasant breath, stained teeth, and clothing that smells of smoke; the addictive nature of cigarettes; and cost issues. Probe for the use of street drugs; for instance, marijuana and inhalants (aerosol sprays, solvents, glue) can cause a cough. After your initial history questions, it would be best for Pedro's father to wait in the waiting room so that you can explore these and other adolescent issues with Pedro.

**QUESTION 3.** What adolescent issues would you also explore at this visit?

**A.** *YES.* Family relationships are important to explore, as conflicts can arise during the adolescent years as teens struggle for independence. Peer and school issues are also primary concerns. Often the visit for a sports physical will be the teen's only health care visit for the year, so this may be the only opportunity for counseling and anticipatory guidance. If indicated, determine if psychosocial factors are influencing respiratory symptoms, as strong emotional expressions, such as fear, anger, hard crying, or laughing, can sometimes precipitate wheezing or coughing.

**B.** *YES.* Pedro's weight is appropriate for his height; however, exploration of eating patterns is appropriate, as nutrition sometimes suffers in adolescence as a result of poor eating habits or overconsumption of high-fat foods. Nutritional guidance regarding healthy food choices, maintaining adequate calcium intake, and safe weight management may be indicated. Also, rhinitis, cough, and wheezing may be precipitated by food allergies. Thus, it would be important to question whether Pedro has noted any of these symptoms associated with certain foods.

**C.** *NO.* A discussion regarding contraception is not indicated at this time unless when asking about peer relationships it is discovered that Pedro has begun dating and is currently sexually active. In that case, it would be necessary to provide counseling regarding pregnancy and sexually transmitted disease (STD) prevention.

**D.** *NO.* It is unlikely that Pedro is concerned about plans after high school, as he is currently a high school sophomore; this issue is more relevant to high school juniors and seniors. Other school issues may be sources of psychological stress, however, so questions about how Pedro likes school, his classes, and his interests may uncover situations requiring further counseling.

**E.** *YES.* Adolescents frequently dispense with seat belt use. Ask Pedro what percentage of the time he wears a seat belt and provide safety counseling as appropriate. Pedro may be taking driver's education and have a permit; some of his friends may already have driver's licenses. Discuss responsible driving, requiring passengers to always wear seat belts, and not riding with teens who are poor drivers or who have been drinking.

**QUESTION 4.** What additional physical examination data are needed?

**A.** *YES.* A 2-min orthopedic exam is designed to examine a child's strength and flexibility (see Fig. 15-1A through 15-1L). The examination will further explore Pedro's ability to participate in sports.

**B.** *NO.* Measurement of JVP is not indicated. Jugular venous pressure assesses the heart's efficiency as a pump; elevated JVP is indicative of congestive heart failure.

**C.** *YES.* Because of Pedro's respiratory symptoms, a PEF measurement would be helpful. As expiratory wheezing was noted on physical examination, the PEF may indicate how compromised Pedro's lung function is; however, if symptoms have subsided, the PEF may be normal.

*(text continues on page 150)*

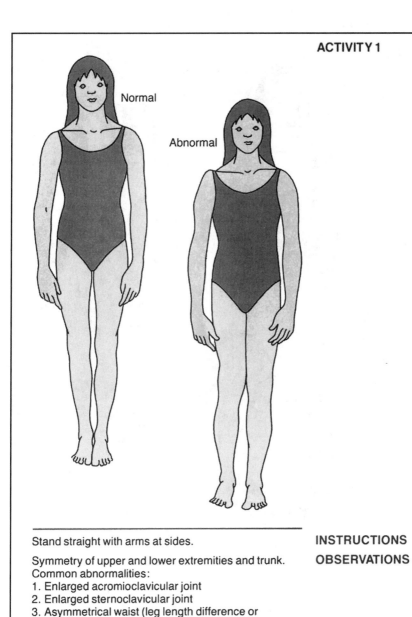

Normal

Abnormal

| | |
|---|---|
| Stand straight with arms at sides. | **INSTRUCTIONS** |
| Symmetry of upper and lower extremities and trunk. | **OBSERVATIONS** |

Common abnormalities:
1. Enlarged acromioclavicular joint
2. Enlarged sternoclavicular joint
3. Asymmetrical waist (leg length difference or scoliosis)
4. Swollen knee
5. Swollen ankle

FIGURE 15-1A.   Two-minute orthopedic exam. Ross Laboratories. *For the Practitioner: Orthopaedic Screening Examination for Participation in Sports.* (1981). No. G437. Columbus, Ohio: Author. Used with permission.

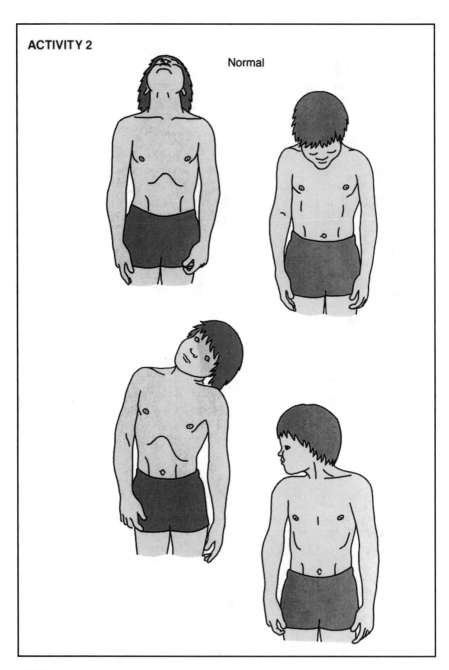

ACTIVITY 2

Normal

FIGURE 15-1B (*Continued*). Used with permission.

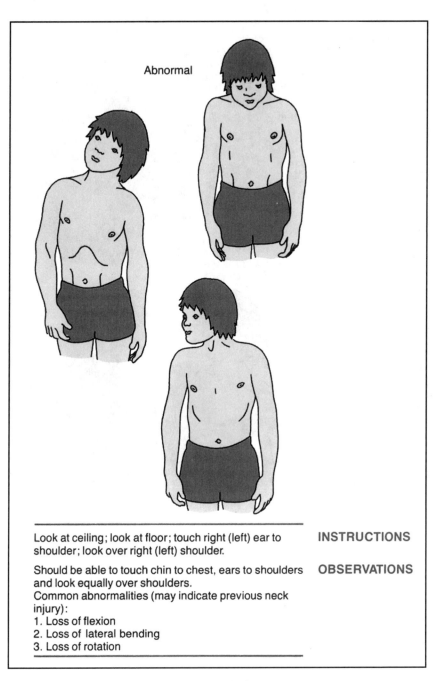

Abnormal

| Look at ceiling; look at floor; touch right (left) ear to shoulder; look over right (left) shoulder. | INSTRUCTIONS |
|---|---|
| Should be able to touch chin to chest, ears to shoulders and look equally over shoulders.<br>Common abnormalities (may indicate previous neck injury):<br>1. Loss of flexion<br>2. Loss of lateral bending<br>3. Loss of rotation | OBSERVATIONS |

FIGURE 15-1B (Continued). Used with permission.

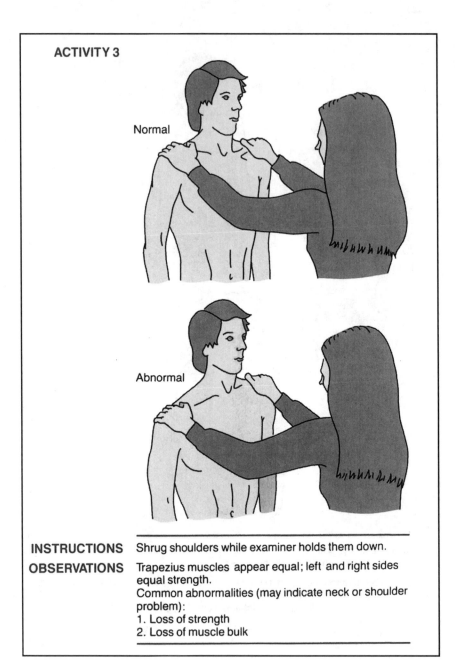

**ACTIVITY 3**

Normal

Abnormal

| | |
|---|---|
| **INSTRUCTIONS** | Shrug shoulders while examiner holds them down. |
| **OBSERVATIONS** | Trapezius muscles appear equal; left and right sides equal strength.<br>Common abnormalities (may indicate neck or shoulder problem):<br>1. Loss of strength<br>2. Loss of muscle bulk |

FIGURE 15-1C (*Continued*). Used with permission.

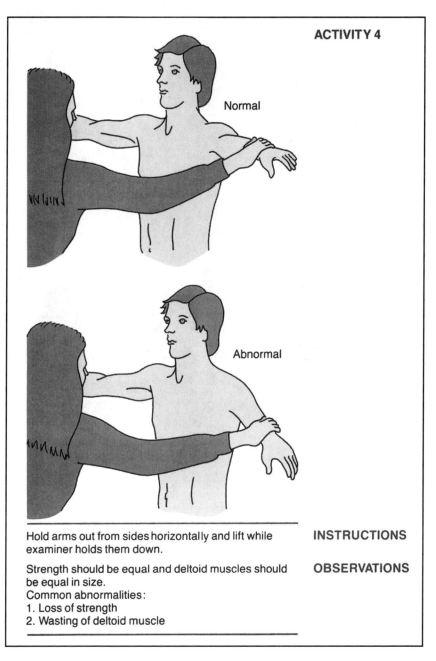

Normal

Abnormal

| | |
|---|---|
| Hold arms out from sides horizontally and lift while examiner holds them down. | **INSTRUCTIONS** |
| Strength should be equal and deltoid muscles should be equal in size.<br>Common abnormalities:<br>1. Loss of strength<br>2. Wasting of deltoid muscle | **OBSERVATIONS** |

FIGURE 15-1D (*Continued*). Used with permission.

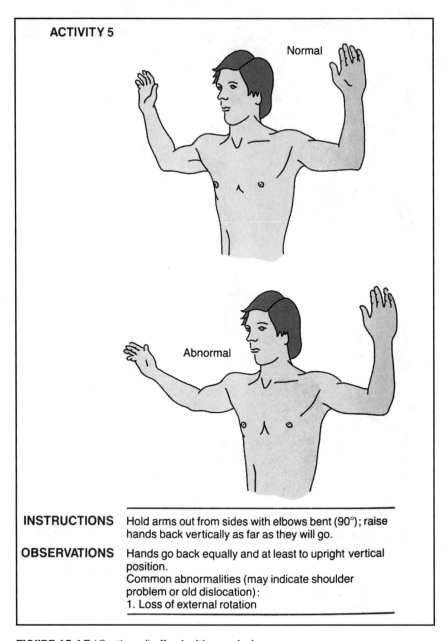

**ACTIVITY 5**

Normal

Abnormal

| | |
|---|---|
| **INSTRUCTIONS** | Hold arms out from sides with elbows bent (90°); raise hands back vertically as far as they will go. |
| **OBSERVATIONS** | Hands go back equally and at least to upright vertical position. |
| | Common abnormalities (may indicate shoulder problem or old dislocation): |
| | 1. Loss of external rotation |

**FIGURE 15-1E** (*Continued*). Used with permission.

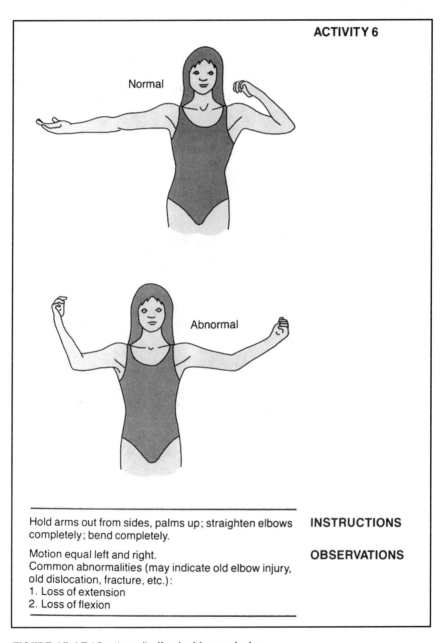

Normal

Abnormal

| | |
|---|---|
| Hold arms out from sides, palms up; straighten elbows completely; bend completely. | **INSTRUCTIONS** |
| Motion equal left and right. Common abnormalities (may indicate old elbow injury, old dislocation, fracture, etc.): 1. Loss of extension 2. Loss of flexion | **OBSERVATIONS** |

FIGURE 15-1F (*Continued*). Used with permission.

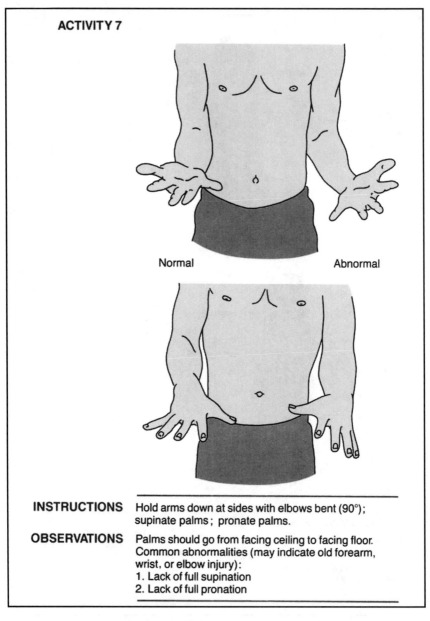

**ACTIVITY 7**

Normal          Abnormal

| | |
|---|---|
| **INSTRUCTIONS** | Hold arms down at sides with elbows bent (90°); supinate palms; pronate palms. |
| **OBSERVATIONS** | Palms should go from facing ceiling to facing floor. Common abnormalities (may indicate old forearm, wrist, or elbow injury):<br>1. Lack of full supination<br>2. Lack of full pronation |

FIGURE 15-1G (*Continued*). Used with permission.

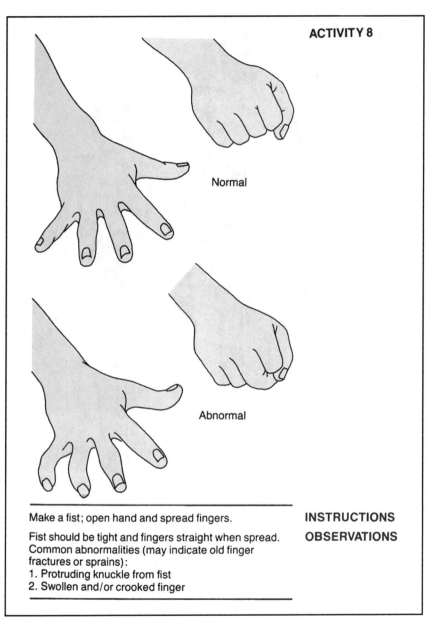

Normal

Abnormal

| | |
|---|---|
| Make a fist; open hand and spread fingers. | **INSTRUCTIONS** |
| Fist should be tight and fingers straight when spread. Common abnormalities (may indicate old finger fractures or sprains):<br>1. Protruding knuckle from fist<br>2. Swollen and/or crooked finger | **OBSERVATIONS** |

FIGURE 15-1H (*Continued*). Used with permission.

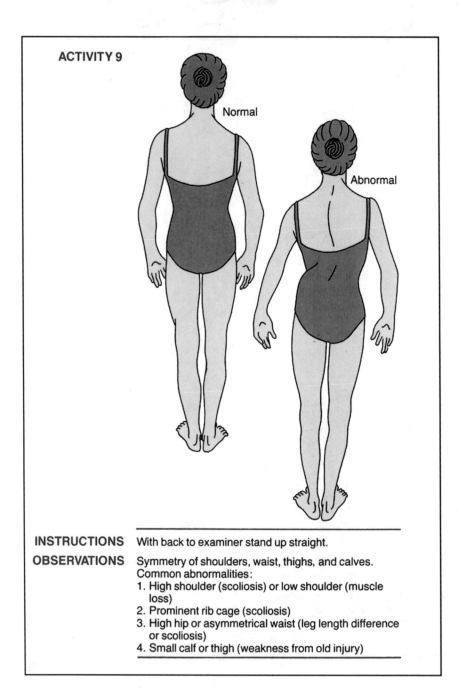

**ACTIVITY 9**

Normal

Abnormal

| | |
|---|---|
| **INSTRUCTIONS** | With back to examiner stand up straight. |
| **OBSERVATIONS** | Symmetry of shoulders, waist, thighs, and calves.<br>Common abnormalities:<br>1. High shoulder (scoliosis) or low shoulder (muscle loss)<br>2. Prominent rib cage (scoliosis)<br>3. High hip or asymmetrical waist (leg length difference or scoliosis)<br>4. Small calf or thigh (weakness from old injury) |

FIGURE 15-1*I* (*Continued*). Used with permission.

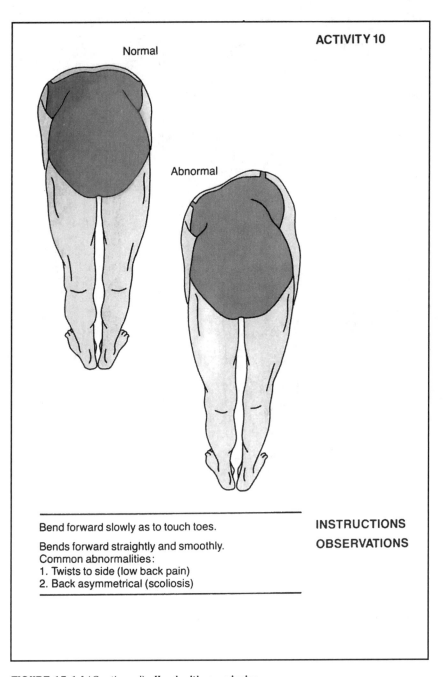

Normal

Abnormal

Bend forward slowly as to touch toes.

Bends forward straightly and smoothly.
Common abnormalities:
1. Twists to side (low back pain)
2. Back asymmetrical (scoliosis)

**INSTRUCTIONS**

**OBSERVATIONS**

FIGURE 15-1J (*Continued*). Used with permission.

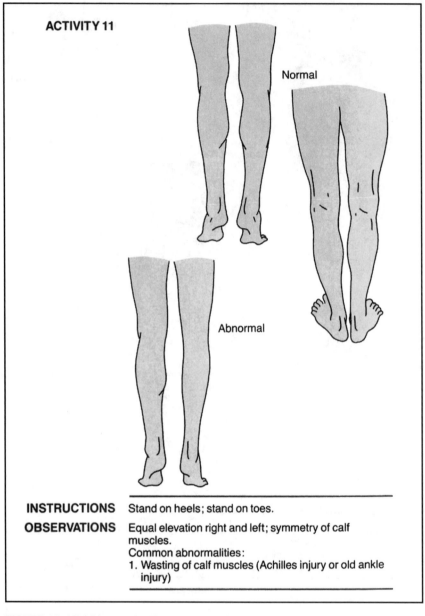

**ACTIVITY 11**

Normal

Abnormal

| | |
|---|---|
| **INSTRUCTIONS** | Stand on heels; stand on toes. |
| **OBSERVATIONS** | Equal elevation right and left; symmetry of calf muscles.<br>Common abnormalities:<br>1. Wasting of calf muscles (Achilles injury or old ankle injury) |

FIGURE 15-1*K* (*Continued*). Used with permission.

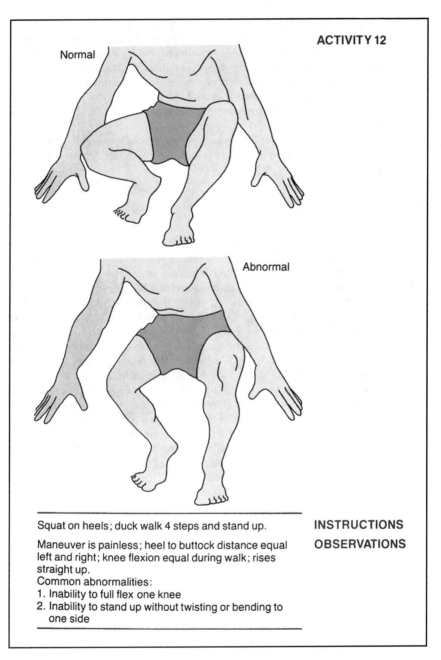

Normal

Abnormal

Squat on heels; duck walk 4 steps and stand up.

**INSTRUCTIONS**

Maneuver is painless; heel to buttock distance equal
left and right; knee flexion equal during walk; rises
straight up.
Common abnormalities:
1. Inability to full flex one knee
2. Inability to stand up without twisting or bending to
   one side

**OBSERVATIONS**

FIGURE 15-L (*Continued*). Used with permission.

Three readings are done, and the best value obtained is compared to a normogram based on gender, height, and age. Ethnicity also influences normal lung function. African Americans have longer legs, shorter trunks, and smaller thoracic diameters than Caucasians for a given height; the normal lung function ranges for Hispanics, Asians, and Native Americans have been less well studied. The most clinically useful standard for ongoing monitoring for any patient is the individual's personal best value.

D. *NO*. Assessment of cranial nerve function is not generally part of the sports physical examination, nor is it related to assessment of respiratory complaints.

**QUESTION 5.** Which of the following would be an appropriate assessment of this patient?

A. *NO*. There is no history of an aspirated foreign body in this case; however, an aspirated object can produce wheezing and shortness of breath and would be part of the differential diagnosis in a young child.

B. *YES*. A history of shortness of breath and wheezing (or cough, chest pain or tightness, or endurance problems) occurring during or just following exercise suggests EIB. Exercise-induced bronchospasm is thought to be caused by a loss of heat, water, or both from the lung during the hyperventilation of exercise. It may occur during exercise, but it typically occurs 5 to 15 min after the activity stops; symptoms subside in another 20 to 30 min. The diagnosis can be established by an exercise free-run test where the child runs or jogs for about 10 min. The PEF is monitored both before and after the test; a decrease of 15 percent or more is indicative of EIB. Exercise may be the only trigger for asthma symptoms in some patients; however, these individuals should be monitored regularly for symptoms indicative of broader asthma involvement. It should be noted that most persons with asthma will experience some degree of EIB.

C. *NO*. An acute respiratory infection can produce wheezing and shortness of breath; however, Pedro has no signs or symptoms of an infection or a history of recent exposure.

D. *NO*. Signs and symptoms of VCD can mimic EIB, and the condition is often misdiagnosed; however, Pedro does not fit the clinical picture of VCD at this time. Symptoms include wheezing, chest tightness, shortness of breath, and cough, commonly associated with exercise, which occur secondary to airflow obstruction as a result of vocal cord adduction during inspiration. Symptoms occur during the day, rather than nocturnally as is common in asthma, and often start and stop abruptly. Inspiratory wheezing, throat tightness, a change in voice quality, and poor response to bronchodilator treatment suggest VCD. It is more commonly noted in female adolescents who are anxious, depressed, or perfectionistic. The diagnosis is best confirmed by direct visualization of the abnormal movement of the vocal cords by fiberoptic rhinolaryngoscopy when symptoms are present; spirometry also shows the presence of truncated inspiratory flow loops. Treatment involves instruction in special breathing techniques to decrease laryngeal tone. The condition can also coexist with asthma and should be considered when asthma is refractory to treatment.

## QUESTION 6.

Management of EIB for Pedro would include which of the following?

A. *YES.* Pedro should take a short-acting $\beta_2$ agonist, such as albuterol (Ventolin, Proventil), 2 puffs, about 10 to 15 min before vigorous exercise. This generally prevents symptoms for 2 to 3 h.

B. *YES.* A lengthy warm-up period before exercise is helpful in reducing symptoms, as is covering the mouth and nose when the air is cold.

C. *NO.* Full participation in sports should be encouraged. Exercise-induced bronchospasm should not limit Pedro's participation in vigorous activity; the condition responds well to $\beta_2$ agonists, which prevent symptoms in over 80 percent of patients.

D. *NO.* A course of oral steroids is not indicated.

**QUESTION 7.** Additional issues that would be important to discuss with Pedro and his father include which of the following?

A. *YES.* School policy generally requires a written medication permission slip signed by the practitioner and the parent to allow medication to be taken during school hours. More schools, particularly high schools, are permitting students with asthma to carry their inhalers with them to allow for prompt access when symptoms occur. Pedro should contact his school nurse, who can apprise him of the school policy and also serve as an advocate for him should any issues arise.

B. *YES.* Pedro's family should inform both his coach and his physical education teacher of his condition, his ability to continue participation in athletics, and that he may need pretreatment with his inhaler before vigorous activity.

C. *YES.* Since Pedro has never used a metered dose inhaler (MDI) before, he needs to be instructed in technique and given a return demonstration. If he has difficulty coordinating inhalation and actuation of the inhaler, a spacer device can be used (see Table 15-1); however, teens may be reluctant to carry a bulky spacer or use it in front of peers. In this case, the newly developed breath-activated MDI may be a more effective option. Currently, pirbuterol (Maxair), a $\beta_2$ agonist similar to albuterol, is available with this new delivery device.

D. *YES.* Pedro should be counseled regarding the sports safety issues of adequate hydration, sufficient warm-up and cool-down, use of sunscreen, and prompt attention to musculoskeletal injuries.

**QUESTION 8.** When should Pedro return for his next appointment?

A. *NO.* Pedro's response to treatment needs to be evaluated so that adjustments can be made as necessary.

B. *YES.* It is important to evaluate the treatment plan in a month or so in order to see if the treatment was effective.

TABLE 15-1    Spacer education

---

Unless you use your inhaler the right way, much of the medicine may end up on your tongue, on the back of your throat, or in the air. Use of a spacer or holding chamber can help this problem.

A spacer or holding chamber is a device that attaches to a metered dose inhaler. It holds the medicine in its chamber long enough for you to inhale it in one or two slow deep breaths. The spacer makes it easy for you to use the medicines the right way (especially if your child is young or you have a hard time using just an inhaler). It helps you not cough when using an inhaler. A spacer will also help prevent you from getting a yeast infection in your mouth (thrush) when taking inhaled steroid medicines.

There are many models of spacers or holding chambers that you can purchase through your pharmacist or a medical supply company. Ask your doctor about the different models.

**How to Use a Spacer**
1. Attach the inhaler to the spacer or holding chamber as explained by your doctor or by using the directions that come with the product.
2. Shake well.
3. Press the button on the inhaler. This will put one puff of the medicine in the holding chamber.
4. Place the mouthpiece of the spacer in your mouth and inhale slowly. (A face mask may be helpful for a young child.)
5. Hold your breath for a few seconds and then exhale. Repeat steps 4 and 5 two more times.
6. If your doctor has prescribed two puffs, wait between puffs for the amount of time he or she has directed and repeat steps 4 and 5.

---

SOURCE: National Institutes of Health; National Heart, Lung, and Blood Institute. (1992). *Teach Your Patients About Asthma: A Clinicians' Guide.* Bethesda, MD: Author.

C. *NO.* This would be too long to wait to evaluate Pedro's response to medication.

D. *NO.* Pedro's response to treatment needs to be evaluated within the next month.

## REFERENCES

Burns, C. E., Barber, N., Brady, M. A., Dunn, A. M. (1996). *Pediatric Primary Care: A Handbook for Nurse Practitioners.* Philadelphia: W. B. Saunders.

Federal Drug Administration. (1995). Regulations restricting the sale and distribution of cigarettes and smokeless tobacco products to protect children and adolescents (Docket No. 95N-0253). *Federal Register 60*(155), 41314–41453.

Landwehr, L. P., Wood, R. P., Blager, F. B., Milgrom, H. (1996). Vocal cord dysfunction mimicking exercise-induced bronchospasm in adolescents. *Pediatrics 98*(5), 971–974.

National Institutes of Health, National Heart, Lung, and Blood Institute. (1997). *National Asthma Education and Prevention Program Expert Panel Report 2: Guidelines for the Diagnosis and Management of Asthma.* NIH Publication No. 97-4051. Bethesda, MD: Author.

# 16

# Date Rape

*Laina M. Gerace*
*Marie L. Talashek*

Rhonda J., an 18-year-old Caucasian college freshman, comes to the student health service following a date rape the night before. She is accompanied by her roommate. Rhonda has a bruise on her face. She is tearful, and states that she is here only because her roommate insisted on bringing her in. Her roommate reports that Rhonda came home late last night, and she heard her showering. Not until this morning did the client tell her roommate that she was raped by a male college student on their first date. The roommate could not convince Rhonda to go to the emergency room of the local hospital, but finally talked her into coming to the student health service.

## CHIEF COMPLAINT

"I want to get checked for a sex disease or AIDS, but I don't want any trouble."

## HISTORY OF THE PRESENT ILLNESS

Rhonda went out on a first date with a college student she had met the day before at a "frat party." According to Rhonda, they went to a bar, had a few drinks, and then went to his fraternity house, where he suddenly cornered her and forced her to have intercourse. He held her down, slapped and punched her, then penetrated her vaginally. After finishing, he ordered her not to tell anyone about the incident. Rhonda did not go to the emergency room after the rape, but went back to the dormitory, where she took a shower.

QUESTION 1. In spite of counseling to the contrary, Rhonda adamantly refuses any police involvement in relation to her rape. Which of the following responses are appropriate? (Select all that apply.)
    A. Insist that she report the rape.
    B. Refuse to examine and treat her.

C. Respect her decision and offer treatment.
D. Call the police despite the client's objections.
E. Save appropriate specimens for legal evidence in case Rhonda changes her mind.

**Question 2.** What additional health history is needed before proceeding to physical examination? (Select all that apply.)
A. Current use of birth control
B. History of sexually transmitted diseases (STDs)
C. History of childhood illnesses
D. General health habits (exercise, diet)

**Question 3.** About 18 h have passed since Rhonda was raped. Which statements about specimen collection *for legal purposes* in rape cases are true? (Select all that apply.)
A. Valid data are not possible after 48 to 72 h.
B. Evidence is best collected with the help of an approved rape evidence collection kit.
C. The police, not the health care provider, collect specimens used for evidence.
D. Each step of the evidence collection process should be recorded.

## PHYSICAL FINDINGS

Crying
Clean and neat in appearance
Vital signs normal
Bruise noted on side of face
Bruise noted on left breast
No abnormalities noted on external vulva, introitus, or cervix
Cultures obtained from cervical and vaginal areas

**Question 4.** What additional data should the practitioner obtain? (Select all that apply.)
A. Examination of rectum and rectal area
B. Combing of pubic area for perpetrator hair
C. Sample of mouth secretions
D. Chest x-ray

**Question 5.** Evaluation of rape complications or preexisting conditions include which of the following? (Select all that apply.)
A. Culture for gonorrhea and chlamydia
B. Venereal Disease Research Laboratory (VDRL) testing
C. Pregnancy assessment
D. Rubella titre
E. Human immunodeficiency virus (HIV) testing

QUESTION 6. What treatment plan should the practitioner offer Rhonda? (Select all that apply.)
A. Prescribe antibiotic therapy
B. Refer for rape counseling
C. Advise to refrain from intercourse until next visit
D. Prescribe vinegar douche
E. Offer HIV testing in 4 weeks

QUESTION 7. Pregnancy is one of Rhonda's concerns, since she is not on birth control, and she requests a pregnancy test. Which interventions are appropriate? (Select all that apply.)
A. Explain that the chance of pregnancy resulting from a rape is low.
B. Offer treatment with the "morning-after pill."
C. Suggest the option of waiting until her next menstrual period is due.
D. Offer a repeat pregnancy test in 7 days.

## ANSWERS

QUESTION 1. In spite of counseling to the contrary, Rhonda adamantly refuses any police involvement in relation to her rape. Which of the following responses are appropriate?
A. *NO.* Since Rhonda is 18, she has the right to decide whether or not to report the rape to authorities. While the practitioner may believe it is best to report the rape, instilling guilt through undue pressuring only adds to Rhonda's distress.
B. *NO.* Rhonda should be examined and treated for complications of rape. The purpose of examination and treatment of rape is to prevent and treat STDs, treat injuries, deal with potential pregnancy, and reduce emotional trauma. While the practitioner also has a role in evidence collection, this is not the only purpose of care.
C. *YES.* Rape is not a medical diagnosis, but rather a legal term. In addition to consenting to examination and treatment, a sexual assault victim must give authorization for the release of information gathered during medical examination to legal authorities.
D. *NO.* Because of Rhonda's objections, the nurse should not call the police at this time. However, because rape is a crime, reporting may be mandatory in jurisdictions that require medical providers to report any injury inflicted in violation of a penal code. The nurse needs to know what the requirements are in the geographical area in which she is practicing. In the absence of an adult's consent or a court order, if reporting the rape is required, the only information the nurse should release to the police is a report of the injury and the client's name and address.
E. *YES.* If the client refuses to sign a release of evidence, the practitioner should save the specimens. Sometimes rape victims change their mind about prosecuting the rape, and in these cases evidence might later be subpoenaed by a court or, in the case of a minor, may later be released with the consent of a parent or guardian.

**Question 2.** What additional health history is needed before proceeding to physical examination?
   A. *YES.* Knowledge of current birth control use is important in planning pregnancy prevention.
   B. *YES.* History of STDs, including HIV infection, is needed for future assessment of rape-induced STDs.
   C. *NO.* There is no need to extend the history into childhood illnesses unrelated to the current problem. However, immunization history will be helpful to determine protection against tetanus and hepatitis B. In Rhonda's case, the student health service should have a record of her immunizations, since most universities and colleges require such a record at admission.
   D. *NO.* There is no need to assess exercise and diet in this case. This line of questioning would unnecessarily burden Rhonda.

**Question 3.** About 18 h have passed since Rhonda was raped. Which statements about specimen collection *for legal purposes* in rape cases are true?
   A. *YES.* After 48 to 72 h, specimens collected are no longer valid for legal purposes. Since Rhonda's rape occurred 18 h ago, specimens would still be valid.
   B. *YES.* Use of a rape evidence collection kit is standard practice, especially in emergency rooms. These kits include comprehensive instructions and forms that assist the health provider in examination of the rape victim and collection of evidence (see Fig. 16-1).
   C. *NO.* The health care provider collects the specimens, but the responsibility for the specimen "custody chain" belongs to the police. Specimens are taken for both diagnostic and forensic purposes. Those specimens for diagnostic purposes are kept at the health facility, whereas specimens for forensic purposes are included in the rape kit and given to law enforcement personnel. In this case the specimens for forensic purposes could be stored at the health care facility for a short period of time in case Rhonda changes her mind about pressing charges against the rapist. Health providers who care for rape victims should obtain handbooks or guidelines disseminated by crime laboratories. These materials clarify the responsibilities of the provider in specimen collection and storage.
   D. *YES.* Evidence collected is invalid unless it is handled properly in accordance with established procedures and guidelines. Use of a rape kit facilitates proper handling of evidence in a step-by-step sequence.

**Question 4.** What additional data should the practitioner obtain?
   A. *YES.* It is standard practice for all rape victims to receive a rectal examination.
   B. *YES.* Clean paper should be placed under the buttocks of the patient and the pubic hair combed toward the paper, collecting all loose hairs on the paper. The paper is folded and placed in a labeled envelope.

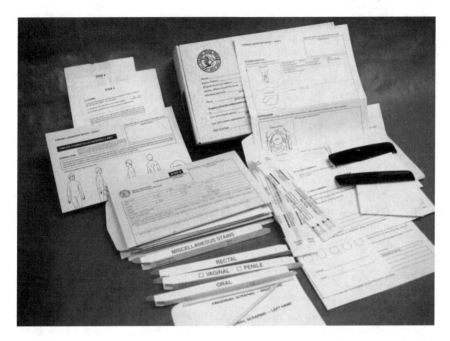

**FIGURE 16-1. Sexual assault evidence collection kit. (Illinois State Police Forensic Science Center at Chicago, 1997.) With permission.**

   C. *NO.* Since there was no oral penetration or oral-genital contact during the rape, it is not necessary to sample mouth secretions.
   D. *NO.* A chest x-ray is irrelevant to this case.

QUESTION 5. Evaluation of rape complications or preexisting conditions includes which of the following?
   A. *YES.* All involved orifices are cultured for gonorrhea and chlamydia.
   B. *YES.* A VDRL test is standard practice in rape follow-up.
   C. *YES.* Urine human chorionic gonadotropin (HCG) pregnancy testing is done to assess current pregnancy status. It is repeated after 7 days to assess rape-related pregnancy. Assessment of pregnancy is done and follow-up testing is offered.
   D. *NO.* There is no reason to assess rubella titer at this time.
   E. *YES.* An HIV test is done and repeated in 3 and 6 months.

QUESTION 6. What treatment plan should the practitioner offer Rhonda?
   A. *YES.* A follow-up visit to assess STD status is important because if a STD is present, a 2- to 3-week follow-up visit is needed to test for cure. Because follow-up cannot be assured, it is advisable to offer antibiotic therapy to all rape victims for treatment of STDs. The CDC treatment

guidelines for gonococcal infections are recommended. Doxycycline 100 mg orally twice a day for 7 days should also be given to treat concurrent infections with *Chlamydia trachomatis.*

B.   *YES.* Rape trauma syndrome is a common aftereffect of rape. Symptoms developing later include nightmares, phobias (especially of being alone), sexual anxieties, and depression or anxiety disorders. Counseling and support should be offered to reduce further trauma and facilitate posttrauma recovery. The practitioner needs to know what resources are available in the community. In the case of Rhonda, the practitioner would most likely refer her to the college counseling center.

C.   *YES.* Intercourse should be refrained from because of the possibility of STD infection.

D.   *NO.* A vinegar douche has no benefit.

E.   *YES.* Even though some debate HIV testing following rape, it is best offered after 3 to 6 months rather than in 4 weeks (the length of time it takes for seroconversion to occur).

**Question 7.** Pregnancy is one of Rhonda's concerns, since she is not on birth control, and she requests a pregnancy test. Which interventions are appropriate?

A.   *YES.* It is reassuring to explain that the chance of pregnancy resulting from a rape is low. Statistically, the chance of pregnancy occurring is 1 to 5 percent.

B.   *YES.* It is recommended that pregnancy prophylaxis be offered to rape victims. Recent court rulings indicate that pregnancy prophylaxis must be offered even if it is contrary to the philosophy of the provider or the institution. It should be explained to Rhonda that this is one of several options for dealing with the problem of potential pregnancy.

C.   *YES.* One way to deal with the possibility of pregnancy is to defer decisions about pregnancy until the next menstrual period is due. However, this will limit further options should a pregnancy result to either carrying to term or having an abortion.

D.   *YES.* A pregnancy test immediately after a rape confirms an existing pregnancy. If that test is negative, a subsequent test 7 days later will determine impregnation due to the rape. This should be explained to Rhonda.

## REFERENCES

Blair, T. M. H., Warner, C. G. (1993). Rape and sexual assault. In T. C. Kravis, C. G. Warner, L. M. Jacobs, Jr. (eds.), *Emergency Medicine.* New York: Raven Press.

Burgess, A. W., Fawcett, J., Hazelwood, R. R., Grant, C. A. (1995). Victim care services and the comprehensive sexual assault assessment tool. In R. R. Hazelwood, A. W. Burgess (eds.), *Practical Aspects of Rape Investigation: A Multidisciplinary Approach.* New York: CRC Press.

Zeccardi, J. A. (1995). Medical exam of the live sexual assault victim. In R. R. Hazelwood, A. W. Burgess (eds.), *Practical Aspects of Rape Investigation: A Multidisciplinary Approach.* New York: CRC Press.

# 17

# Suicidal Thoughts

*Cheryl A. Sullivan*
*Laina M. Gerace*

Todd P. and Mike L. are 18-year-old high school seniors who present themselves to the school health office. Both young men have visited the nurse on several occasions since their freshman year for health screening appointments. They both have regular physical examinations, are in excellent physical health, are on the honor roll, and are active in sports and student government. Mike is desperately seeking help for Todd, whom he describes as exhausted, much quieter than usual, hard to get along with, and not interested in his usual activities.

## CHIEF COMPLAINT

Given by Mike: "Todd is sad, withdrawn, irritable, and making comments about being tired of living."

## HISTORY OF PRESENT ILLNESS

Since Todd is not overtly seeking help for himself, the nurse conducts a client-centered interview that reveals the following data:

Todd reluctantly admits that he has recently had to push himself to go to school and drag himself through the day. He further reports a recent decreased appetite and that he has been sleeping about 12 h a day. He has been upset about his grades and "other stuff." While he usually gets mostly As on his report card, last week he got two Cs. So far his parents have not seen his grades. Todd's father expects him to get all A⁺s, and Todd worries that he will be very disappointed in him.

After pleading for confidentiality, Mike reveals that 3 weeks ago he and Todd engaged in homosexual experimentation, using condoms for protection. Both boys are confused about what happened, but Todd is really afraid of his father's reaction if he finds out "the truth." Todd admits to strong homosexual feelings, which he finds both exciting and confusing, but also highly stressful.

**QUESTION 1.** What differential diagnoses for Todd should be considered at this point? (Select all that apply.)
A. Adjustment disorder
B. Primary hypersomnia
C. Major depressive episode
D. Gender identity disorder
E. Dysthymic disorder

## OBJECTIVE DATA

A complete physical examination and complete blood count (CBC) and differential were normal except for the following:

Vital signs:     Temperature 98.2°F, blood pressure 124/82, pulse 68, respirations 14, height 6'1", weight 185 lb (195 lb 3 months ago)

General survey:  An alert, well-developed, well-groomed male of average height and weight. Distressed, sad, and tearful.

**QUESTION 2.** Questions related to which of the following areas are needed to help differentiate the diagnosis? (Select all that apply.)
A. Length of time symptoms have been present
B. Presence of recurrent thoughts of death or suicidal ideation, plans, or attempts
C. Level of interest/pleasure in activities previously enjoyed
D. Degree of distress about social, academic, and family relationships
E. Presence of cross-gender identification

## SUBJECTIVE DATA

Todd reluctantly admits that his symptoms of sadness, hopelessness, hypersomnia, suppressed appetite, and irritable mood have been present every day for most of the day for the past 3 weeks. When questioned directly, Todd reveals that he thinks about "offing" himself at times, especially when he thinks about facing his father's disappointment in him. "I feel so guilty," he says. When asked about the pattern of excessive sleepiness, Todd says that this developed along with his feelings of depression and hopelessness. "I sleep to avoid things," he explains. This is the first time Todd has experienced these symptoms.

**QUESTION 3.** Questions related to which of the following areas would help to further assess Todd's risk for suicide? (Select all that apply.)
A. Degree of hopelessness
B. Use/abuse of alcohol and or drugs
C. Accessibility of firearms
D. Existence of a specific plan, method, time, and place to commit suicide
E. Family history of suicidal behavior

## ASSESSMENT

QUESTION 4. What is the appropriate diagnosis for Todd? (Select all that apply.)
A. Adjustment disorder with depressed mood
B. Major depressive disorder, single episode
C. Body dysmorphic disorder
D. Primary hypersomnia

## PLAN

QUESTION 5. Maintaining confidentiality, the usual approach in the care of adolescents, may need to be abandoned with respect to which of the following areas? (Select all that apply.)
A. Self-destructive behaviors
B. Homosexual experimentation
C. Sexual history
D. Family relationships

QUESTION 6. What interventions are appropriate for Todd? (Select all that apply.)
A. Antidepressant medication
B. In-depth individual psychiatric assessment
C. Family therapy
D. Hospitalization
E. Means restriction

## ANSWERS

QUESTION 1. What differential diagnoses for Todd should be considered at this point?
A. *YES.* The essential feature of an adjustment disorder is the development of clinically significant emotional or behavioral symptoms in response to an identifiable psychosocial stressor. Todd's symptoms seem to be related to an episode of homosexual experimentation and his awareness of homosexual feelings.
B. *YES.* While hypersomnia is less likely as a diagnosis, it still should be ruled out. Todd admits that recently he has had to push himself to go to school, drags himself through the day, and can't get enough sleep. The data suggest that excessive sleepiness (hypersomnia) is causing him significant daytime fatigue which is an essential feature of this disorder. Additionally, Todd reports a lowering in his usual grades. Low-level alertness as a result of excessive sleepiness may be contributing to his drop in school performance by leading to poor efficiency, concentration, and memory. Hypersomnia typically begins between the ages of 15 and 30 years.
C. *YES.* Mike describes a change in Todd's behavior that warrants consideration of this disorder: sadness, decreased interest in his usual activities, irritability, and suicidal remarks. Todd provides further data suggestive

of this disorder: hypersomnia, fatigue, decreased appetite, loss of energy, and distress about school and his relationship with his father. These symptoms have lasted for over 2 weeks, which is an essential feature of a major depressive episode.

D. *NO*. The components that must be present to make this diagnosis are clearly not evident. While Mike reveals that both he and Todd are confused and upset about their recent homosexual experimentation, gender identity disorder refers to confusion about being male or female. There is no evidence to support the idea that Todd is confused, experiencing discomfort in the male role, or preoccupied with traditionally feminine activities.

E. *NO*. Data revealed by Mike and Todd suggest that Todd's symptoms represent a recent change in behavior and that Todd has not been chronically depressed. The same symptoms that are suggestive of depression would, if chronically present (several years) for most of the day, more days than not, suggest dysthymic disorder.

QUESTION 2. Questions related to which of the following areas are needed to help differentiate the diagnosis?

A. *YES*. An essential feature and critical data for differentiating the DSM-IV diagnostic categories is the length of time symptoms are present. For a diagnosis of adjustment disorder, the symptoms must develop within 3 months after the onset of an identifiable stressor. For a diagnosis of primary hypersomnia, the essential feature is excessive sleepiness for at least 1 month. To assign a DSM-IV diagnosis of major depressive episode, symptoms must have been present during the same 2-week period and represent a change in previous functioning. For a diagnosis of dysthymic disorder, a depressed or irritable mood must be present for most of the day on most days for at least 2 years.

B. *YES*. It is not uncommon for adolescents to experience sad times or to have occasional thoughts of suicide. However, recurrent thoughts of death, preoccupation with thoughts of committing suicide, and expressions of suicidal thoughts are often features of an adjustment disorder or a major depressive episode and represent precursors to suicide that must be taken seriously. Many adolescents who are in significant distress do not seek help or overtly express thoughts of suicide. As Todd's confidant, Mike is an excellent source of information. Mike's statement that Todd is tired of living warrants further exploration and must be taken seriously.

C. *YES*. Mike's statement that Todd is not interested in his usual activities warrants further assessment to clarify the extent of the change. A markedly diminished interest or pleasure in all or almost all activities nearly every day is common in depression.

D. *YES*. A diagnostic feature of any psychiatric disorder is the presence of clinically significant distress or impairment in social or other important areas of functioning.

E. *NO*. The data do not suggest that further information is needed to clarify Todd's level of comfort with his gender. Gender identity disorder is characterized by strong and persistent cross-gender identification accompanied by persistent discomfort with one's assigned sex. Further, Todd's homosexual experimentation is not a diagnosis, nor are homosexual relationships considered psychopathological.

**QUESTION 3.** Questions related to which of the following areas would help to further assess Todd's risk for suicide?
  **A.** *YES.* Studies have shown that degree of hopelessness is even more predictive of suicidal behavior than a specific diagnosis of depression. Failure to mobilize problem-solving strategies is at the heart of suicidal thinking. To explore Todd's degree of hopelessness, the nurse might ask him how he thinks he should solve his problems. If Todd has no ideas about solutions to his problems and expresses hopelessness, the nurse should ask, "Have you thought about harming or perhaps killing yourself?" If Todd says yes and seems comfortable (rather than uncomfortable) with being suicidal, his risk for suicide is higher. Patients with reasons for not committing suicide (such as not wanting to hurt family or having religious prohibitions) are at lower risk.
  **B.** *YES.* Use and abuse of alcohol and other drugs are associated with higher suicidal risk. Substance abuse increases the risk of overdosing and also impairs judgment, leading to risky behaviors.
  **C.** *YES.* Accessibility of firearms makes means of suicide more readily available. Suicidal males, especially, are more likely to use firearms to kill themselves. Even children under the age of 15 have killed themselves with guns. Rates of overall firearm-related deaths among children and adolescents in the United States (both homicide and suicide) is higher than in any other economically comparable country.
  **D.** *YES.* The more specific the suicidal plan, the more likely the person is to implement it. Todd has been depressed and miserable. If he acknowledges that he wants to kill himself, he should be asked how, when, and where he plans to commit suicide.
  **E.** *YES.* Research has shown that a family history of completed suicide is a risk factor.

**QUESTION 4.** What is the appropriate diagnosis for Todd?
  **A.** *YES.* Adjustment disorder with depressed mood is a diagnosis given when there is a clear psychosocial precipitant and the predominant manifestations of the adjustment problem are symptoms of depressed mood, tearfulness, or feelings of hopelessness. Adjustment disorders are associated with increased risk of suicide attempts and suicide. Todd is disturbed and confused about his sexual orientation and experimentation, and his distress about his sexual orientation is a clear precipitant to his depression. He also has suicidal thoughts.
  **B.** *NO.* In Todd's case, differentiating between adjustment disorder with depressed mood and major depressive disorder is a clinical judgment. Because Todd does not have a previous history of depression, and because there is such a clear psychosocial stressor present, adjustment disorder with depressed mood is a better choice for diagnosis. Major depressive disorder could be assigned, though, if Todd's symptoms are

severe enough: (1) being depressed most of the day nearly every day for over 2 weeks, (2) experiencing loss of pleasure, (3) sleeping excessively, (4) experiencing daily fatigue and loss of energy, (5) having trouble concentrating, and (6) being preoccupied with suicidal ideation. Further, for a major depressive episode, these symptoms cause clinically significant distress and social impairment and are not due to physiological effects of a substance or due to bereavement. If the clinical judgment is that Todd's symptoms are more severe than adjustment disorder with depressed mood, then this diagnosis could be given.

C. *NO.* The essential feature of body dysmorphic disorder is inordinate preoccupation with a defect in personal appearance, either an imagined defect or a slight anomaly. Complaints usually involve imagined or slight flaws of the face or head, such as acne, wrinkles, scars, complexion, facial asymmetry, size or shape of the nose, or other similar things. Todd has none of these complaints.

D. *NO.* Additional subjective data do not support the diagnosis of primary hypersomnia. The excessive sleepiness experienced by Todd seems to be secondary to his psychosocial stressor and depressed mood.

**QUESTION 5.** Maintaining confidentiality, the usual approach in the care of adolescents, may need to be abandoned with respect to which of the following areas?

A. *YES.* There is a duty to inform key people when someone is suicidal. In Todd's case, he is thinking about killing himself and is depressed. The practitioner needs to notify Todd's parents of his suicidality. In addition, since Todd is being seen in a school situation, the principal and the school counselor should be notified. The fact that this information is being shared with others should be told to Todd in a caring manner.

B. *NO.* Todd's homosexual experimentation is a private matter and should not be divulged to anyone else without Todd's permission.

C. *NO.* Sexual history is considered confidential.

D. *NO.* Unless Todd reports family violence and abuse, his concerns about his relationship with his father are confidential.

**QUESTION 6.** What interventions are appropriate for Todd?

A. *NO.* If a nonmood disorder seems to be contributing to a depression, the nonmood disorder should be treated first. In Todd's case, the adjustment disorder related to his homosexual feelings and experimentation is a clear precipitant to his depression and suicidality. Addressing the adjustment problems should be the first step in treating the depressed mood. Further, Todd is still functioning and is not experiencing any psychotic symptoms. He is able to verbalize his distress and confusion, making him amenable to individual counseling to work through the problem.

B. *YES.* Referring Todd for an in-depth individual psychiatric assessment is indicated. Adolescence can be a stormy time, and dealing with homosexuality in a culture that in many ways is disapproving can be very difficult. Adjustment disorder, while a passing condition, does place

Todd at serious suicidal risk. Suicide is the third leading cause of death in adolescents, and adolescent suicide rates have tripled over the last 40 years, from 4 per 1,000,000 to 13.2 per 1,000,000. It is important to assess more closely the nature and depth of Todd's depression (including family history) plus any underlying personality disorder.

C. *NO.* Because of Todd's concerns about his father's potential reactions to his grades and sexual orientation, family therapy is contraindicated at this time. In addition, more information is needed as to why Todd seems so concerned with his father's response. Also, Todd is just beginning to grapple with his homosexual feelings and, since family therapy is designed to foster open and honest family communication, this is not a good time for him to reveal his feelings in a family setting.

D. *NO.* Suicidal thoughts are not a reason for hospitalization. Many adolescents have suicidal ideas that can be dealt with by giving additional support and a caring approach. Evaluating the patient's resources (family, best friend, other caring adults) and contacting them on behalf of the patient (with the patient's knowledge) are the best lines of prevention for suicide. Hospitalization is indicated if suicidal risk factors are high (family history, previous attempts, engaging in highly risky behaviors, a specific plan and means) or if there is no support that can be mobilized for the patient.

E. *YES.* Means restriction refers to removal of methods of suicide (pills, firearms, and the like) from the patient's environment. The health care provider has a duty to inform key people about the patient's suicidality and teach them about their role in providing a safe environment. In Todd's case, the family should be told something like: "Your son has symptoms of depression. He is sad, upset, and has suicidal thoughts. You need to help him through this crisis and give him support. It is especially important for you to keep the environment safe. Please lock up or remove all guns, pills, and other dangerous items." The provider should follow up later to see if the family has complied with these requests.

## REFERENCES

American Psychiatric Association. (1994). *Diagnostic and Statistical Manual of Mental Disorders IV*, 4th ed. Washington, DC: Author.

Araoz, D. L., Carrese, M. A. (1996). *Solution-Oriented Brief Therapy for Adjustment Disorders: A Guide for Providers under Managed Care*. New York: Brunner/Mazel.

Buzan, R. D. (1996). Assessment and management of the suicidal patient. In J. L. Jacobson, A. M. Jacobson (eds.), pp 451–455. *Psychiatric Secrets*. Philadelphia: Hanley & Belfus.

Centers for Disease Control and Prevention. (1997). Rates of homicide, suicide, and firearm-related death among children in 26 industrialized countries. *JAMA 227*(9), pp 704–705.

Community Action for Survival. (1996). *Team Up to Save Lives: What Your School Should Know about Preventing Youth Suicide*. CD-ROM. Chicago: University of Illinois at Chicago and Ronald McDonald Charities.

U.S. Department of Health and Human Services. (1993). *Depression in Primary Care: Detection and Diagnosis*. Rockville, MD: U.S. Dept. of Health and Human Services.

# 18

# Urinary Tract Infection

*Susan A. Fontana*
*Marie L. Talashek*

Carla R. is a 15-year-old Hispanic female who has been brought to the clinic today by her father, a local farmer in a nearby rural community. The school nurse told Carla to visit her health care provider because she had asked to use the bathroom frequently during class that morning.

## CHIEF COMPLAINT

Carla complains of "burning inside" when she urinates since this morning.

## HISTORY OF PRESENT ILLNESS

Carla first noticed discomfort with urination upon arising to empty her bladder around 7:00 A.M. Otherwise, she did not notice anything unusual about her urine. She denies any fever, chills, back pain, or previous history of urinary tract infection (UTI). She reports that she is still "going steady" with the same boy that she told you about on her last visit, but denies coitus.

## PAST HISTORY

Her medical record shows that her last visit was 6 months ago for a sports physical. Allergy to penicillin with a reaction characterized by a "body rash" was reported at age 8. No hospitalizations or surgeries. Medications: Poly-Vi Fluor vitamins, since the water supply is from a well on their farm.

QUESTION 1. Which of the following historical information must be obtained from Carla? (Select all that apply.)
A. Presence of vaginal discharge
B. Presence of any external irritation on urination
C. Sexual history
D. Recent history of a sexually transmitted disease (STD)

QUESTION 2. What risk factors, if present in Carla's history, would raise the likelihood that this is a subclinical pyelonephritis? (Select all that apply.)
  A. History of multiple UTIs in childhood
  B. History of three or more UTIs in the past year
  C. Symptoms present for 7 to 10 days prior to seeking care
  D. Diagnosis of acute pyelonephritis in the past year

QUESTION 3. What is the best way to manage Carla's father's presence during the encounter?
  A. Include him in the history taking, but ask him to wait in the waiting room during the physical examination.
  B. Ask him to stay in the waiting room during the history taking and physical examination.
  C. Include him in the history taking and encourage his presence during the physical examination.
  D. Ask his preference and conduct the encounter accordingly.

## OBJECTIVE DATA

Vital signs: Temperature 98.7°F, blood pressure 118/76 right arm sitting.
General: Shy teenager; appears anxious but not in any distress.
Abdomen: Flat contour. Active bowel sounds. No bruits. Mild suprapubic tenderness. No costovertebral angle tenderness. No organomegaly.
Laboratory: Clean catch urine specimen, 8 to 10 white blood cells (WBCs) per high-power field (HPF) with 1+ bacteria. No blood, protein, glucose.

QUESTION 4. Which laboratory findings in urine can be used to confirm the diagnosis of lower urinary tract bacterial infection? (Select all that apply.)
  A. Urine culture with >$10^2$ organisms/mL
  B. 5 to 10 WBCs per HPF
  C. 0 to 2 red blood cells (RBCs) per HPF
  D. 3+ bacteria

QUESTION 5. A pelvic examination would be included in the physical examination of a female with dysuria if it was associated with which of the following symptoms? (Select all that apply.)
  A. Suprapubic tenderness with palpation
  B. Vaginal discharge
  C. Fever
  D. Onset of sexual activity

QUESTION 6. Which of the following are indications for performing a urine culture? (Select all that apply.)
  A. Female age 15
  B. Physical findings that include flank pain
  C. History of renal calculi
  D. History of diabetes or other medical complications

## ASSESSMENT

**QUESTION 7.** Based upon the history and clinical findings, what is Carla's most likely diagnosis?
A. Subclinical pyelonephritis
B. Bacterial vaginosis
C. Lower urinary tract infection
D. Vesicoureteral reflux (VUR)

**QUESTION 8.** Which organism is responsible for the majority of lower urinary tract infections and subclinical pyelonephritis?
A. *Escherichia coli*
B. *Staphylococcus saprophyticus*
C. Enterococci
D. *Staphylococcus aureus*
E. Group B streptococci

## PLAN

**QUESTION 9.** Benefits of single-dose antibacterial therapy with any of several antibacterials include which of the following? (Select all that apply.)
A. Improved compliance
B. Lower rate of relapse
C. Less chance of an allergic reaction
D. Generally lower cost than with multidose therapies with the same agent
E. Applicable to most patients

## ANSWERS

**QUESTION 1.** Which of the following historical information must be obtained from Carla?
A. *YES.* The presence of vaginal discharge would help to support vaginal infection as the cause of the dysuria.
B. *YES.* External irritation is associated with a vaginal etiology and would prompt the clinician to pursue a more detailed review of systems relative to the genitalia.
C. *YES.* Information on risk factors such as new sexual partners or a partner with a penile discharge would be helpful in considering chlamydia and/or gonococcal pathogens as the cause of urethritis. Carla denies sexual intercourse.
D. *YES.* Other etiologies of dysuria are gonococcal urethritis and chlamydia urethritis. These would be suggested by a history of gonorrhea or an intercurrent chlamydia cervicitis.

**QUESTION 2.** What risk factors, if present in Carla's history, would raise the likelihood that this is a subclinical pyelonephritis?
A. *YES.* A history of multiple UTIs in childhood is a risk factor for subclinical pyelonephritis.
B. *YES.* Patients who have had three or more UTIs in the past year are at risk for subclinical pyelonephritis.

C. *YES.* Patients who have had symptoms for 7 to 10 days prior to obtaining care are more likely to have a subclinical pyelonephritis.

D. *YES.* A history of acute pyelonephritis in the past year increases the likelihood of subclinical pyelonephritis. Additional risk factors for subclinical pyelonephritis include a history of urinary tract pathology, immunocompromised health status, and indigent inner-city residence.

QUESTION 3. What is the best way to manage Carla's father's presence during the encounter?

A. *YES.* Carla's father may be helpful in obtaining details about his daughter's early childhood. However, conducting the physical examination alone with Carla affords privacy and confidentiality, which are important for establishing a therapeutic relationship with the adolescent. For example, in several states adolescents who are 14 or older are not required to have parental consent for treatment of STDs. The clinician needs to be aware of laws related to treating adolescents, which can vary by state.

B. *NO.* Include Carla's father in the health history as needed.

C–D. *NO.* Any of these arrangements could undermine the adolescent's need for privacy and confidentiality. Adolescents may be reluctant to share sensitive aspects of their history in the presence of parents or guardians because of fear of reprisal, embarrassment, or both.

QUESTION 4. Which laboratory findings in urine can be used to confirm the diagnosis of lower urinary tract bacterial infection?

A. *YES.* The diagnostic criteria for significant bacteriuria have been liberalized from $>10^5$ colony-forming units (CFU) of bacteria in an asymptomatic individual on one or more urine cultures to $>10^2$ CFU in a symptomatic female or $>10^3$ CFU in a symptomatic male.

B. *YES.* The presence of pyuria is the most important diagnostic parameter and may be as low as 2 to 5 WBCs per HPF in a spun sediment of a symptomatic individual.

C. *NO.* The presence of 0 to 2 RBCs per HPF is considered within normal limits.

D. *YES.* However, the presence of bacteria via dipstick without pyuria is indicative of contamination from the perineal area. Urine specimens need to be examined within 2 h or be refrigerated.

QUESTION 5. A pelvic examination would be included in the physical examination of a female with dysuria if it was associated with which one of the following symptoms?

A. *NO.* Suprapubic tenderness with palpation is indicative of lower urinary tract infection and would not by itself necessitate a pelvic examination.

B. *YES.* If a women complains of vaginal discharge or has a history of pelvic inflammatory disease, a pelvic examination should be performed.

C. *NO.* Fever is strongly suggestive of an upper urinary tract infection, but by itself would not necessitate a pelvic exam.

D. *YES.* Urinary tract infections are common in young women initiating sexual intercourse.

**QUESTION 6.** Which of the following are indications for performing a urine culture?
  A. *NO.* However, urine cultures are indicated in girls younger than 5 years of age and in all boys, irrespective of age.
  B. *YES.* Flank pain is highly suggestive of upper urinary tract infection, in which a urine culture is indicated.
  C. *YES.* A history of renal calculi or other renal abnormalities justifies a urine culture.
  D. *YES.* Persons with a history of diabetes, recent instrumentation of the urinary tract, recent hospitalization, prolonged symptoms prior to seeking care, compromised immune function, or an indwelling catheter should have a urine culture performed, since these factors may be associated with infection.

**QUESTION 7.** Based upon the history and clinical findings, what is Carla's most likely diagnosis?
  A. *NO.* Carla does not have any of the risk factors for subclinical pyelonephritis.
  B. *NO.* Carla complains of internal rather than external discomfort, which is most consistent with a urinary rather than vaginal etiology.
  C. *YES.* The sudden onset of Carla's symptoms without signs or symptoms of acute pyelonephritis is consistent with lower urinary tract infection.
  D. *NO.* Vesicoureteral reflux signifies retrograde passage of urine from the bladder to the ureter. A voiding cystourethrogram is used to establish the diagnosis. The incidence of UTI is increased in the presence of VUR. Approximately 40 to 50 percent of infants with UTI have a history of VUR. These percentages decrease to about 25 percent in school-age children and 10 to 15 percent in adolescents.

**QUESTION 8.** Which organism is responsible for the majority of lower urinary tract infections and subclinical pyelonephritis?
  A. *YES. Escherichia coli* accounts for 80 to 90 percent of first UTIs.
  B–D. *NO.* The remainder of infections are caused by other gram-negative enteric bacilli (proteus, klebsiella, enterobacter) and gram-positive cocci (enterococci, *S. epidermidis*). Residents in nursing homes typically present with infections caused by proteus and a sixfold increase of klebsiella and pseudomonas compared to counterparts living at home.
  E. *NO.* Group B streptococci are implicated in serious bacterial infection/occult bacteremia in children less than 3 months of age.

**QUESTION 9.** Benefits of single-dose antibacterial therapy with any of several antibacterials include which of the following?
  A. *YES.* Single-dose therapies have excellent compliance.
  B. *NO.* The frequency of relapse is higher with single-dose therapies than with longer regimens.
  C. *YES.* There is a reduced chance of allergic reactions with single-dose therapies.
  D. *YES.* Cost is lower with single-dose therapies with the same agent. In addition, a 3-day course of antibiotics provides nearly the same results

as conventional 7- to 10-day therapies while significantly reducing side effects, emergence of resistant organisms, cost, and poor compliance. Other benefits of single-dose and 3-day regimens compared to the conventional regimens are that treatment failures can be identified earlier and patients switched to more effective agents.

E.   *NO.* Patients with diabetes, a history of relapses, or more than three UTIs in the past year and immunocompromised persons are suboptimal candidates for shortened therapies and are best treated with longer, more conventional therapies.

## REFERENCES

Burns, C. E., Barber, N., Brady, M. A., Dunn, A. M. (1996). *Pediatric Primary Care: A Handbook for Nurse Practitioners.* Philadelphia: W. B. Saunders.

French, M. (1995). UTI in the elderly. *Advance for Nurse Practitioners 3*(11), 25–28.

Goroll, A. H., May, L. A., Mulley, A. G., Jr. (eds.). (1995). *Primary Care Medicine: Office Evaluation and Management of the Adult Patient,* 3d ed. Philadelphia: J. B. Lippincott.

Rubin, R. H. Voss, C., Derksen, D. J., Gateley, A., Quenzer, R. W. (1996). *Medicine: A Primary Care Approach.* Philadelphia: W. B. Saunders.

# V

## YOUNG ADULT

# Introduction

*Arlene Miller*

The years between ages 25 and 44 encompass young adulthood, which includes the developmental tasks defined by Erikson as intimacy vs. isolation and generativity vs. stagnation. Issues that have an important impact on mental and physical health during young adulthood include managing the implications of intimacy and sexuality in interpersonal relationships, dealing constructively with stress, and balancing multiple roles, such as being a worker, spouse or partner, and parent. Conflicts regarding alternative adult lifestyles must be addressed or resolved, such as remaining single or childless, being divorced, or maintaining a relationship with a same-sex partner. Developing a sense of responsibility for one's actions, particularly those that are health-related, is an important component of successful participation in health promotion and preventive behavior, and should be encouraged by health care providers during this time.

The initiation of young adulthood varies among social and cultural groups in the United States, where, particularly in urban areas and among affluent cultures, the ages 18 to 24 approximate a period of older adolescence or youth. This represents sanctioned time before adult responsibilities must be assumed, and corresponds to being a college student or serving a career apprenticeship. During this transitional period, identity development, including self-image and self-concept, begins to stabilize. Establishment of independence is symbolized by moving away from home. The peer group recedes in social importance. More mature relationships are characterized by emotional intimacy with chosen partners, as well as reciprocity and interdependence with parents. Career choices are made, and issues relating to values, religion, and ethics are contemplated.

Screening for early diagnosis of cardiovascular and several other chronic diseases is initiated during young adulthood. The American College of Physicians and the American Academy of Family Physicians recommend annual hypertension screening for individuals aged 18 and older. For men, total blood cholesterol screening should begin at age 35. For women who are sexually active, annual Papanicolaou testing is recommended by the American College of Obstetricians and Gynecologists. The American Academy of Family Physicians, however, suggests that this can be decreased to at least once every 3 years for women with low risk who have had at least three normal annual Pap smears. Contraception to prevent unintended pregnancy should be discussed at primary care visits. Rubella serology or vaccination and maintenance of adequate folic acid (vitamin $B_6$) are also recommended for women who are of childbearing age. For high-risk individuals, annual screening for syphilis, gonorrhea, chlamydia, and HIV/AIDS infection is recommended. To prevent sexually transmitted diseases, avoidance of high-risk sexual behavior and the use of condoms and/or female barrier methods with spermicide are important components of counseling during primary care visits for all sexually active adults. Hepatitis B and/or hepatitis A vaccine should be given to susceptible individuals, particularly those who are health care workers or at risk of these potentially sexually and blood-borne transmitted diseases. Hepatitis B may also be problematic for immigrants from Southeast Asia and other regions.

Screening and counseling should also address alcohol use, tobacco cessation, modification of dietary fat and cholesterol, initiating or continuing regular physical activity, injury prevention, and dental health. Maintaining adequate calcium intake (1200 to 1500 mg/day) throughout young adulthood may increase bone mineral density and may reduce the risk of postmenopausal osteoporosis in women.

The case studies chosen for this chapter include situations seen in sexually active women in primary care settings: normal pregnancy and contraception. Substance abuse is a lifestyle problem that crosses the boundaries of socioeconomic groups in this country, and the inclusion of a case study regarding hepatitis emphasizes the increasing number of immigrants and refugees who enter the United States and are in need of general and specialized health care services. The other case studies, headache, gastritis, and thyroid disease, cover health problems commonly seen in primary care settings.

## REFERENCES

Erikson, E. H. (1982). *The Life Cycle Completed.* New York: Norton.

Miller, A., Wilbur, J., McDevitt, J. (1997). Health promotion: The perimenopausal to mature years (45–64). In K. Allen, J. Phillips (eds.), *Women's Health across the Lifespan: A Comprehensive Perspective,* 55–71. Philadelphia: J.B. Lippincott.

Murray, R. B., Zentner, J. P. (1997). *Nursing Assessment and Health Promotion: Strategies through the Life Span,* 6th ed. Stamford, CT: Appleton & Lange.

Stevens-Long, J. (1990). Adult development: Theories past and future. In R. Nemeroff, C. Colarusso (eds.), *New Dimensions in Adult Development,* 125–169. New York: Basic Books.

Woolf, S., Jonas, S., Lawrence, R. (eds.). (1996). *Health Promotion and Disease Prevention in Clinical Practice.* Baltimore: Williams & Wilkins.

U.S. Preventive Services Task Force. (1996). *Guide to Clinical Preventive Services,* 2nd ed. Baltimore: Williams & Wilkins.

# COLOR PLATES*

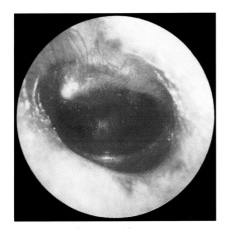

**PLATE 1** (Fig. 1-1)
Tympanic membrane.

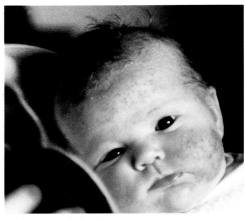

**PLATE 2** (Fig. 6-1)
Infantile eczema.

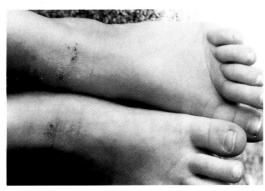

**PLATE 3** (Fig. 6-2)
Current skin lesions.

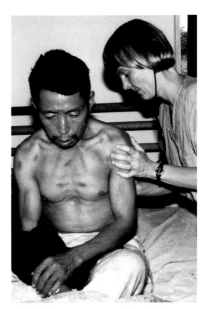

**PLATE 4** (Fig. 11-1)
Skin coining.

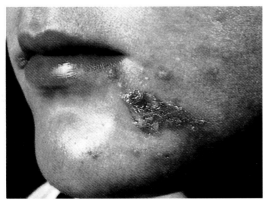

**PLATE 5** (Fig. 12-1)
Skin findings.

* The figures in each plate have been double-numbered in order to indicate the chapter in which they are cited and the order of their citation therein.

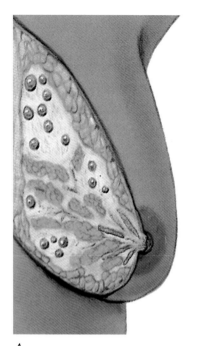

A

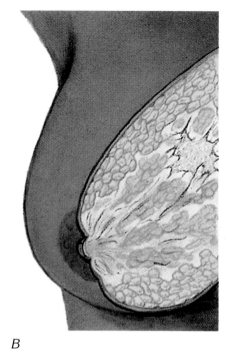

B

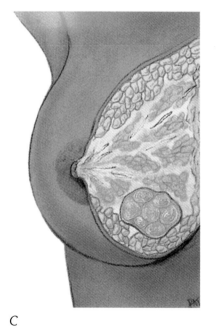

C

**PLATE 6**
(Fig. 28-1A) Benign breast disease.
(Fig. 28-1B) Cancer.
(Fig. 28-1C) Fibroadenoma.
For complete legends to Plates 6A–C,
see Fig. 28-1A–C.

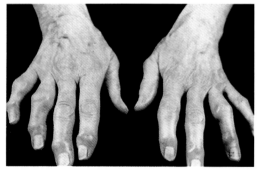

**PLATE 7** (Fig. 37-1) Degenerative joint disease: Heberden nodes at the distal inter-phalangeal joints and Bouchard nodes at the proximal interphalangeal joints.

# 19

# Substance Abuse

*Marie L. Talashek*
*Laina M. Gerace*

George F., a 40-year-old Latino lawyer, has sought help at the request of his law firm partners. They have been concerned about his decline in productivity over the past 6 months. Mr. F. states that he isn't sleeping well, has difficulty concentrating, is tired, and has lost interest in work. He is an extremely competent lawyer, and over the past 10 years he has become a partner in a very prestigious law firm.

## CHIEF COMPLAINT

"I just want to be productive at work like I used to be; maybe you can give me something to get my energy back."

## HISTORY OF PRESENT ILLNESS

Six months ago Mr. F.'s partners began expressing concern about his behavior at the firm's cocktail parties and social events; they also expressed concern that his effectiveness and productivity at work were declining. It was around this time that he reports noticing his fatigue and other symptoms. He admits that he started drinking more about 3 years ago, when his wife died of metastatic breast cancer.

QUESTION 1. What additional historical information is required to evaluate an alcohol problem? (Select all that apply.)
A. Past and current use of alcohol
B. Amount, type, and frequency of consumption
C. Under what conditions he drinks
D. Outcomes of alcohol use

**QUESTION 2.** What additional historical information is needed to evaluate Mr. F.? (Select all that apply.)
  A. Tobacco use
  B. Other drug use
  C. Family history
  D. Review of systems (ROS)
  E. Impact of wife's death

## PAST HISTORY

Mr. F. smokes one pack of cigarettes a day, drinks the equivalent of 2 oz of alcohol each day, and began experimenting with cocaine 3 years ago. Over the past 6 months he has been using cocaine as a way to help him complete projects at work and as self-treatment for his malaise. He snorts cocaine, but denies freebase or intravenous cocaine use. His father had an alcohol problem. He has not sought help to resolve grief and has been socially isolated since the death of his wife. He has had neither a close relationship nor sexual intercourse with a woman since the death of his wife. They had no children. He has never experienced legal problems related to alcohol or cocaine use. The ROS is noncontributory except for a problem with sleeping and symptoms of irritability and racing pulse rate when using cocaine.

**QUESTION 3.** In which components of the physical examination might you find substance-related problems? (Select all that apply.)
  A. Vital signs
  B. Skin
  C. Abdomen
  D. Head, eyes, ears, nose, and throat (HEENT)
  E. Neurological

## ASSESSMENT

**QUESTION 4.** What is your preliminary diagnosis based on the history and physical findings?
  A. Experimental substance use
  B. Social-recreational substance use
  C. Substance abuse
  D. Substance dependence
  E. Depression

**QUESTION 5.** What laboratory tests can support your diagnosis of substance abuse? (Select all that apply.)
  A. Complete blood count (CBC) with liver enzymes
  B. Hemoglobin electrophoresis
  C. Toxicology screen
  D. Lipid profile
  E. Uric acid

## LABORATORY FINDINGS

Elevated gamma-glutamyl/transferase (GGT), triglycerides, and cholesterol support your diagnosis.

## PLAN

A plan of care is a joint decision between the patient and the health care provider.

**QUESTION 6.** What intervention alternatives are appropriate to consider at this time? (Select all that apply.)
A. Inpatient detoxification
B. Trial of abstinence or controlled use
C. Consultation with an alcohol/substance specialist
D. Family meeting
E. Referral to Alcoholics Anonymous (AA) or Rational Recovery (RR)

**QUESTION 7.** If Mr. F. refuses to seek help from an addiction counselor or attend a self-help group but is willing to attempt a trial of abstinence, what should be included in the plan of care? (Select all that apply.)
A. Negotiate a plan of total abstinence from alcohol and drugs for the next 4 weeks.
B. Negotiate a GGT and urine drug screen for 4 weeks hence
C. Encourage stress-relieving techniques
D. Discuss referral for grief counseling

## ANSWERS

**QUESTION 1.** What additional historical information is required to evaluate an alcohol problem?
A. *YES.* Past and current use of alcohol are both important. Age at initiation is important because it identifies years of use. Problem drinkers will often report enjoying the feeling they had the first time they drank and the ability to drink more than their contemporaries. These effects from drinking provide positive reinforcement to continue drinking.
B. *YES.* Amount, type, and frequency of consumption are all needed to assess the actual amount of alcohol being consumed. A standard drink consists of 1½ oz of distilled spirits (whiskey, gin, vodka, etc.), 5 oz of wine, or 12 oz of beer. Each provides 1 oz of alcohol. The National Institute of Alcohol Abuse and Alcoholism (NIAAA) indicates that individuals who drink moderately do not development alcohol-related health problems. Moderate consumption is considered to be no more than 7 oz of alcohol per week for men and 5 oz of alcohol per week for women. According to the U.S. Preventive Task Force, the definition of heavy drinking or hazardous drinking in asymptomatic people is variable. One definition of hazardous drinking is five or more drinks per day for men and three or more drinks per day for women or frequent intoxication.

C. *YES*. Identifying under what conditions Mr. F. drinks will provide information about his level of tolerance and physical addiction. Drinking to decrease tremulousness is indicative of physical dependence. A report of becoming intoxicated on a lesser amount of alcohol than was previously the case indicates liver damage. Routine use of the CAGE questionnaire (C, feel the need to cut down on drinking; A, annoyed at someone who criticizes your drinking; G, feel guilty about drinking; E, need an eye-opener drink in the morning) allows identification of patients who have a physical dependence on alcohol.

D. *YES*. Outcomes of alcohol use are indicative of level of addiction. Blackouts, the term used to describe amnesia about what happened while drinking, occur later in the course of alcohol dependence. Lack of control is indicated by continued alcohol consumption in the face of serious problems such as driving under the influence, marital discord, or threatened loss of employment or friends.

**QUESTION 2.** What additional historical information is needed to evaluate Mr. F?

A. *YES*. The nicotine in tobacco is addictive. The pharmacological and behavioral processes of nicotine addiction are similar to those in cocaine and heroin addiction. Tobacco and alcohol are often coaddictions.

B. *YES*. Use of substances other than alcohol and nicotine should always be investigated. There are four categories of substance use: experimental use, social-recreational use, substance abuse, and substance dependence.

C. *YES*. Research supports a genetic predisposition for alcoholism. Studies show that adolescent sons of alcoholics react differently to alcohol than do sons of nonalcoholics. Twin studies also lend credence to a genetic predisposition for alcoholism.

D. *YES*. The ROS is important in order to identify nonsubstance causes for decreased energy and to identify symptoms that may be substance-related, such as gastritis or depression.

E. *YES*. Mr. F.'s pattern of alcohol use changed around the time of his wife's death. Did he receive any grief counseling, and what sort of support system does he have in addition to what is provided by the partners in his law firm?

**QUESTION 3.** In which components of the physical examination might you find substance-related problems?

A. *YES*. Borderline hypertension is related to alcohol abuse, and so alcohol use should always be investigated when working up a patient with elevated blood pressure (BP). Decreasing alcohol use can bring the blood pressure back to normal. Weight loss is often a problem with cocaine use and is a finding of later-stage alcoholism. During cocaine use the pulse rate is rapid and often irregular. For the early abuser, the physical examination usually offers few clues.

B. *YES*. A thorough review of the skin can reveal findings about the route of drug administration and the amount of physical damage. However, for the early nonintravenous (non-IV) drug abuser, the skin may offer few clues. Skin color such as jaundice indicates possible alcoholic liver disease. Alcohol abuse is also related to acne rosacea, spider angioma, and palmar erythema. Track marks, ecchymosis, and skin infections like cellulitis are often caused by IV drug use. Burns on the fingers are often indicative of careless smoking.

C. *YES*. For the early abuser, the abdomen offers few clues. However, the abdomen should be examined for fluid retention, organomegaly, tenderness, and increased bowel sounds associated with gastritis. Ascites is a finding of late-stage alcoholism, whereas gastritis often occurs earlier in the disease.

D. *YES*. The HEENT examination yields important clues to substance use and abuse. Nystagmus is present during intoxication. Sniffing cocaine leads to irritation of nasal mucosa and bleeding, and with high levels of use the nasal cartilage can be destroyed. Inhalation of cocaine can also lead to inflammation of the throat.

E. *YES*. Alcohol is a central nervous system depressant; heavy use leads to slurred speech, lack of coordination, flaccid muscles, decreased sexual functioning, blackouts, and ultimately coma. However, lower levels of alcohol use can act as a behavioral stimulant. Cocaine stimulates both the central and peripheral nervous system. Cocaine prevents reuptake of a neurotransmitter, thus causing an excess of neurotransmitter in the synapse, which continues to stimulate the postsynaptic receptors. Increases in the sensitivity of the postsynaptic receptor sites caused by cocaine leave the user alert and confident. Enzymatic action eventually breaks down the entrapped neurotransmitters, causing dysphoria, specifically anhedonia, irritability, and restlessness. Cocaine is often used repeatedly to overcome these feelings.

**QUESTION 4.** What is your preliminary diagnosis based on the history and physical findings?

A. *NO*. The use in this case is more than experimental use or initial use.

B. *NO*. Social-recreational use involves repeated occasional use, controlling the dose and time of use. Mr. F. has moved beyond this stage, because he has lost control, and his use interferes with both his social and business functions.

C. *YES*. Abuse, as defined by the *Diagnostic and Statistical Manual* of the American Psychiatric Association (DSM-IV), is a maladaptive pattern of substance use leading to clinically significant impairment or distress manifested by one or more of the following occurring during the same 12 months:

1. Recurrent substance use resulting in a failure to fulfill major role obligations at work, school, or home. Mr. F. is being seen at the urging of his partners because his productivity has decreased.
2. Recurrent substance use in situations in which it is physically hazardous. This is not reported by Mr. F.
3. Recurrent substance-related legal problems. Legal problems have not been reported.

4. Continued substance use despite having persistent or recurrent social or interpersonal problems caused or exacerbated by the effects of the substance. Mr. F.'s problem drinking was first brought to his attention 6 months ago, and he has continued to drink in spite of concerns shown by his law partners. He also has not dealt effectively with the grief from the death of his wife.

D. *NO.* Substance dependence, according to DSM-IV, is a maladaptive pattern of substance use leading to clinically significant impairment or distress, as manifested by three or more of the following occurring at any time in the same 12-month period:

1. Tolerance as defined by either a need for markedly increased amounts of the substance to achieve intoxication or the desired effect or markedly diminished effect with continued use of the same amount of the substance.
2. Withdrawal as manifested by either withdrawal syndrome for the substance or taking the substance to relieve or avoid withdrawal symptoms.
3. Taking the substance in larger amounts or over a longer period than was intended.
4. A persistent desire or unsuccessful efforts to cut down or control substance use.
5. Spending a great deal of time in activities necessary to obtain the substance or recover it from its effects.
6. Giving up or reducing important social, occupational, or recreational activities because of substance use.
7. Continuing substance use despite knowledge of having had a persistent or recurring physical or psychological problem that was likely to have been caused or exacerbated by the substance. Findings do not indicate that Mr. F. is physically dependent on alcohol or drugs.

E. *NO.* He does not have the classic signs of depression. However, symptoms of depression are common for cocaine users between drug use episodes, and alcohol abusers often feel depressed about family and work problems caused by drinking. Symptoms of substance abuse often mirror those of psychiatric disorders. It is important for the patient to be substance-free for at least a month prior to making a psychiatric diagnosis, to ensure accuracy of the diagnosis.

**Question 5.** What laboratory tests can support your diagnosis of substance abuse?

A. *YES.* Macrocytic anemia and increased mean corpuscular volume (MCV) are sometimes evident early in alcoholism, and an unexplained decreased hematocrit may also be present. Liver enzymes are important, because they give information for diagnosis early in the disease and can be used later in the disease to assess the degree of liver damage. The GGT can suggest problem drinking; it has a sensitivity between

.35 and .60 and a specificity of .85. The GGT will be decreased after a month of decreased alcohol consumption. Other causes of elevated GGT include some medications, trauma, diabetes, and heart or kidney or biliary tract disease. Other liver enzymes are generally insensitive to early drinking; however, they will all be abnormal with later-stage alcoholism.

B. *NO.* Hemoglobin electrophoresis is of no value in this case because there is no indication of a hemoglobinopathy.

C. *YES.* A toxicology screen provides information about current use but not about abuse. Random toxicology screening is done in some work settings to detect heavy users of drugs and to discourage casual use of drugs at the work site. It is important to have the procedures explained in detail in the employee handbook. Blood or urine specimens should be divided into two samples so that retesting can be done if the first analysis is positive for one or more drugs.

D. *YES.* Both triglycerides and cholesterol can be elevated with alcohol use.

E. *YES.* Uric acid can be elevated with alcohol abuse.

QUESTION 6. What intervention alternatives are appropriate to consider at this time?

A. *NO.* It is unlikely that 2 oz of alcohol a day will lead to withdrawal symptoms. Cocaine users crave cocaine, but those who use cocaine intranasally do not experience physical dependence or withdrawal from the drug.

B. *YES.* A trial of abstinence from cocaine and alcohol may be all that is required to convince the patient that he has a problem and needs treatment. Some patients refuse to join a peer support group; therefore, the primary care provider assumes management of their substance use. It is important to tie the insomnia, difficulty concentrating, tiredness, loss of interest in work, and abnormal laboratory findings to alcohol and cocaine use.

C. *YES.* A referral for consultation with an alcohol/substance specialist should be made. Patients who administer cocaine intranasally generally enter remission after referral for treatment of substance use with psychotherapy or behavioral therapy. However, caregivers should be prepared to deal with patients who refuse to follow up on such a referral.

D. *NO.* A family meeting is not appropriate in this case, because Mr. F. is responding to the concerns of his partners. Family interventions are most appropriate for patients who do not admit that they have a problem. Input from the family is an effective means for moving the patient toward treatment.

E. Referral to AA or RR is appropriate for this case. RR, a self-help organization, has a cognitive orientation. The emphasis is on self-examination rather than the twelve-step focus on a higher being that is integral to AA. Members of AA are assigned a sponsor from the group, and supportive exchanges between meetings are encouraged. This is not the case with RR; rather, there are group facilitators who make referrals to professionals as needed. Success rates are similar with these interventions.

**QUESTION 7.** If Mr. F. refuses to seek help from an addiction counselor or attend a self-help group but is willing to attempt a trial of abstinence, what should be included in the plan of care?
   A. *YES.* Negotiate a plan of total abstinence from alcohol and drugs for the next 4 weeks. Contract with Mr. F. that if he changes his mind about a referral to a substance abuse counselor or support group, he will contact you earlier than 4 weeks, and that he should call if he needs to talk to you prior to the 4-week evaluation. Use of drugs in the management of cocaine abuse is not as effective as counseling.
   B. *YES.* It is important to negotiate a GGT and urine drug screen for the fourth-week appointment. The GGT should be lower after abstaining from alcohol for 4 weeks, and the urine toxicology screen can identify current drug use.
   C. *YES.* It is important to encourage Mr. F. to engage in stress management. A program of walking is an excellent first step. Yoga is another relaxation technique that alleviates stress. If Mr. F. has a sport that he enjoys, but has not been engaging in it because of work, encourage him to become active again. Aerobic activities will help him sleep better, and will replace the time spent using alcohol or drugs.
   D. *YES.* It is important for Mr. F. to deal with the death of his wife. Grief counseling may be a helpful adjunct to therapy for substance use.

## REFERENCES

Brown, R. L., Talashek, M. L. (1992). *Developing Clinical and Teaching Skills on Screening, Assessment, and Brief Intervention for Alcohol and Drug Problems.* AMERSA National Meeting, Preconference Workshop, Nov. 12, 1992.

Donovan, D. M., Marlatt, G.A. (1993). Behavioral treatment. In M. Galanter (ed.), *Recent Developments in Alcoholism,* Vol. 11, *Ten Years of Progress,* 397–411. New York: Plenum Press.

Galanter, M., Egelko, S., Edwards, H. (1993). Rational recovery: Alternative to AA for addiction? *Am J Drug Alcohol Abuse 19,* 499–510.

Mendelson, J. H., Mello, N. K. (1996). Drug therapy: Management of cocaine abuse and dependence. *N Engl J Med 334,* 965–972.

Naegle, M. A. (1996). Alcohol and other drug abuse: Identification and intervention. *American Association of Occupational Health Nursing Journal 44,* 454–464.

Neinstein, L. S, Heischober, B. S. (1996). Miscellaneous drugs: Stimulants, inhalants, opiates, depressants, and anabolic steroids. In L. S. Neinstein (ed.), Adolescent *Health Care: A Practical Guide,* 3d ed., 1052–1056. Baltimore: Williams & Wilkins.

# 20

# Normal Pregnancy

*Patricia A. Furnace*
*Marie L. Talashek*

Maria G., a 25-year-old Latina, has an appointment today for her initial prenatal visit. It is her first visit with the private rural practice. She had a positive human chorionic gonadotropin (HCG) test 2 days ago. Maria and her husband are both excited about the pregnancy; this is their first child. Their families live approximately 4 h away and are also excited about the first grandchild for each set of grandparents. Mr. and Mrs. G. are employed in the neighboring city; she as an administrative assistant and he as an engineer.

## CHIEF COMPLAINT

"I did a home pregnancy test 2 days ago that was positive."

## HISTORY OF PRESENT ILLNESS

Mrs. G. has had nausea every day for 2 weeks. She has noticed breast tenderness for the past 3 weeks. Fatigue has been a problem for 1 week.

## PAST MEDICAL HISTORY

Mrs. G's history is negative for diabetes mellitus, hypertension, asthma, cardiovascular disease, hepatitis, thyroid dysfunction, kidney disease, seizure disorder, liver disease, phlebitis, blood transfusion, tuberculosis, or exposure to sexually transmitted diseases.

| | |
|---|---|
| Habits: | Denies smoking and street drugs. Wears seat belts 100 percent of the time, and walks 30 min three times per week. Caffeine limited to iced tea two to four glasses daily. |
| Medications: | Tylenol once a month for headaches. |
| Dietary supplements: | None. |
| Herbs: | None. |

| Allergies: | None. |
|---|---|
| Family history: | Negative for any genetic or chromosomal problem. |
| Nutritional assessment: | Twenty-four-hour diet recall. |
| | Breakfast—Orange juice, cereal with skim milk; lunch—turkey and Swiss cheese sandwich, carrot sticks, apple, and iced tea; supper—hamburger, cole slaw, peaches, skim milk; snacks—crackers and cheese. |

QUESTION 1. What additional subjective information should be obtained at this time? (Select all that apply.)
A. Alcohol use
B. Previous obstetrical and gynecologic history
C. Immunization history
D. Menstrual history
E. Occupational exposure to hazards

QUESTION 2. Which of the following common discomforts of pregnancy would you expect a woman to experience during the first trimester? (Select all that apply.)
A. Low backache
B. Edema
C. Physiologic leukorrhea
D. Nausea and vomiting
E. Physiologic urinary frequency

## PHYSICAL FINDINGS
Vital signs: Blood pressure 118/64 left arm sitting, temperature 36.5°C (98.4°F), pulse 72, respirations 16, height 5 ft 4 in, Weight 124 pounds.

The physical examination is normal. Changes indicative of pregnancy include the following:

| Breasts: | Generalized tenderness with no palpable masses. |
|---|---|
| Pelvic: | |
| External: | No lesions or exudate. |
| Vagina: | Normal rugae. |
| Cervix: | Nulliparous, bluish in color. |
| Bimanual: | Eight-week-size uterus; anteflexed. Nonpalpable adnexa. Adequate pelvis. |
| Rectal: | Hemoccult negative. No masses or areas of tenderness. |
| Laboratory: | A urine dipstick is negative for glucose and protein. |

QUESTION 3. Which of the following best describes the enlargement of a gravid anteflexed uterus at 8 weeks gestation? (Select all that apply.)
A. Nonpalpable
B. Palpable below the symphysis pubis; slightly enlarged, about the size of an orange

C. Palpable 15 cm above the symphysis pubis
D. Palpable at umbilicus

## ASSESSMENT

**QUESTION 4.** Which of the following would be an appropriate assessment for this patient?
A. High-risk pregnancy
B. Single intrauterine pregnancy
C. Hyperemesis gravidarum
D. Unconfirmed pregnancy

## PLAN

**QUESTION 5.** Which of the following laboratory tests would be appropriate to obtain at the initial first-trimester prenatal visit? (Select all that apply.)
A. Hemoglobin and hematocrit
B. Rubella screen
C. Maternal serum alpha-fetoprotein (MSAFP)
D. Blood type; Rh factor and antibody screen
E. One-hour glucose screen

**QUESTION 6.** Management of first-trimester nausea and vomiting would be accomplished with which of the following? (Select all that apply.)
A. High fat content in diet
B. Change to less stressful job
C. Small, frequent meals
D. Vitamin $B_6$
E. Exercise 20 min three to five times per week

**QUESTION 7.** Return appointments should be scheduled according to which schedule?
A. Once a month until delivery
B. One visit each in the first, second, and beginning of the third trimester, then every two weeks starting at 36 weeks until delivery
C. Whenever she feels she needs to be seen, as this is a healthy time of life
D. Once a month until 30 weeks, every two weeks until 36 weeks, then once a week until delivery.

**QUESTION 8.** Additional laboratory tests this client can expect to complete during her pregnancy would include which of the following?
A. No additional blood work is recommended after the first trimester.
B. One-hour postprandial glucose screen at 24 to 28 weeks.
C. All the laboratory tests done at the initial visit will be repeated early in the third trimester.
D. She will need testing for the specific infectious diseases of cytomegalovirus, toxoplasmosis, and herpes simplex.

## ANSWERS

**QUESTION 1.** What additional subjective information should be obtained at this time?

**A.** *YES.* A history of alcohol use is important information to obtain, because prenatal alcohol use places the infant at high risk for mental retardation and fetal alcohol syndrome. Substance use can contribute to learning disabilities later.

**B.** *YES.* Previous obstetrical and gynecologic history is needed to assess risk for problems with this pregnancy. This is Mrs. G.'s first pregnancy; however, women who have had more than two abortions (spontaneous or induced), a preterm delivery, infertility treatment, or a surgically scarred uterus are at greater risk of problems.

**C.** *YES.* Rubella status is important because contracting this disease during pregnancy may result in congenital problems for the fetus. Overall risk of congenital rubella syndrome is 20 to 25 percent if maternal infection occurs in the first trimester, and less than 1 percent if the infection occurs during the second or third trimester. Some immunizations are administered postexposure to protect the mother. Hepatitis A immune serum globulin can be used for postexposure prophylaxis. Hepatitis B immune globulin for postexposure prophylaxis can be given along with hepatitis B vaccine initially, then alone at 1 and 6 months. Tetanus immune globulin can be given for postexposure prophylaxis. Varicella immune globulin would need to be given within 96 h of exposure to protect against maternal, not congenital, infection.

**D.** *YES.* Knowledge of the date of her last normal menstrual period (LNMP) allows the provider to determine the estimated date of delivery (EDD). If the LNMP is unknown, an ultrasound should be ordered. Obstetric ultrasound in the first trimester provides a good indication of the EDD.

**E.** *YES.* Knowledge of exposure to occupational and environmental hazards allows the provider to assess the risk for the pregnancy and make appropriate recommendations to reduce the risk. Hazards may be physical (heat, lifting, and violence) or chemical (pesticides, plastic, secondary smoke, and carbon tetrachloride).

**QUESTION 2.** Which of the following common discomforts of pregnancy would you expect a woman to experience during the first trimester?

**A.** *NO.* Low backache is not common during the first trimester. It usually occurs during the second and third trimesters because of the change in the center of gravity and concomitant lordosis.

**B.** *NO.* Edema frequently occurs during the third trimester. Dependent edema is due to impeded venous return. Generalized edema of the hands and face may be an indication of preeclampsia or eclampsia. Edema is not a common finding in the first trimester.

**C.** *YES.* Physiologic leukorrhea is the presence of increased vaginal discharge without accompanying signs or symptoms of vaginitis. It occurs during the first trimester of pregnancy.

D. *YES.* Nausea and vomiting are common during the first trimester because of pregnancy hormonal changes. If nausea and vomiting become intractable, dehydration resulting in electrolyte imbalance and weight loss can occur.

E. *YES.* Urinary frequency is often present in the first and third trimesters of pregnancy. It is caused by compression of the bladder by the gravid uterus, effects of pregnancy hormones, and vascular congestion of the pelvis.

QUESTION 3. Which of the following best describes the enlargement of a gravid anteflexed uterus at 8 weeks gestation?

A. *NO.* A gravid uterus would be palpable at 8 weeks.

B. *YES.* A gravid uterus would be palpable at this size at 8 weeks gestation.

C. *NO.* The uterine fundus would be palpable at 15 cm above the symphysis pubis at approximately 15 weeks gestation. However, in obese women, palpation of the uterine fundus is more difficult.

D. *NO.* The fetus would be palpable at the umbilicus at approximately 20 weeks gestation.

QUESTION 4. Which of the following would be an appropriate assessment for this patient?

A. *NO.* There is no information from the history or physical examination that would indicate that this pregnancy is at risk.

B. *YES.* The positive pregnancy test along with physical examination findings of an 8-week-size uterus indicates a single intrauterine pregnancy.

C. *NO.* Mrs. G. has had nausea, but she has not had problems with recurrent or intractable vomiting.

D. *NO.* The pregnancy was confirmed with a positive pregnancy test, HCG.

QUESTION 5. Which of the following laboratory tests would be appropriate to obtain at the initial first-trimester prenatal visit?

A. *YES.* Hemoglobin and hematocrit are obtained to screen for anemia.

B. *YES.* A rubella screen is done to assess immune status. If a woman has not been immunized or had the disease, she is at risk for developing rubella if she is exposed. Rubella causes specific congenital problems for the fetus depending on gestational age at the time of exposure. Nonimmune pregnant woman should avoid exposure. Postpartum vaccination should be done, and pregnancy should be avoided for 3 months.

C. *NO.* The best time to screen MSAFP for neural tube defects is at 15 to 20 weeks gestation.

D. *YES.* Blood typing, Rh factor, and antibody screen should be obtained initially in the first-trimester visit. If the mother is Rh negative, antenatal and postpartum RhoGAM needs to be administered to prevent isoimmunization.

E. *NO.* The 1-h glucose screen is done in the third trimester of pregnancy. However, screening in the second trimester would be indicated if Mrs. G. had a history of gestational diabetes or glucosuria, or a first-degree relative with diabetes. This patient has none of these risk factors.

**QUESTION 6.** Management of first-trimester nausea and vomiting would be accomplished by which of the following?
   **A.** *NO.* High-fat foods usually increase nausea during pregnancy. A low-fat diet will help with nausea and vomiting.
   **B.** *NO.* Job stress has not been shown to be a factor in managing nausea.
   **C.** *YES.* Food in the stomach helps prevent nausea, provided the food is taken as small, frequent meals.
   **D.** *YES.* Vitamin $B_6$ in divided doses up to 200 mg a day is helpful in managing nausea and vomiting.
   **E.** *NO.* Rest, sleep, and relaxation are more helpful in managing nausea than exercise. Some women require no further intervention than rest.

**QUESTION 7.** Return appointments should be scheduled according to which schedule?
   **A.** *NO.* Monthly visits would be scheduled until 30 weeks, then more frequent visits are necessary to detect any potential problems and assess the growth and development of the fetus.
   **B.** *NO.* Weekly visits are scheduled from 36 weeks until delivery.
   **C.** *NO.* While pregnancy is a normal condition, problems occasionally arise, and unfortunately not all potential problems have early warning signs. Pregnancy-induced hypertension and gestational diabetes are two problems that may not have early warning signs.
   **D.** *YES.* Visits at this frequency allow for early detection of potential problems and allow for assessment of the growth and development of the fetus.

**QUESTION 8.** Additional laboratory tests this client can expect to be completed during her pregnancy would include which of the following?
   **A.** *NO.* Some states mandate additional testing for syphilis in the third trimester. Antibody screen and hemoglobin/hematocrit are frequently repeated early in the third trimester.
   **B.** *YES.* Universal screening for gestational diabetes mellitus is not necessary. However, screening should be based on the risk of the population in that clinical setting. This patient is at risk because of her ethnic background. Ethnic groups with higher risk include Asians, Hispanics, and Native Americans.
   **C.** *NO.* The initial laboratory tests do not all need to be repeated. The rubella screen, hepatitis B screen, gonorrhea culture, and chlamydia culture will not change unless the woman is exposed to these or is immunized against rubella during the pregnancy. Good history taking will indicate the need for additional testing later in pregnancy.
   **D.** *NO.* Specific infectious disease testing should be completed only if the woman is at risk. There is no consensus on screening for cytomegalovirus and toxoplasmosis except in endemic areas. A culture of the actual lesion is recommended for herpes simplex virus.

# REFERENCES

Carlson, K. J., Eisenstat, S. A. (eds.). (1995). *Primary Care of Women.* St. Louis: Mosby-Yearbook.

Cunningham, F. G., MacDonald, P. C., Gant, N. F., Leveno, K. J., Gilstrap, L. C., Hankins, G. D. V., Clark, S. L. (1997). *Williams Obstetrics,* 20th ed. Stamford, CT: Appleton & Lange.

Johnson, C. A., Johnson, B. E., Murray, J. L., Apgar, B. S. (eds.), (1996). *Women's Health Care Handbook.* Philadelphia: Hanley & Belfus.

Noble, J., Greene, H. L., Levenson, W., Modest, G. A., Young, M. (1996). *Textbook of Primary Care Medicine,* 2d ed. St. Louis: Mosby-Yearbook.

Star, W. L., Shannon, M. T., Sammons, L. N., Lommel, L., Gutierrez, Y. (1990). *Ambulatory Obstetrics: Protocols for Nurse Practitioners/Nurse-Midwives,* 2d ed. San Francisco: School of Nursing, University of California, San Francisco.

# 21

# Contraception

*Judith McDevitt*
*Marie Lindsey*

Latisha is a 24-year-old African American female who has come to the HMO for her annual examination. She is a programmer putting in long hours on software projects and has her own apartment in a nearby complex. Her tympanic temperature is 36.3°C (97.9°F), blood pressure is 114/76 (right arm sitting), height is 67 in, and weight is 135 lb. Her last menstrual period started Monday and lasted 4 days.

## CHIEF COMPLAINT

"I want to change my birth control method."

## HISTORY OF PRESENT ILLNESS

For the past few years, Latisha has been so busy with school and work that she has never had time for a boyfriend. She relied on condoms for the occasional sexual encounters she did have. Now there is someone new in her life, and it is becoming a serious relationship. Latisha wants to use something more reliable than condoms so that she will not have to worry every month about accidentally getting pregnant.

## PAST HISTORY

Latisha has received all her health care from the HMO since she got her first job 3 years ago. She has always been in good health, and since her last annual examination she has had only two mild colds. She has never been hospitalized or had surgery, has no allergies, and takes no medicines regularly. In her sexual history, Latisha says that she has had three partners before, the first when she was 18. She says she has only vaginal intercourse with males and had never had a sexually transmitted disease (STD) or abnormal Papanicolaou (PAP) smear. She questioned her new boyfriend about

STDs, and he said he has never had one. She denies vaginal or urinary symptoms today as well as fever, chills, or pelvic pain. Latisha has never been pregnant, and she says, "I'm too busy for that right now! Maybe in a few years!"

**QUESTION 1.** Which of the following additional historical information must be obtained from Latisha or updated from her previous history? (Select all that apply.)
  A. General health history
  B. Menstrual history
  C. Contraceptive history
  D. Risk assessment for hormone use

Latisha has been in good health all her life except for the usual childhood illnesses. She had her first period when she was 12. For years her periods have been regular, coming about every 28 days and lasting 4 to 5 days. Flow is light to moderate, with mild cramps at the beginning. She has no spotting between periods and has never had unexplained abnormal vaginal bleeding. The only problem she has with her periods is that she feels bloated and "kind of moody" for 2 or 3 days at the end of her cycle. She tried the pill for 2 months when she was 18, but she stopped because she kept spotting and she was breaking up with her boyfriend anyway. Since then she has used condoms, but she is worried about how reliable they are. Her blood pressure has always been normal, and she has never had thromboembolic disease or a deep vein thrombosis, ischemic heart disease, stroke, insulin-dependent diabetes, migraine, breast cancer or other estrogen-dependent tumor, liver disease or tumor, or kidney or heart disease. She smokes four or five cigarettes a day. Her two sisters and her father are all in good health, but her mother had a mild heart attack at the age of 53 and is now on medication for high cholesterol.

**QUESTION 2.** What factors in Latisha's health history contraindicate use of hormones for contraception? (Select all that apply.)
  A. Spotting during previous oral contraceptive use
  B. Feeling bloated and moody before her periods
  C. Smoking
  D. Her mother's cardiovascular disease
  E. None

## PHYSICAL FINDINGS

Skin:      Warm, dry, intact, turgor good. No lesions, birthmarks, or edema. Color uniformly medium brown.
Hair:      Normal texture, female distribution, no pest inhabitants.
Head, ears, eyes, nose, throat:      Normocephalic, no lesions or lumps. Extraocular movements intact, no nystagmus. Conjunctivae clear, sclerae white, no lesions or redness. Pupils equal, round, reactive to light and accommodation. Pinnas no masses or tenderness, canals clear, tympanic membranes pearly gray, landmarks intact. No sinus tenderness, nares patent, mucosa pink, no lesions. Oral

mucosa pink, no lesions, teeth in good repair. Pharynx pink, no exudate, tonsils 1+.

Neck:     No masses, tenderness, or lymphadenopathy. Trachea midline, thyroid nonpalpable.

Spine:     Normal spinal profile.

Lungs:     Clear to auscultation.

Heart:     $S_1$, $S_2$ normal, no $S_3$ or $S_4$, regular rate and rhythm, no murmur.

Breasts:     Moderate size, left slightly larger than right; no dimpling, retractions, or lesions. Nodular, granular consistency bilaterally; no tenderness or masses. No nipple discharge. No axillary lymphadenopathy.

Abdomen:     Soft, rounded, liver span 7 cm at midclavicular line by percussion. Liver, spleen, and kidney nonpalpable, nontender. No inguinal lymphadenopathy.

## PELVIC

External genitalia:     No infestations, swelling, lesions, or redness. Urethra, Bartholin's and Skene's glands intact.

Vagina:     Pink, no lesions, flocculent white secretions without odor, pH 4.2.

Cervix:     Pink, no lesions, no discharge. No cervical motion tenderness.

Uterus:     Small, firm, mobile, smooth, nontender, anteverted.

Adnexae:     Right ovary 3 × 2 × 1 cm, nontender; left ovary 3 × 2 × 2 cm, nontender.

Rectal:     Rectal wall intact, no masses or tenderness. Brown stool present, guaiac negative.

QUESTION 3. Which of the following tests should be done today? (Select all that apply.)
- A. Pap smear
- B. Screening tests for chlamydia and gonorrhea
- C. Wet prep
- D. Lipid screen

## ASSESSMENT

Latisha's Pap smear was reported satisfactory for evaluation, within normal limits. Screening tests for both chlamydia and gonorrhea were negative. Serum cholesterol was 183 mg/dL, and triglycerides were 123 mg/dL.

## TREATMENT

QUESTION 4. Latisha is requesting contraception that would be more reliable than the condoms she is currently using. Based on the assessment, which contraceptives can Latisha use that would be more reliable? (Select all that apply.)
- A. Condoms and spermicide
- B. Oral contraceptive
- C. Implanted or injected progestin-only methods
- D. Intrauterine device (IUD)
- E. Diaphragm with spermicide

**QUESTION 5.** After the different options and their advantages, disadvantages, and cautions are explained, Latisha decides that she would like to try the pill again. Given her family and menstrual history, which oral contraceptive would be the most appropriate for Latisha? (Select all that apply.)
   A. The minipill
   B. A low-estrogen pill (20 $\mu$g of ethinyl estradiol)
   C. A monophasic pill with low progestational activity
   D. A pill with a newer progestin such as desogestrel or norgestimate

**QUESTION 6.** After selecting a pill, what should be included in the teaching plan? (Select all that apply.)
   A. When to start and how to take the pill
   B. Side effects and precautions in using the pill
   C. Danger signals when using the pill
   D. Condom use
   E. Smoking cessation and healthy lifestyle

## ANSWERS

**QUESTION 1.** Which of the following additional historical information must be obtained from Latisha or updated from her previous history?
   A. *YES.* A health history is an essential screening tool. It should include childhood diseases and immunization status; allergies; hospitalizations; injuries, violence, or abuse; medications; use of alcohol, tobacco, caffeine, or illicit drugs; sleep, exercise, and diet patterns; family medical history; review of systems; and social data such as family and partner relationships, economic status, coping and stress management, and responses to care and compliance.
   B. *YES.* A menstrual history is essential for providing appropriate contraceptive care, since some methods affect menstrual patterns and symptoms. Questions should cover the date of the last menstrual period, the usual interval between menses, the duration, amount, and characteristics of flow, symptoms associated with menses, and whether there is spotting between periods.
   C. *YES.* The contraceptive history provides further essential information for appropriate contraceptive care. Ask about what contraceptives were previously used, how long they were used, whether there were any complications or side effects, and whether Latisha and her partner were satisfied with the method.
   D. *YES.* Because hormonal methods are so highly effective, they should be considered as a possible choice for Latisha. First, however, it must be determined whether she has any risk factors that would contraindicate their use, just as it must be determined for any other method. The estrogen component poses most of the risks associated with hormonal methods. Because estrogens promote blood clotting, estrogen-containing oral contraceptives should not be used in women who have a history of, or who currently have, thrombophlebitis or thromboembolic disorder, cerebrovascular accident, or coronary artery disease. Estrogen use should be

avoided during an illness or surgery requiring immobilization or a long leg cast. Estrogen use should also be avoided in women with breast cancer and those who have an estrogen-dependent tumor because it may promote tumor growth, and it should be avoided in pregnant women because exogenous estrogens may cause birth defects. Estrogen use requires caution and careful monitoring in women over 35 who are heavy smokers, women whose migraine headaches began after they started oral contraceptives, and women with certain medical conditions including asthma, hypertension, diabetes, sickle cell or sickle cell–hemoglobin C disease, gallbladder disease, congenital hyperbilirubinemia, or current or past cardiac or renal disease. A history of gestational diabetes or pre-diabetes and a family history of hyperlipidemia or fatal heart attack in a first-order relative under age 50 are other situations in which estrogen should be used with caution. Because estrogen interferes with the establishment of lactation, use should be avoided for 6 weeks postpartum. Both estrogens and progestins affect liver function and should not be used in women with hepatic adenoma or liver cancer, or in women whose liver function is currently impaired. Interactions with other drugs must be considered when prescribing estrogen or progestins. Finally, because exogenous hormones can mask an underlying problem, unexplained vaginal bleeding is an absolute contraindication for both estrogen and progestin use until the cause of the bleeding has been diagnosed.

**QUESTION 2.** What factors in Latisha's health history contraindicate use of hormones for contraception?

A. *NO.* The most common reason for spotting is missed pills. Even with perfect use, however, spotting and breakthrough bleeding are very common side effects during the first 1 to 3 months of oral contraceptive use, while the endometrium is adjusting to the amounts of estrogen and progesterone in the contraceptive. These side effects are the major reason why women discontinue using the pill, but they can be managed by switching to a pill with greater endometrial activity if this becomes necessary.

B. *NO.* Feeling bloated and moody before the onset of menses is a characteristic of Latisha's menstrual cycle that actually could be alleviated by placing her on the appropriate hormonal contraceptive. Some women have an increased or decreased sensitivity to their own natural sex hormones, and the symptoms in Latisha's case suggest a sensitivity to progesterone.

C. *NO.* Women using estrogen-containing contraceptives should be strongly advised not to smoke, but the risk of a heart attack is related to both age and the number of cigarettes smoked per day. Latisha is under 25 and smokes less than ½ pack of cigarettes per day, so she does not have the risks associated with heavy smoking or being over 35. Also, because she smokes only four to five cigarettes per day, her habituation to nicotine may be minimal. Smoking cessation might not be as difficult for her as it would be for a heavy smoker. As part of health promotion for Latisha, her smoking history should be assessed further and an appropriate smoking cessation intervention should be offered.

D. *NO.* Latisha's mother was over 50 at the time of her heart attack. However, her mother's hyperlipidemia may have preceded her heart attack and may indicate a possible hereditary predisposition to atherosclerotic disease.

E. *YES.* Latisha has no contraindications for contraceptive hormones.

**QUESTION 3.** Which of the following tests should be done today?

A. *YES.* Pap tests to screen for abnormal cervical cytology are recommended for all women with a cervix who currently are or have been sexually active. How often a Pap should be done depends on the patient's risk for cervical cancer and whether she has had an abnormal Pap. Risk factors for cervical cancer include a history of human papillomavirus (HPV) infection; multiple sexual partners; onset of sexual activity at age 17 or younger; having a sexual partner with HPV or a history of HPV exposure; drug, alcohol, or tobacco use; and immunosuppressive disease or therapy.

B. *YES.* Screening tests for both chlamydia and gonorrhea are recommended by all major authorities for patients at high risk for infection. Having a new partner or multiple partners, age under 25, and being unmarried are risk factors associated with infection. Actual risk depends on the number of risk factors and the local epidemiology of these infections.

C. *NO.* A wet prep would screen for vaginal infection, including sexually transmitted vaginal infection, but Latisha has no signs or symptoms of infection, her pH of 4.2 is in the normal acidic range, and the physical examination is entirely normal. There is no need to screen her further.

D. *YES.* Latisha's mother, a first-degree relative, did have a heart attack at the age of 53 and has had hyperlipidemia for an unknown length of time. Some progestins in oral contraceptives appear to lower high-density lipoproteins (HDLs), and a decline in HDLs has been related to an increased incidence of ischemic heart disease. Conversely, the estrogens in oral contraceptives act to increase HDLs. Depending on the composition of the oral contraceptive prescribed and individual response to it, the lipid profile may or may not be adversely affected. In the light of her family history, knowing Latisha's baseline cholesterol and triglycerides would be helpful, both for determining her appropriateness for oral contraceptives and for identifying whether early lifestyle modifications to lower cholesterol should be recommended. However, HMO coverage of these tests must also be taken into consideration.

**QUESTION 4.** Latisha is requesting contraception that would be more reliable than the condoms she is currently using. Based on the assessment, which contraceptives can Latisha use that would be more reliable?

A. *YES.* Latisha could have more effective contraception if she started using a spermicide along with the condoms and was careful to use the condoms consistently and correctly every time (see Fig. 21-1A–C). About 12 percent of women using condoms alone experience an unintended pregnancy in a year of typical use (which includes not using condoms some of the time). If condoms are used consistently and correctly every time, only about 3 percent experience an unintended pregnancy. The best scenario, however, occurs when condoms are used consistently and correctly together with a vaginal spermicide such as contraceptive film, suppository, or foam. Mathematical modeling suggests that these two methods used together have a 0.1 percent accidental pregnancy rate, similar to that with hormonal methods or sterilization.

**B.** *YES.* Latisha has no absolute contraindications to use of oral contraceptives, all of which are highly effective, reversible, and safe for most women. Oral contraceptives containing both estrogen and a progestin have a 0.1 percent failure rate when used consistently and correctly. Progestin-only oral contraceptives have a slightly higher failure rate, 0.5 percent. Oral contraceptives can be used to alleviate menstrual cycle problems and to improve acne and other medical conditions. They protect against pelvic inflammatory disease as well as ovarian and endometrial cancer, and they prevent ectopic pregnancy.

**C.** *POSSIBLY.* Latisha has no diagnoses that would contraindicate using these methods, and both are highly effective. Implanted levonorgestrel capsules (Norplant) have a failure rate of 0.09 percent, and injected medroxyprogesterone acetate (Depo-Provera) has a failure rate of 0.3 percent. A common side effect of these progestin-only methods, however, is gaining weight or feeling bloated, probably due to the increased appetite that many women experience. Since cyclic episodes of feeling bloated are already a problem for Latisha, an implanted or injected progestin-only method may not be the best choice for her.

**D.** *NO.* Intrauterine devices, although highly effective for contraception, are generally not recommended for nulliparous women like Latisha because they tend not to tolerate an IUD as well and because there is a slight risk of introducing an infection during insertion that could adversely affect fertility in the future. Other methods should be considered first.

**E.** *NO.* Diaphragms with spermicide are less effective than condoms alone, Latisha's current method. About 18 percent of typical diaphragm users have an accidental pregnancy during a year of use. Even with perfect use, the failure rate is 6 percent.

**QUESTION 5.** After the different options and their advantages, disadvantages, and cautions are explained, she decides that she would like to try the pill again. Given her family and menstrual history, which oral contraceptive would be the most appropriate for Latisha?

**A.** *NO.* Although the progestin-only pill, or "minipill," does not have the problem of weight gain or feeling bloated that implanted or injected progestin-only methods do, it has a very small margin of error and pills must be taken exactly on time. There is a chance of ovulation if the pill is taken only 3 h late. This is a good choice for women who are breast feeding or who cannot take estrogen, but it is not indicated in Latisha's case.

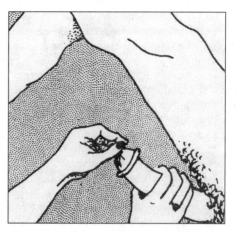

A

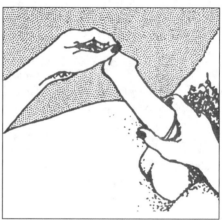

B

FIGURE 21-1. Instructions for correct condom use.
A. Unroll the condom a small amount and put it on the erect penis before beginning intercourse. The rolled rim of the condom should be on the outside of the condom. (Either partner can apply the condom.)
B. Unroll the condom all the way down to the base of the erect penis. Leave a space at the top of the condom by pinching the tip of the condom as it is unrolled.
C. Soon after ejaculation and while the penis is still erect, the penis is withdrawn while holding the rim of the condom against the base of the penis. Wrap used condom in tissue paper for disposal and wash any spilled semen from hands or body parts. (Illustrated by Judith L. Hanlon.)

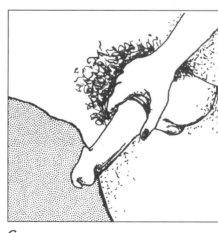

C

B. *NO.* The last time Latisha was on oral contraceptives, spotting was the problem, not nausea. Nausea is an estrogen-mediated side effect that can be minimized by using a low-estrogen pill, but there is no particular indication for doing this in Latisha's case. Using a low-estrogen pill can also worsen spotting and breakthrough bleeding.

C. *YES.* Oral contraceptives have differing levels of endometrial, progestational, and androgenic activity, and the amounts of estrogen and progestin they contain may be the same throughout the cycle (monophasic pill) or may vary during the cycle (multiphasic pill). Which pill to prescribe depends on the physical examination and laboratory results, whether there are contraindications for use, the patient and family health history, and the patient's menstrual characteristics and hormone sensitivity. Latisha is in good health, her examination was normal, and she has light to moderate flow and mild cramps with her menses. She does feel bloated and moody before the onset of menses, which suggests a sensitivity to progesterone. A pill with low progestational activity is recommended, and prescribing a monophasic pill may alleviate mood changes that may be related to the varying doses of progestin in multiphasic oral contraceptives. Monophasic pills with low progestational activity include Ortho-Cyclen, Modicon, and Brevicon.

D. *YES.* The newer progestins such as desogestrel or norgestimate produce a more favorable lipid profile, increasing HDL and decreasing LDL cholesterol. They are similar in their efficacy, cycle control, and acceptability to patients. Although it is not yet known if improving lipid profiles by using these progestins will make a difference clinically in the long term, their use is appropriate when the lipid profile is a potential or actual concern. Given Latisha's family history of cardiovascular disease and hyperlipidemia in a first-degree relative, prescribing a pill with a newer progestin is recommended. Pills containing the newer progestins include Desogen, Ortho-Cept, and Ortho-Cyclen.

QUESTION 6. After selecting a pill, what will be included in the teaching plan?

A. *YES.* When to start and how to take the pill is essential information. There are several different schedules that may be chosen for starting the pill. Latisha is on day 5 of her cycle, since her last period started Monday and this is now Friday. She can start the pill today, so that she will always be starting her next pack on a Friday, or she can wait until Sunday and start the pill then. Many women use the Sunday start because it is easy to remember and the withdrawal bleed during the fourth week of each cycle will tend to occur during the week rather than on the weekend. The pill prevents ovulation and is very effective if taken at the same time every day. If she is using a 28-day pack (3 weeks of hormones and 1 week of inert pills), Latisha should take 1 pill a day at the same time until she finishes the pack and then begin the next pack immediately. If she is using a 21-day pack (3 weeks of hormone only), she should wait 1 week after finishing a pack before beginning the next pack.

B. *YES.* Side effects and precautions in using the pill must also be covered. Two common side effects when starting the pill are nausea and menstrual changes, both of which usually resolve within one to three cycles. If nausea is a problem, the patient can try taking the pill with food or at bedtime. Spotting and breakthrough bleeding are more likely if pills are forgotten or not taken on time, which often happens during the first weeks of use. Having a regular routine will make it easier to take pills on time. The pill may be less effective if doses are missed, if other medications are being taken, or if there are episodes of diarrhea or vomiting. In these instances, backup contraception is advisable. Patients should be provided with specific information, including written instructions, on how to handle these problems. Having patients return during the third pack of pills is recommended so that follow-up can be done and any problems assessed and handled.

C. *YES.* All patients should be taught the warning signals of using the pill, most of which are related to the hypercoagulability associated with the estrogen component. These signals have the acronym ACHES, which stands for *a*bdominal pain (severe); *c*hest pain (severe), cough, shortness of breath; *h*eadache (severe), dizziness, weakness, or numbness; *e*ye problems (vision loss or blurring, speech problems); and *s*evere leg pain (calf or thigh). Patients experiencing these problems or developing depression, jaundice, or a breast lump should seek medical attention promptly. Patients should be sure to inform any clinician they see that they are on oral contraceptives.

D. *YES.* All pill users should have a backup method to use when needed, and the most common backup is condoms. Because Latisha will be starting the pill on day 5 or 7 (Friday or Sunday), it is possible that she may ovulate this cycle. She should use condoms throughout this first pack of pills. Also, oral contraceptives do not protect against human immunodeficiency virus or STD infection. For safer sex practices, consistent condom use is recommended unless the sexual relationship is mutually monogamous and the partners are known to be free of infection at the onset of the relationship.

E. *YES.* This visit provides an excellent opportunity for disease prevention and health promotion through healthy lifestyle. Offering information about smoking cessation, nutrition, and exercise will promote cardiovascular health and is recommended.

## REFERENCES

Caufeld, K. A. (1998). Controlling fertility. In E. Q. Youngkin, M. S. Davis (eds.), *Women's Health: A Primary Care Clinical Guide,* 161–221. Norwalk, CT: Appleton & Lange.

Dickey, R. P. (1994). *Managing Contraceptive Pill Patients,* 8th ed. Durant, OK: Essential Medical Information Systems.

Hatcher, R. A., Trussell, J., Stewart, F., Stewart, G. K., Kowal, D., Guest, F., Cates, W., Jr, Policar, M. S. (1994). *Contraceptive Technology,* 16th rev. ed. New York: Irvington.

Stifel, E. N., Anderson, J. (1997). Contraception. In J. Rosenfeld, N. Alley, L. S. Acheson, J. B. Admire (eds.), *Women's Health In Primary Care,* 289–313. Baltimore: Williams & Wilkins.

# 22

# Hepatitis

*Bernard P. Tadda*
*Marie Lindsey*

Thai N. is a 28-year-old Amerasian male who presents to this small-town practice for the first time. His last complete physical was 10 years ago when he came to the United States as a refugee from Vietnam with his mother, two brothers, and one sister. He considers himself to be in good health.

## CHIEF COMPLAINT

"I gave blood during a blood drive 2 weeks ago. Yesterday I got a letter from the blood bank telling me I have hepatitis B."

## HISTORY OF PRESENT ILLNESS

The letter that Thai received from the blood bank after donating blood states that his blood was positive for hepatitis B surface antigen (HBsAg). He has no past history of hepatitis or liver problems. He denies nausea, vomiting, fatigue, skin changes, or weight loss. He smokes about 5 to 6 cigarettes per day. He describes himself as a social drinker and denies any past or present street drug use.

## PAST MEDICAL HISTORY

Thai was hospitalized for 1 week in Vietnam at the age of 5 for a high fever but does not know any of the details. He also received an injury during a car accident about 3 years ago; he had some cuts and bruises, but he did not go to the hospital. The review of systems is unremarkable.

## SOCIAL HISTORY

Thai works the evening shift in a local factory and is taking some classes at a junior college during the day. He is engaged to a young woman from

Vietnam and will be getting married in 6 months. They are sexually active, and she has no symptoms of liver problems. They rely on her use of oral contraceptives for birth control and never use condoms.

**QUESTION 1.** What additional history would be helpful in evaluating Thai's health status? (Select all that apply.)
A. In-depth history of alcohol/drug use and medication use, including patterns of consumption
B. Constitutional symptoms of malaise and fatigue, as well as gastrointestinal disturbances
C. Color of urine and feces
D. Hepatitis B immunization

**QUESTION 2.** Which of the following laboratory tests should be ordered to evaluate Thai's liver function status? (Select all that apply.)
A. Aspartate aminotransferase (AST), alanine aminotransferase (ALT), and gamma-glutamyltransferase (GGT)
B. Hepatitis profile, including indices for hepatitis A, B, and C
C. Urinalysis (UA)
D. Fasting blood glucose

**QUESTION 3.** Which of the following is true about hepatitis A? (Select all that apply.)
A. There is a vaccine available to help protect against this disease.
B. People who have had this disease may develop a carrier state.
C. It is spread by food or water.
D. It is usually spread by blood contact or intravenous (IV) drug use.

## PHYSICAL FINDINGS

A complete physical examination was performed and revealed the following:

| | |
|---|---|
| Skin: | No open lesions. No skin color changes or evidence of IV drug use noted. |
| Eyes: | Pupils equal, round, reactive to light and accommodation, sclerae white, noninjected; fundus: grossly within normal limits. |
| Abdomen: | Soft, nontender, no masses or organomegaly; bowel sounds active in all quadrants. |
| Genitalia: | No lesions or penile discharge. |

**QUESTION 4.** Because this patient does not have skin or scleral icterus, which of the following conclusions can be drawn? (Select all that apply.)
A. The report from the blood center was probably a "false positive."
B. The blood center result identified an old hepatitis infection that is of no concern now.
C. He is not contagious.
D. He is at no risk for chronic liver disease.

## ASSESSMENT

**QUESTION 5.** The laboratory results indicate a reactive (positive) HBsAg, suggesting which of the following? (Select all that apply.)
A. He does not have hepatitis A.
B. He has probably used IV drugs.
C. He could have an active case or be a carrier of hepatitis B.
D. He should be considered infectious.

## PLAN

**QUESTION 6.** Because of his reactive HBsAg result, Thai should tell his fiancée which of the following? (Select all that apply.)
A. She should have a blood test to see if she has antibodies to hepatitis B.
B. She should start the hepatitis B vaccine series as soon as possible.
C. She is at no risk because hepatitis B is spread by contaminated food and water.
D. She needs the hepatitis B immunoglobulin injection as soon as possible.

**QUESTION 7.** If the laboratory results were also positive for antibodies to hepatitis C (anti-HCV), Thai should be told which of the following? (Select all that apply.)
A. He has an case of active hepatitis C.
B. There is a 50 percent chance of chronic liver problems.
C. He has immunity to hepatitis C and does not need to be concerned about this infection.
D. He will need a liver biopsy immediately to rule out hepatocellular carcinoma.

**QUESTION 8.** What other precautions should Thai take until his status is known? (Select all that apply.)
A. He should not share toothbrushes or razors with anyone.
B. He may continue his normal sexual activity.
C. He should avoid foods that are high in lactose.
D. He should refrain from drinking any alcoholic beverages.

**QUESTION 9.** If Thai were found to be an asymptomatic hepatitis B carrier, what would be the appropriate follow-up treatment? (Select all that apply.)
A. He should be told that he has an increased risk for developing hepato-cellular carcinoma or chronic infection later in life.
B. He should be told that he will never be able to donate blood.
C. He should have his liver enzymes monitored on a periodic basis for any sign of liver problems.
D. Because he is a carrier and does not have active disease, he needs to be cautioned only about transmitting the disease to others.

# ANSWERS

**Question 1.** What additional history would be helpful in evaluating Thai's health status?

A. *YES.* As excessive use of alcohol and many other recreational drugs can also cause liver damage, it is important to obtain this information so that patients can be counseled as to the importance of avoiding these drugs. High dosages of some over-the-counter (OTC) medications such as acetaminophen (Tylenol) can cause liver damage and, therefore, need to be avoided. Another reason for avoiding nonessential medications is that their metabolism may be altered in the patient with unstable liver disease.

B. *YES.* The spectrum of illness in acute viral hepatitis is broad, and many patients have no recognized clinical illness. Those who do have symptoms may present with transient gastrointestinal or upper respiratory symptoms suggestive of a nonspecific viral infection, such as diminished appetite, nausea, malaise, fatigue, 1 or 2 days of a low-grade fever, and an aching discomfort in the upper abdomen. Jaundice is uncommon in hepatitis A or C, more common in hepatitis B, and fairly common in hepatitis D and E.

C. *YES.* With acute hepatitis and injury to the liver, the urine may become darker in appearance (tea-colored) and the feces may become lighter (clay-colored); therefore, these symptoms would indicate an icteric form of the illness.

D. *YES.* Hepatitis B immunization does not cause a positive HBsAg. Therefore, if Thai had been immunized, the positive HBsAg result suggests that he had already been exposed to the disease prior to the immunization. This information may provide clues regarding when the disease was transmitted to the patient.

**Question 2.** Which of the following laboratory tests should be ordered to evaluate Thai's liver function status?

A. *YES.* Elevated results of the AST, ALT, and GGT would indicate whether Thai has active liver disease. Furthermore, an elevated GGT suggests excessive alcohol intake, information that would affect subsequent counseling.

B. *YES.* Patients presenting with one form of hepatitis should be evaluated for other forms of the disease. However, different forms of hepatitis are spread in different ways. Hepatitis A is most commonly spread via the fecal-oral route, transmitted through contaminated food and water or by persons working in neonatal units, preschools, day care centers, or other sites where workers are exposed to feces. Sexual or parental transmission of hepatitis A is uncommon. Hepatitis E is also transmitted via the fecal-oral route and is largely a water-borne infection. Hepatitis B, C, and D are generally transmitted either sexually or parenterally; however, of the three forms, hepatitis B is considered to be transmitted sexually far more often than hepatitis C or D.

C. *YES.* Urine bilirubin and urobilinogen levels can reveal asymptomatic liver disease. Bilirubin in the urine often precedes clinical icterus or may occur without jaundice in anicteric or early hepatitis, early obstruction, or liver metastases. Increased urobilinogen in urine may be present in hepatitis in the preicteric stage or, alternatively, in the recovery stage.

D. *NO.* A fasting blood glucose is not indicated and would provide no additional information for the given history and physical.

**Question 3.** Which of the following is true about hepatitis A?

A. *YES.* The hepatitis A vaccine, with the brand name Havrix, is available for prophylaxis against hepatitis A. The recommended dose for adults is one intramuscular injection of 1440 ELISA units, with a recommended booster in 6 to 12 months.

B. *NO.* Hepatitis A, which is generally transmitted via the fecal-oral route, does not promote any type of carrier state.

C. *YES.* Hepatitis A is spread by contaminated food and water and is excreted via an infected person's feces. Proper food-handling procedures and good personal hygiene decrease transmission.

D. *NO.* Parenteral transmission of hepatitis A appears to be rare because of its brief period of viremia. In rare cases, there have been reported outbreaks among homosexual men.

**Question 4.** Because this patient does not have skin or scleral icterus, the following conclusions can be drawn.

A. *NO.* As it is common for those infected with hepatitis to be asymptomatic, there is no reason to assume that the blood bank's result was a false positive.

B. *NO.* The blood bank would conduct several hepatitis B tests to confirm the stage of the disease. Even an old hepatitis infection would be a source of concern, as it may indicate that the patient is in a carrier state.

C. *NO.* Hepatitis B has a long incubation period (from 45 to 160 days); therefore, even serologic testing may not reveal an infection in its earliest stages before symptoms appear. Furthermore, it is not uncommon for those in a carrier state to be entirely asymptomatic. Therefore, a patient's appearance is not an indication of his or her ability to transmit the disease.

D. *NO.* That the patient shows no current symptoms of hepatitis is not an indication of the effect this infection will eventually have on his liver. Persons infected with hepatitis B are at risk for subsequent fulminant hepatitis, bridging necrosis, and hepatocellular carcinoma.

**Question 5.** The laboratory results indicate a reactive (positive) HBsAg, suggesting which of the following? (Select all that apply.)

A. *NO.* The presence of the HBsAg does not rule out the possibility that he may also have a hepatitis A infection.

B. *NO.* The presence of the HBsAg indicates an infection that was probably spread via blood contact, but it does not imply that the route was necessarily IV drug use.

**C.** *YES.* The presence of the HBsAg could indicate either an acute infection *or* a carrier state. In the United States, less than 1 percent of those infected with hepatitis B continue to carry the antigen after their illness. In some other countries, such as Vietnam, the percentage may be greater than 10 percent.

**D.** *YES.* Regardless of whether his illness is in an early stage or a carrier stage, a positive HBsAg indicates an infectious state.

**QUESTION 6.** Because of his reactive HBsAg result, Thai should tell his fiancée which of the following?

**A.** *YES.* The easiest way to check Thai's fiancee's immune status is to test for antibodies to the surface antigen of hepatitis B (anti-HBs). Anti-HBs signal late convalescence or recovery from infection and remain in the blood to provide immunity. If a person has received the hepatitis B vaccination, the anti-HBs will also show a reactive titer. If Thai's fiancée is negative for anti-HBs, tests for HBsAg and liver enzymes should also be performed to determine the presence and stage of the disease.

**B.** *NO.* The vaccine may not be necessary if Thai's fiancée already has immunity to hepatitis B. *Active* immunization is the measure of choice for protection against hepatitis B infection. Protective efficacy rates are about 90 to 95 percent. In the three-dose schedule, after the initial injection, a second injection is given at 1 month and a third 6 months from the first. In the four-dose schedule, the third dose is given 2 months after the first, and the fourth is given 12 months after the first. The four-dose schedule may provide more rapid protection in some persons. Since Thai's fiancée is also Vietnamese, it is likely that she may have been infected prior to her relationship with Thai.

**C.** *NO.* Hepatitis B is spread by body fluids, not by contaminated food and water.

**D.** *NO.* *Passive* immunoprophylaxis with hepatitis B immunoglobulin (HBIG) should not be given until her immune status has been determined by testing for antibodies to the surface antigen of hepatitis. Administration of HBIG is indicated for postexposure prophylaxis in three situations: (a) after accidental inoculation, ingestion, or splashing onto mucous membranes or contact with hepatitis B-positive blood or secretions of nonvaccinated persons, (b) for the sexual contacts of the acutely infected patient, and (c) concomitantly with hepatitis B vaccine for neonates of HBsAg-positive mothers.

**QUESTION 7.** If the laboratory results were also positive for antibodies to hepatitis C (anti-HCV), Thai should be told which of the following?

**A.** *NO.* The mere presence of the antibody does not confirm an active infection.

**B.** *YES.* Approximately 50 percent of those infected with hepatitis C will go on to have chronic liver problems.

**C.** *NO.* An anti-HCV test may be positive in acute *or* chronic hepatitis C or indicate a possible HCV carrier state or some past HCV infection. Further testing and follow-up will be needed.

D. *NO*. A liver biopsy is not indicated immediately. The decision to seek further diagnostics depends upon many factors, including his liver function status and the presence of any symptoms.

**QUESTION 8.** What other precautions should Thai take until his status is known?
A. *YES*. To reduce the risk of body fluid contact, Thai should not share his toothbrushes or razors, as they may be contaminated with his blood.
B. *NO*. Sexual activity should be avoided until the status of both Thai and his fiancée is known. While condoms do provide some protection against transmission of disease, there remains the risk of their breaking or falling off during coitus.
C. *NO*. Lactose intake is not a concern related to hepatitis.
D. *YES*. Since alcohol can have detrimental effects on the liver, he should not drink any alcoholic beverages.

**QUESTION 9.** If Thai were found to be an asymptomatic hepatitis B carrier, what would be the appropriate follow-up treatment?
A. *YES*. The risk for developing hepatocellular carcinoma or chronic infection later in life is greater in those infected in infancy or early childhood.
B. *YES*. Hepatitis B carriers are ineligible to donate blood.
C. *YES*. Elevated liver enzymes may signify early complications of liver disease, including hepatic carcinoma.
D. *NO*. While Thai does need to be instructed regarding precautions against transmitting the disease to others, he also needs to understand the importance of regular monitoring of his health status.

## REFERENCES

Dienstag, J. L. (1995). Management of hepatitis. In A. Goroll, L. May, A. Mulley (eds.), *Primary Care Medicine: Office Evaluation and Management of the Adult Patient,* 3d ed., 399–412. Philadelphia: J. B. Lippincott.

Dienstag, J. L., Isselbacher, K. J. (1998). Acute viral hepatitis. In A. S. Fauci, E. Braunwald, K. H. Isselbacher, J. D. Wilson, J. B. Martin, D. L. Kasper, S. L. Hauser, D. L. Longo (eds.), *Harrison's Principles of Internal Medicine,* 14th ed., 1676–1692. New York: McGraw-Hill.

Dindzans, V. (1992). Viral hepatitis. *Postgrad Med, 92*(4), 43–52.

Koff, R. S. (1996). Liver. In J. Noble (ed.), *Textbook of Primary Care Medicine,* 616–621. Chicago: Mosby.

Uphold, C., Graham, M. (1993). *Clinical Guidelines in Family Practice.* Gainesville, FL: Barmarrae Books.

Wallach, J. (1996). *Interpretation of Diagnostic Tests.* Boston: Little, Brown.

# 23

# Headache

*Marie Lindsey*
*Marie L. Talashek*

Marjorie J. is a 38-year-old Caucasian female who obtains her routine care at a rural family practice center. She is married and the mother of two teenage boys, and she works full-time as a telephone operator. Her last health care visit was 9 months ago for her annual examination and Papanicalaou test; the results of both were normal. She has been urged by her family to seek care for her recurring headaches.

## CHIEF COMPLAINT

"I've been having bad headaches for the past 4 months."

## HISTORY OF PRESENT ILLNESS

Approximately 4 months ago, Mrs. J. had her first episode of what has become a recurrent syndrome. Initially, the pain was a unilateral throbbing over her right eye and temple, accompanied by photophobia and nausea. Since that time, the pain has recurred about three times a month, but may affect either the right or the left eye and temple. The pain usually occurs in the late morning or early afternoon. Her treatment has consisted of two 325-mg tablets of aspirin at the onset of pain, applying a cold towel to her forehead, and lying down. These measures provide minimal relief, and she must rest for 2 to 3 hours before the pain goes away.

Between headache episodes, Mrs. J. has experienced a dull pain over her shoulder, neck, and scalp, and these areas are painful to touch, responding only slightly to two tablets of aspirin. These episodes are often accompanied by early morning awakening. She recalls that her mother also experienced painful headaches that required bed rest. She is concerned that the pain is increasing in frequency and thus interfering with her work and family life.

Mrs. J. has regular menstrual periods every 28 days, and the headaches are not consistent with any particular time during her menstrual cycle. She uses a diaphragm for birth control.

## PAST MEDICAL HISTORY

Mrs. J. has no history of head trauma or loss of consciousness, is taking no medication, has had no surgeries or hospitalizations, and has no known allergies to medications, plants, animals, or foods.

QUESTION 1. Based on the information provided thus far, which headache type is Mrs. J. most likely to have? (Select all that apply.)
  A. Sinus
  B. Intracranial mass lesion
  C. Migraine
  D. Hypertension
  E. Temporomandibular joint (TMJ) dysfunction
  F. Giant cell arteritis (temporal arteritis)

QUESTION 2. What other information should be obtained to help arrive at the correct diagnosis? (Select all that apply.)
  A. Diet history
  B. Eye symptoms
  C. Prodromal symptoms
  D. Chest pain
  E. Timing of symptoms

## PHYSICAL EXAMINATION

Vital signs:  Temperature 36.6°C (98.6°F), pulse 72, respirations 20, blood pressure 118/72, height 5 ft 5 in, weight 120 lb.

General:  Cooperative white female in no apparent distress. Oriented ×3; excellent historian.

Head:  No lesions, swelling, or tenderness of scalp. No swelling, tenderness, or bruits of temporal arteries bilaterally.

Eyes:  Pupils equal, round, reactive to light and accommodation. No lacrimation or other discharge. Conjunctivae clear and moist; sclerae white, corneas clear. Visual acuity, visual fields, and extraocular movements all intact. Funduscopic: Disk margins sharp, no arteriovenous narrowing or crossing, no exudates or hemorrhages.

Nose:  No rhinorrhea; nares moist and pink.

Mouth:  Facial appearance symmetrical; no TMJ tenderness or clicking.

Neck:  No nuchal rigidity. No masses or swelling of throat. No carotid bruits.

Thorax:  Pulse—regular rate and rhythm; $S_1 > S_2$ at apex. No $S_3$, $S_4$, murmurs, or clicks. Lungs clear.

Musculo-skeletal:  Diffuse tenderness of posterior neck and upper back noted. No joint tenderness. Full range of motion of all extremities. Muscle strength strong and equal.

Neurological:  Cranial nerves II to XII intact. Gait and tandem, heel, toe, and heel-toe walk all steady. Deep tendon reflexes all 2+ bilaterally. Sharp/dull discrimination intact bilaterally. Rapid hand/foot movement intact.

**QUESTION 3.** Mrs. J. appears to have symptoms of both migraine and muscle contraction (tension-type) headaches. What are other symptoms of muscle contraction headache? (Select all that apply.)
  A. Acute onset
  B. Occipital and frontal sites
  C. Worsens through the day
  D. Situationally related

**QUESTION 4.** Which of the following diagnostic tests clearly should be ordered for Mrs. J. (Select all that apply.)
  A. Computerized axial tomography (CAT) scan
  B. Magnetic resonance imaging (MRI)
  C. Lumbar puncture
  D. Sinus films
  E. None of the above

## ASSESSMENT

Combined headache.

**QUESTION 5.** Which of the following are features of combined headache? (Select all that apply.)
  A. It is thought to be related to both vascular and muscle contraction abnormalities.
  B. Patients with combined headache rarely have a family history of headache.
  C. Patients with combined headache often go "doctor shopping."
  D. The treatment can exacerbate symptoms.

**QUESTION 6.** Which of the following are appropriate medications for Mrs. J.'s combined headaches? (Select all that apply.)
  A. Nonsteroidal anti-inflammatory drugs (NSAIDs)
  B. β-Adrenergic blockers and calcium channel blockers
  C. Ergotamine agents
  D. Antidepressants
  E. Narcotics

**QUESTION 7.** If Mrs. J.'s symptoms did not respond to the medications noted in Question 6, which of the following are other medications used in the treatment of migraine, contraction, or combined headache? (Select all that apply.)
  A. Combination sedative-analgesic medications
  B. Anticonvulsants
  C. Serotonin antagonist
  D. Selective serotonin receptor agonist

**QUESTION 8.** Which of the following other measures or issues should be considered in treating Mrs. J.'s headaches? (Select all that apply.)
A. Avoidance of precipitating factors
B. Exercise
C. Relaxation techniques
D. Psychotherapy
E. Avoidance of chronic pain syndrome

## ANSWERS

**QUESTION 1.** Based on the information provided thus far, which headache type is Mrs J. most likely to have?
A. *NO.* Mrs. J.'s symptoms do not appear to be related to sinusitis, in which pain is typically frontal; is described as deep, dull, and aching; and is often accompanied by sinus tenderness. Sinusitis is more likely to follow an upper respiratory illness or otitis media and often presents with purulent nasal discharge. True sinusitis produces a headache that is characteristically acute in onset, worse on awakening, better on standing, and worsening again as the day progresses. Because the pain of sinusitis is sometimes described as throbbing in quality and can worsen on bending over, it may be mistaken for migraine or the headache of an intracranial mass lesion.
B. *NO.* Headache pain caused by an intracranial mass lesion may be localized to the site of the lesion. Characteristically the pain in-creases in duration and severity over several months. The pain is associated with subtle changes in mental status or development of focal neurological deficits. Initially, the discomfort may be lessened by lying down, but as intracranial pressure increases, lying down may actually exacerbate the headache, as may straining with stooling, coughing, or bending over. As intracranial pressure increases, a more generalized headache may develop. Examples of intracranial mass lesions include brain tumor, brain abscess, subdural hematoma, and pseudotumor cerebri.
C. *YES.* Mrs. J.'s symptoms described thus far are, indeed, indicative of migraine headaches. Therefore, the possibility of migraines should be thoroughly pursued.
D. *NO.* Hypertension headaches are typically occipital, with a dull, achy quality that is worse in the morning and gets better as the day progresses.
E. *NO.* While TMJ dysfunction headaches resemble Mrs. J.'s symptoms somewhat, the presentation is typically different. The usual description is a chronic dull, aching, unilateral discomfort about the jaw, behind the eyes and ears, and even down the neck into the shoulders. Jaw pain, clicking sounds, and difficulty opening the mouth in the morning are characteristic. Chewing may exacerbate the symptoms; locking of the jaw is common.
F. *NO.* The scalp pain of giant cell arteritis (temporal arteritis) is usually considered more of a scalp tenderness that often localizes to the

involved vessel and occurs with hair combing. Mrs. J.'s scalp pain, however, is associated with a dull pain over the shoulders and neck. Many patients with giant cell arteritis complain of burning or piercing pain. Jaw (masticatory muscle) claudication is another common presentation of giant cell arteritis.

**QUESTION 2.** What other information should be obtained to help arrive at the correct diagnosis?

A. *YES.* Diet history and a thorough alcohol, drug, and medication history must be obtained. Precipitants of migraines can include ingestion of tyramine- or tryptophan-rich foods. The list of such foods includes ripe cheeses, fermented foods, pickles, red wine, some citrus fruits, chocolate, monosodium glutamate, and Nutrasweet. Alcohol in any form may trigger a cluster headache. Sudden caffeine withdrawal is known to cause headaches. Medication history is critical because a number of agents can trigger nonspecific headaches, including indomethacin, nifedipine, cimetidine, captopril, nitrates, atenolol, trimethoprim-sulfamethoxazole, and oral contraceptives.

B. *YES.* Different types of headaches can cause eye symptoms. More than 50 percent of cluster headache patients complain of an intense, nonthrobbing, unilateral headache "behind the eye" that is accompanied by ipsilateral lacrimation, nasal stuffiness, and facial flushing. These symptoms help distinguish cluster headaches from migraines, which are also often unilateral. Migraine headaches often present with the eye symptoms of photopsia (twinkling, flashing lights or colors), scotomata (blind spots), fortification (zigzag patterns), metamorphopsia (visual distortion of objects), hemiopsia, diplopia, and photophobia. The most feared complication of giant cell arteritis is blindness, which is often preceded by diplopia (50 percent risk). Once visual impairment occurs, the progression to total visual loss happens quickly over several hours.

C. *YES.* Prodromal symptoms are a distinguishing feature of migraines, this is one of five phases through which an attack may progress: prodrome, aura, headache, termination, and postdrome. The prodrome phase is characterized by lassitude, irritability, difficulty concentrating, and nausea. Patients with the aura phase often report visual complaints, as well as vertigo, aphasia, or even hemiplegia. The headache is typically unilateral and throbbing, though it may begin as a dull sensation and take a while to reach maximum intensity. Headache termination usually occurs within 24 h, but sometimes not until 48 h. The postdrome phase includes feelings of fatigue, sleepiness, or irritability.

Migraine used to be designated as "classic" if unilateral and accompanied by aural symptoms and as "common" if bilateral and without aura. It is now usually accepted that migraine has three main types: (1) classic, or unilateral headache of short duration, (2) common, or bilateral headache of longer duration, and (3) complicated, or headache with hemiparesis or an ophthalmic plegia.

D. *NO.* Chest pain is not generally a symptom of any of the major types of headache.

E. *YES.* The classic presentation of cluster headaches is that the patient is awakened during the first period of sleep with rapid eye movements (90 min from onset of sleep). Headaches from vascular bleeds typically are preceded by physical exertion. Headache pain of sinusitis is severe upon awakening, improves with standing, and may worsen later in the day. The muscle contraction (tension-type) headache is most severe later in the afternoon.

**QUESTION 3.** Mrs. J. appears to have symptoms of both migraine and contraction (tension-type) headaches. What are other symptoms of contraction headache?

A. *NO.* Muscle contraction headaches tend to develop gradually and worsen throughout the day.

B. *YES.* Occipital and frontal sites are usually both involved in contraction headaches. In fact, typically patients complain of a "tight band" on the head, a pressure, a feeling that the head is in a vise, a fullness, a tightness, or a feeling that the head will explode. Such symptoms usually involve the whole head and often the neck and upper shoulders. At times, however, the symptoms may be just bitemporal or involve the face and jaws bilaterally or both sides of the neck and upper trapezius areas only. If the disturbance is unilateral in any or all of these regions, the cause may be TMJ syndrome.

C. *YES.* Muscle contraction headaches are often chronic. Headaches decrease with sleep and rest, then recur the next day. This pattern may go on for days, weeks, or months, so that some patients report headaches occurring daily.

D. *YES.* Attacks of muscle contraction headaches most often develop while the situation causing the disturbance exists, in contrast to migraine headache, which tends to follow the causative event. Muscle contraction headaches often coexist with poorly designed workstations that require sitting or standing in faulty alignment while trying to accomplish tasks in a timely manner.

**QUESTION 4.** Which of the following diagnostic tests clearly should be ordered for Mrs. J.?

A. *NO.* However, patients complaining of the worst headache ever, especially if accompanied by meningeal signs or evidence of intracranial pressure, would require immediate hospitalization, at which time a CAT scan would be obtained.

B. *NO.* In light of a normal physical examination and a nonworrisome history (e.g., no head trauma or the "worst headache ever"), a positive MRI is extremely rare in patients with chronic headaches. the MRI is an appropriate diagnostic test in a few instances of normal physical and neurologic examinations. These include headaches of new onset (<6 months) with an etiology that is not apparent from a thorough history and physical, persistent headaches that worsen over time and do not resemble contraction headaches, a history of aural symptoms or loss of consciousness suggestive of seizures, recurrent personality changes, or a change in the character of chronic headaches.

C. *NO.* However, in patients presenting with meningeal irritation (e.g., fever, nuchal rigidity, exaggerated and symmetric deep tendon reflexes, opisthotonos, sinus arrhythmias, irritability, photophobia, diplopia, delirium), a lumbar puncture should follow a CAT scan.

D. *NO.* As Mrs. J. does not present with a history of an upper respiratory infection or subsequent sinus symptoms, sinus films would be inappropriate.

E. *YES.* Mrs. J's symptoms do not warrant any particular diagnostic tests.

**QUESTION 5.** Which of the following are features of combined headache?

A. *YES.* Combined headache, sometimes called mixed headache or, in Europe, vasomotor headache, is thought to be related to both vascular and muscle contraction abnormalities working together at the same time in the same person. This headache type may be present constantly during every waking hour, and has the symptoms of tightness, pressure, and discomfort characteristic of muscle contraction (tension) headaches, plus the pulsatile, painful quality of migraine headaches, which at times leads to nausea and vomiting. The elements of combined headaches might be further distinguished if patients keep a headache diary to help pinpoint precipitants.

B. *NO.* Patients with combined headaches often have a family history of migraine.

C. *YES.* Patients with combined headaches tend to go from one provider to the next to seek help, often accumulate drugs, and develop dependency-addiction syndromes. The persistent complaint of pain usually results in the ordering of many different tests, the results of which are negative. As a result, providers are likely to assume that the patient is neurotic or malingering, an attitude that only promotes frustration in the patient and augments the symptoms.

D. *YES.* Patients with combined headaches may fall into a vicious cycle of inappropriate treatment and perpetuated symptoms, a trap from which they may or may not wish to be released. These patients use multiple drugs for relief, which only leads to a continual state of headache because such drugs lead to rebound headaches when their effect has worn off. It is not just heavy narcotic pain relievers that have this effect, but the more common remedies as well—aspirin, caffeine, sedatives, tranquilizers, decongestants—and the more potent therapies such as barbiturates, propoxyphene (Darvon), pentazocine (Talwin), bromides, codeine, and oxycodone. In fact, since headache is a major feature of withdrawal symptoms from these remedies, the treatment may result in a patient's being diagnosed as having chronic headaches, which simply invites more inappropriate treatment.

**QUESTION 6.** Which of the following are appropriate treatments for Mrs. J.'s combined headaches.?

A. *YES.* Combined headache often responds well to the treatment recommended for tension-type headaches. Nonsteroidal anti-inflammatory drugs, including aspirin, are actually very useful in the treatment of either migraine or tension headaches. Acetaminophen may also be helpful. It is possible that Mrs. J. did not receive relief from aspirin simply because she did not take it in sufficient doses or in a prophylatic manner.

B. *YES.* β-Adrenergic blockers have been used to treat many types of headaches for years. Calcium channel blockers are not usually recommended for tension-type headaches; however, they are often used as prophylactic migraine therapies.

C. *YES.* Although ergotamine agents (Ergostat and others) would not be first-line treatment for combined headache, they may have a place in severe attacks with strong migraine symptoms.

D. *YES.* Tricyclic antidepressants are sometimes used in the treatment of either migraine or tension-type headaches. Providers should explain to patients that antidepressants are often used for chronic pain syndromes unrelated to clinical depression.

E. *NO.* As there are so many other medications available, it is rarely necessary to use narcotics for the treatment of headaches.

**QUESTION 7.** If Mrs. J.'s symptoms did not respond to the medications noted in Question 6, which of the following are other medications used in the treatment of migraine, contraction, or combined headache?

A. *YES.* Combination sedative-analgesic medications are sometimes prescribed for contraction headache; however, their addictive potential requires that they be used cautiously.

B. *YES.* Some anticonvulsant medications may be used to treat migraine headaches. However, it is important that patients understand that the use of an anticonvulsant in this situation does not imply that they have a seizure disorder. Furthermore, the provider must be aware that the dosage of anticonvulsants often varies from that used to control seizures.

C. *YES.* The serotonin antagonist methysergide (Sansert) is sometimes used for severe headaches refractory to other drugs.

D. *YES.* One of the newest drugs to treat migraines is a selective serotonin 5-hydroxytryptamine 1D receptor agonist, sumatriptan succinate (Imitrex).

**QUESTION 8.** Which of the following other measures or issues should be considered in treating Mrs. J.'s headaches?

A. *YES.* Keeping a careful headache diary may be helpful in identifying precipitating factors (e.g., nitrites, monosodium glutamate, salt, cheese, chocolate, red wine, stress, etc.) for headaches. Avoidance of known precipitating factors could be the only treatment necessary.

B. *YES.* Regular aerobic exercise has been demonstrated to decrease the frequency and severity of headaches for some patients.

**C.** *YES.* Like aerobic exercise, relaxation techniques (e.g., diaphragmatic breathing, progressive deep muscle relaxation, mental imagery) have been demonstrated to decrease the frequency and severity of headaches for some patients. Other modalities in this category, such as massage, acupressure, biofeedback, hypnosis, and acupuncture, have yet to receive scientific support to warrant the same endorsement as relaxation techniques. However, these modalities offer few risks and probably pose no contraindications for interested patients. Generally, younger patients are more receptive to modalities of this nature than older patients.

**D.** *YES.* In some situations, psychotherapy is recommended for the patient who clearly has significant psychosocial and coping problems. The provider may need to offer this approach very diplomatically, so that the patient does not feel that his or her symptoms are simply being dismissed or not being taken seriously by the provider.

**E.** *YES.* Patients with combined headache face the real risk of developing chronic pain syndrome that is refractory to treatment, especially if they are using multiple drugs. The agents that bring relief may lead to rebound headache when their effects have worn off. This may compel the patient to take the medications all the more frequently and in higher doses. The provider must monitor headache patients carefully (and probe for evidence of "clinic hopping") so that medications are prescribed in sufficient doses to provide relief without propelling the patient into a vicious cycle of overtreatment.

## REFERENCES

Barker, L., Burton, J., Zieve, P. (eds.). (1995). *Principles of Ambulatory Medicine,* 4th ed. Philadelphia: Williams & Wilkins.

Gorall, A., May, L., Mulley, A. (1995). *Primary Care Medicine: Office Evaluation of the Adult Patient.* Philadelphia: J. B. Lippincott.

Noble, J. (ed.). (1996). *Textbook of Primary Care Medicine,* 2d ed. St. Louis: Mosby.

Rucker, L. (ed.). (1997). *Essentials of Adult Ambulatory Care.* Baltimore: Williams & Wilkins.

Uphold, C., Graham, M. (1993). *Clinical Guidelines in Family Practice.* Gainesville, FL: Barmarrae Books.

# 24

# Gastritis

*Susan A. Fontana*
*Marie L. Talashek*

Eric L., a 35-year-old African American male, is a regular patient of an urban family practice clinic. His last checkup (2 years ago) was normal, including a cholesterol level of 170 mg/dL. He is married with three school-age children and is employed as a division sales representative for a national computer network. In addition, he is an avid runner and fisherman.

## CHIEF COMPLAINT

"My stomach has been aching and burning, off and on for the past 2 months."

## HISTORY OF PRESENT ILLNESS

Eric points to his epigastric area and says that the aching and burning occur after meals about three or four times a week and on the weekends when he has a few drinks with his family and/or friends. He expresses concern that the pain might be due to an ulcer, and he would like some medicine prescribed for the discomfort. Eric also experiences sour belches and has noted this more often after going to bed at night. His symptoms are usually relieved with antacids. He does not recall any particular food that precipitates the discomfort. He denies any nausea, vomiting, diarrhea, constipation, melena, or weight loss or gain. He has noticed that his symptoms occur more frequently when the demands at work are heavy and he is feeling stressed. He denies tobacco or illicit drug use and states that he is conscientious about maintaining a professional image. He denies taking any medications other than ibuprofen one to two times monthly for muscle aches after a strenuous workout. His responses to the CAGE questionnaire indicate that he has never felt the need to Cut down on his drinking, been Annoyed by others criticizing his drinking, felt Guilty about drinking, or needed an Eye-opener drink the first thing in the morning. There is no family history of alcoholism or other substance abuse.

## PAST HISTORY

The past history was noncontributory.

QUESTION 1. The cardinal symptom of gastroesophageal reflux disease (GERD) is as follows:
A. Epigastric pain or tenderness
B. Heartburn or a burning sensation beneath the sternum
C. Weight loss
D. Dysphagia and odynophagia

QUESTION 2. Extraesophageal symptoms of GERD include which of the following? (Select all that apply.)
A. Classic angina
B. Chronic cough with episodes worse at nighttime
C. Asthma, especially nocturnal
D. Chronic sore throat and/or hoarseness
E. Erosion of tooth enamel

QUESTION 3. The two major causes of peptic ulcer disease are *Helicobacter pylori* infection and use of aspirin or other nonsteroidal anti-inflammatory drugs (NSAIDs); however, other factors include which of the following? (Select all that apply.)
A. Psychological stress
B. Smoking
C. Depression
D. Caffeine-containing beverages
E. Alcohol use

## OBJECTIVE DATA

Vital signs:   Blood pressure 136/84 right sitting; pulse 88, regular sinus rhythm; respiration 16 breaths/min.

General:   Middle-aged male slightly overweight in no distress.

Skin:   Warm, intact without any lesions or rashes.

Abdomen:   Flabby. Active bowel sounds. No bruits. Nontender without any palpable masses. No organomegaly.

Rectal:   Prostate smooth, rubbery. Hemoccult negative stool.

Laboratory:   Complete blood count—hematocrit 43 percent (42 to 52 percent), hemoglobin 16.3 g/dL (13.0 to 18.0), mean corpuscular volume (MCV) 83 $\mu m^3$ (86 to 98), others within normal limits.

Liver panel—gamma-glutamyltransferase (GGT) 85 units/L (5 to 38), aspartate aminotransferase (AST) 21 units/L (10 to 40), alanine aminotransferase (ALT) 28 units/L (10 to 55), alkaline phosphatase 83 units/L (45 to 115).

*Note:* Reference ranges for men are provided in parentheses.

QUESTION 4. Which laboratory findings can be used to support a clinician's suspicion of alcohol abuse? (Select all that apply.)
A. MCV increased
B. GGT increased
C. ALT increased
D. Ratio of AST/ALT 2:1 or more

QUESTION 5. If findings from Eric's history and physical examination disclosed dysphagia, significant weight loss, or occult blood loss, which further diagnostic studies would be warranted? (Select all that apply.)
A. Barium swallow
B. Upper GI series
C. Endoscopy
D. Twenty-four-hour esophageal pH monitoring

## ASSESSMENT

QUESTION 6. The diagnosis of GERD in this patient is supported by which of the following? (Select all that apply.)
A. Burning that occurs frequently, postprandially, and nocturnally
B. Sour or hot belches
C. Lack of epigastric tenderness or mass on physical examination
D. Discomfort that occurs shortly after lying down, i.e., at bedtime.
E. Alcohol abuse.

## PLAN

QUESTION 7. Which of the following lifestyle interventions control symptoms related to GERD? (Select all that apply.)
A. Dieting to return to ideal weight in overweight patients
B. Eating the main meal close to evening or bedtime
C. Limiting alcohol-containing beverages to no more than one to two drinks per day
D. Keeping the head of the bed elevated with blocks or bricks for nighttime sleep
E. Decreasing or stopping tobacco use

QUESTION 8. Which of the following foods are known to cause heartburn or reduce lower esophageal sphincter (LES) pressure? (Select all that apply.).
A. Tomatoes
B. Chocolate
C. Bananas
D. Fatty foods
E. Coffee and caffeine-containing drinks

**QUESTION 9.** H$_2$-antagonist drugs are the mainstay of pharmacologic treatment for patients who require additional measures beyond lifestyle modification to control their symptoms. Which of the following are considerations in the use of these drugs? (Select all that apply.)
- **A.** Must be given at least twice daily.
- **B.** Standard doses achieve better control of symptoms than do lower doses.
- **C.** Therapy should be continued for 8 to 12 weeks.
- **D.** Combination therapy with prokinetic or other drugs is best reserved for use in the elderly.

## ANSWERS

**QUESTION 1.** The cardinal symptom of reflux disease is:
- **A.** *NO.* Epigastric pain or tenderness suggests peptic ulcer disease (PUD) or gallbladder disease, which causes pain in the right subcostal area.
- **B.** *YES.* Heartburn or a burning sensation beneath the sternum is the cardinal symptom of GERD. Explore what the patient means by "heartburn," since it may be different from the clinical definition.
- **C.** *NO.* Weight loss is not a symptom of gastritis, GERD, or PUD. If it is present with other GI symptoms, it suggests a gastric malignancy.
- **D.** *NO.* These esophageal symptoms are not specific for GERD. Esophageal pain may be referred to the base of the neck, midline of the back, and upper abdomen.

**QUESTION 2.** Extraesophageal symptoms of GERD include which of the following?
- **A.** *YES.* Unexplained chest pain is an atypical manifestation of GERD. It must be differentiated from other causes of chest pain, such as myocardial ischemia, pericarditis, costochondritis, or referred pain.
- **B.** *YES.* Chronic cough, especially when manifested as nocturnal coughing episodes, is an extraesophageal symptom of GERD.
- **C.** *YES.* Asthma is an extraesophageal symptom of GERD and may be more difficult to treat.
- **D.** *YES.* Chronic sore throat is an atypical manifestation of GERD and may not respond promptly to therapeutic interventions. Hoarseness caused by acid irritation of the vocal cords may be a manifestation of GERD.
- **E.** *YES.* Erosion of the teeth by acid is another extraesophageal symptom.

**QUESTION 3.** The two major causes of peptic ulcer disease are *Helicobacter pylori* infection and use of aspirin or other NSAIDs; however, other factors include which of the following:
- **A.** *YES.* Reseach indicates that the incidence of chronic stress is higher in ulcer patients than in controls. In response to stress, there is an increase in gastric acid production.

B. *YES.* Impaired prostaglandin production can be demonstrated in the gastric mucosa of smokers. Also, there are epidemiologic data to support that ulcers are more likely in smokers than in nonsmokers.

C. *YES.* Depression appears to exacerbate PUD in some individuals. Since anxiety and depression often coexist, the mechanism may be related to acid hypersecretion.

D. *YES.* Caffeine has been implicated as a factor in PUD because it stimulates gastric acid secretion.

E. *YES.* Alcohol can alter the mucosal barrier, which results in gastritis. Beer is known to be a potent stimulant of gastric acid secretion.

QUESTION 4. Which laboratory findings can be used to support a clinician's suspicion of alcohol abuse?

A. *YES.* The MCV is often increased in chronic alcohol abuse and indicates a toxic effect of alcohol on developing erythroblasts.

B. *YES.* The GGT is raised by alcohol and hepatotoxic drugs and is useful to monitor drug toxicity and alcohol abuse. Since levels return to normal after short periods of abstinence, the GGT can be used to monitor sobriety.

C. *NO.* Alanine transaminase, formerly known as serum glutamate pyruvate transaminase, is found in liver tissue, kidney, heart, and skeletal muscle tissue. An isolated ALT value is not clinically significant.

D. *YES.* The ratio of AST, formerly called serum glutamic-oxaloacetic transaminase, to ALT is useful in differentiating various types of liver disease. Aspartate transaminase greater than ALT (2:1) often indicates alcohol abuse, whereas elevated ALT levels predominate in hepatitis.

QUESTION 5. If findings from Eric's history and physical examination disclosed dysphagia, significant weight loss, or occult blood loss, which diagnostic studies would be warranted?

A. *YES.* A barium swallow would be indicated in a patient with dysphagia. In the absence of this symptom, the information provided by this test is limited.

B. *YES.* A GI series is indicated for patients over the age of 40 or in patients with severe or prolonged symptoms. This can be used to exclude the presence of complications (i.e., ulcers, strictures), anatomic abnormalities, gastric lesions, and motility disorders.

C. *YES.* Endoscopy, though not required for most patients, is the initial test of choice for identifying esophagitis and detecting Barrett's esophagus, which places the patient at risk for adenocarcinoma.

D. *NO.* Twenty-four-hour pH monitoring is expensive, not universally available, and usually not indicated. It is reserved for patients with extraesophageal symptoms who do not respond to therapy.

QUESTION 6. The diagnosis of GERD in this patient is supported by which of the following?

A. *YES.* Most often GERD presents with heartburn (retrosternal pain or discomfort). The discomfort is typically worse after meals.

B. *YES.* Sour or hot belches are words often used by patients to describe gastric or duodenal contents refluxed into the esophagus.

C. *YES.* A lack of epigastric tenderness or mass on physical examination is helpful in differentiating GERD from other conditions, such as peptic ulcer disease or a gastric malignancy.

D. *YES.* Pain that occurs shortly after the patient slouches or lies down is a common complaint of patients with GERD.

E. *NO.* Although the GGT was slightly elevated, other laboratory findings and the CAGE do not support a chronic problem with alcohol. Two or more positive CAGE responses indicate a problem and require immediate follow-up. It would be prudent to reassess at future intervals.

**QUESTION 7.** Which of the following lifestyle interventions control symptoms related to GERD?

A. *YES.* Losing weight will reduce intraabdominal pressure and is a useful adjunct to improving symptoms. Also, avoiding tight-fitting clothes will reduce pressure on the abdomen.

B. *NO.* Eating a large meal in the evening or lying down or exercising immediately after dinner will exacerbate symptoms.

C. *YES.* Alcohol and smoking decrease lower esophageal sphincter (LES) pressure. Also, certain drugs decrease LES pressure, such as theophylline, calcium channel blockers, and anticholinergics.

D. *YES.* Raising the head of the bed will make it less likely that stomach contents will flow into the esophagus.

E. *YES.* Nicotine decreases LES pressure.

**QUESTION 8.** Which of the following foods are known to cause heartburn or reduce LES pressure?

A. *YES.* Tomatoes, peppermints, and other foods irritate the damaged epithelium.

B. *YES.* Chocolate decreases LES tone and allows stomach contents to enter the esophagus and irritate the esophageal mucosa.

C. *NO.* Fruits other than citrus types do not aggravate heartburn.

D. *YES.* Fatty foods lower LES pressure, which relaxes the sphincter and allows acid to flow upward, or reflux, into the esophagus.

E. *YES.* Caffeine stimulates acid secretion, which can further irritate the epithelium.

**QUESTION 9.** $H_2$-antagonist drugs are the mainstay of pharmacologic treatment for patients who require additional measures beyond lifestyle modification to control their symptoms. Which of the following are considerations in the use of these drugs?

A. *YES.* Prescription $H_2$ blockers taken twice daily at full dosage are known to achieve the best results. These medications do not have to be taken just before or after meals. Another option is to prescribe a promotility drug that contracts the LES, clears the esophagus, or hastens gastric emptying. For patients with GERD associated with esophagitis, proton pump inhibitors are the most effective agents.

**B.** *YES.* Efficacy is dose dependent.

**C.** *YES.* Therapy should continue for 8 to 12 weeks, although adequate healing may not occur until 16 to 20 weeks after symptom control. Patients may need continued therapy if they do not make the necessary lifestyle changes. Failure to respond to regular doses of these drugs should lead to referral to a specialist in gastroenterology.

**D.** *NO.* Combination therapy with promotility agents is best avoided in the elderly, who are at greatest risk from drug interactions and potentially serious side effects.

## REFERENCES

Castell, D. O., Richter, J. E., Spechler, S. J. (1996). Achieving better outcomes for patients with GERD. *Patient Care 30*(8), 20–43.

Gorol, A. H., May, L. A., Mulley, A. G. (eds.). (1995). *Primary Care Medicine: Office Evaluation and Management of the Adult Patient,* 3d ed. Philadelphia: J.B. Lippincott.

Rubin, R. H., Voss, C., Derksen, D. J., Gateley, A., Quenzer, R. (1996). *Medicine: A Primary Care Approach.* Philadelphia: W. B. Saunders.

# 25

# Thyroid Disease

*Marie Lindsey*
*Ricki S. Witz*

Theresa H., a 35-year-old Caucasian woman, has been coming to the same family practice center on a regular basis for 10 years. Her last appointment, a well-woman examination, was 9 months ago. She has been divorced for 4 years and is the mother of two children, ages 7 and 10. Her ex-husband is not involved in their lives. Her usual state of health has been good: She seeks care for only preventive examinations and an occasional upper respiratory infection. She is employed full time as an assembly line worker, a job requiring long hours of standing, much upper arm movement, and fine motor activity. Although she hates being away from her children, lately she has been working 4 to 10 h of overtime per week because she needs the extra income.

## CHIEF COMPLAINT

"I haven't felt good since I got a cold 2 months ago."

## HISTORY OF PRESENT ILLNESS

Two months ago, Theresa had a cold, characterized by symptoms of rhinitis, slight sore throat, and slight cough. She may have had a fever, but she did not check her temperature with a thermometer. Those symptoms resolved with no treatment. She continued to feel fatigued and developed joint pain and anterior neck pain, which was amplified when she yawned. She thought the neck and joint pain might be related to the long periods of time she stands in one position at work. She tried to improve her body mechanics and posture by doing neck exercises while on the assembly line and by changing the type of shoes she wore while at work. These measures did not provide any relief; however, the occasional use of ibuprofen 400 mg did seem to alleviate both her neck and joint pain. Although Theresa felt feverish at the time she exhibited the upper respiratory symptoms, she now often feels cold. She has also noticed that her hair, normally thick and easy to manage, has become thinner.

## PAST MEDICAL HISTORY

Theresa's past medical history was unremarkable.

## FAMILY HISTORY

Her father, age 65, has diabetes and hypertension. Her mother, age 62, takes iron supplements for anemia. Her maternal grandmother, who died at age 70, had a history of a goiter.

QUESTION 1. Information on which of the following symptoms should be elicited at this time? (Select all that apply.)
- A. More about her neck pain
- B. More about the changes in the condition of her hair
- C. Changes in the condition of her skin
- D. Fluctuations in weight

## PHYSICAL FINDINGS

Vital signs:   Temperature 36.5°C (98.4°F); pulse 84, regular; respirations 16; blood pressure 100/70; height 5 ft 3 in; weight 155 lb.

Skin:   Uniformly white in color, soft, smooth, warm and clammy; without edema, lesions, or rashes.

Head, eyes, ears, nose, throat:
Hair: Fine; thin, but no areas of alopecia.
Nails: Smooth, pink, brisk capillary refill, no clubbing.
Face: Symmetrical, no edema, lesions, muscular weakness, or involuntary movements.
Eyes: Pupils equal, round, reactive to light and accommodation; sclerae white, no retinopathy, no exophthalmos or ptosis.
Mouth: Pharynx pink, moist. Tonsils present. No redness, swelling, lesions, or exudate.
Neck: Trachea midline. Thyroid gland asymmetrical: left side enlarged, hard, tender, but no discrete nodules palpated. No bruits over thyroid or carotids; carotid pulses of normal amplitude bilaterally. Full range of motion. No lyphadenopathy.

Joints:   Full range of motion of all extremities; no swelling or redness.

Neurologic:   Deep tendon reflexes all +2; cranial nerves II to XII grossly intact; rapid alternating movements intact.

QUESTION 2. Which of the following are other clinical features associated with hyperthyroid conditions? (Select all that apply.)
- A. Exophthalmos
- B. Restlessness
- C. Bradycardia
- D. Diarrhea

QUESTION 3. Which of the following are other clinical features associated with hypothyroid conditions? (Select all that apply.)
A. Dry, rough skin
B. Peripheral edema
C. Rapid, bounding pulse
D. Sluggishness

QUESTION 4. In light of the above findings, which of the following laboratory tests would be essential in establishing a diagnosis? (Select all that apply.)
A. Erythrocyte sedimentation rate (ESR)
B. Serum thyroid-stimulating hormone (TSH)
C. Serum free thyroxine (free $T_4$)
D. Serum total thyroxine (total $T_4$)
E. Serum total triiodothyronine ($T_3$)
F. Radioactive iodine uptake (RAIU)

## ASSESSMENT

Theresa's laboratory results were positive for an elevated free $T_4$ level, a low TSH level, and an elevated ESR of 52.

QUESTION 5. Which one of the following diseases is most likely, considering Theresa's symptoms, her laboratory results, and her tender, asymmetrically enlarged thyroid gland?
A. Primary myxedema
B. Hashimoto's thyroiditis
C. Graves' disease
D. Subacute thyroiditis

## TREATMENT

QUESTION 6. What is the standard treatment for Theresa's condition? (Select all that apply.)
A. Nonsteroidal anti-inflammatory medications
B. Prednisone
C. β-adrenergic blockers
D. Iodine
E. Antithyroid drugs
F. Synthetic or natural thyroid hormones

## ANSWERS

QUESTION 1. Information on which of the following symptoms should be elicited at this time?
A. *YES. Anterior* neck pain is seen in thyroid conditions and sometimes in fibromyalgia syndrome. The only other common etiology of anterior neck pain would be trauma or significant strain to the anterior neck. Theresa's assembly line work, which requires upper extremity move-

ment and fine motor coordination, is more likely to cause strain on the *posterior neck* and trapezius muscles, rather than anterior neck pain. It would be also be important to distinguish Theresa's previous pharyngitis symptoms (discomfort inside the posterior oral cavity) from her current complaint.

**B.** *YES.* As the anterior neck pain indicates possible thyroid disease, other thyroid symptoms should be pursued. Fine, thin, silky hair is often associated with hyperthyroid conditions. Coarse, brittle hair, even slight alopecia, and hair loss of lateral eyebrows is often associated with hypothyroid conditions.

**C.** *YES.* As the anterior neck pain indicates possible thyroid disease, associated changes in the skin should be explored. Hyperthyroid conditions often present with excessive sweating and warm, smooth, moist skin. Pruritus may be present as a result of increased blood flow to the skin. Patients with Graves' disease, the most common cause of hyperthyroidism in North America, may present with dermopathy of the distal lower extremities, which may range from slight discoloration to elephantiasis. Hypothyroid conditions often present with cool, very dry skin.

**D.** *YES.* Fluctuations in weight are common in thyroid conditions. Hyperthyroid conditions are often associated with weight loss, despite an increase in appetite. Hypothyroid conditions are often associated with weight gain, despite a decrease in appetite.

**QUESTION 2.** Which of the following are other clinical features associated with hyperthyroid conditions?

**A.** *YES.* Ophthalmopathy is common in many hyperthyroid conditions, but exophthalmos (abnormal protrusion of the eyeball) is a sign specific to Graves' disease. Ophthalmopathy is the result of enlarged extraocular muscles due to inflammatory infiltrate of mucopolysaccharides, which causes proptosis (downward displacement of eyeball) by displacing the eye forward, and orbital edema by compressing orbital veins. Manifestations range from mild periorbital edema and conjunctival inflammation to extraocular muscle dysfunction, corneal injury, and optic nerve damage. The lid lag and stare of hyperthyroidism may exacerbate the eye appearance and make the ophthalmopathy look more severe than it actually is. Other eye complaints may include pain, diplopia, proptosis, and blurred vision. Exophthalmos should be distinguished from the periorbital edema that is often present with *hypo*thyroid conditions, in which there is a puffiness of the eyelids and the entire face, resulting in a dulled facial expression.

**B.** *YES.* Restlessness, nervousness, anxiety, irritability, and shakiness or tremor are often associated with hyperthyroid conditions, as a result of increased sympathetic tone.

**C.** *NO.* Bradycardia is associated with hypothyroid conditions. The increased sympathetic tone related to hyperthyroidism often leads to tachycardia and palpitations, and may advance to shortness of breath, arrhythmias, congestive heart failure, and pericardial effusion.

**D.** *YES.* Frequent defecation, diarrhea, nausea, vomiting, and abdominal pain may occur in hyperthyroid conditions.

**QUESTION 3.** Which of the following are other clinical features associated with hypothyroid conditions?
   **A.** *YES.* Dry, coarse, and cold skin, as well as decreased sweating, is commonly seen in hypothyroid patients, whereas hyperthyroid patients are more likely to present with warm, moist, smooth (velvety) skin and increased sweating.
   **B.** *YES.* Edema can be present in either hypothyroid or hyperthyroid conditions. Graves' disease, a hyperthyroid condition, can present with a non-pitting edema, which is really a type of infiltrative dermopathy. This type of edema is sometimes referred to as pretibial myxedema and is an uncommon autoimmune disorder present in fewer than 5 percent of patients with Graves' disease. The term *pretibial myxedema* should not be confused with primary myxedema, which is another term for advanced hypothyroidism. Pretibial myxedema is characterized by localized dermal accumulation of mucopolysaccharides (the same infiltrate as in the orbits of ophthalmopathy), most commonly over the tibial surface. It may present as diffuse nonpitting lesions of the anterior lower leg or as sharply circumscribed lesions or plaques. An elephantiasis form is rare. The lesions are usually nontender and usually resolve spontaneously. Rarely, they may cause pain or ulcerate. Patients with severe forms of hypothyroidism may also present with a generalized nonpitting edema, which is accompanied by dry, waxy, pale skin.
   **C.** *NO.* A rapid, bounding pulse resulting from increased sympathetic tone is associated with hyperthyroid states. Hypothyroid patients are likely to be bradycardic.
   **D.** *YES.* Sluggishness, fatigue, lethargy, and slow speech are common clinical features of hypothyroidism. A related, but less common feature of hypothyroidism is depression.

**QUESTION 4.** In light of the above findings, which of the following laboratory tests would be essential in establishing a diagnosis?
   **A.** *YES.* An ESR is a nonspecific test used to detect the presence and intensity of an inflammatory process. Fluctuations in the ESR are more significant than a single abnormal occurrence, because the ESR is often higher when the disease is active and lower when the intensity of the disease decreases. The ESR may be increased in either hyper- or hypothyroid conditions. In the Wintrobe method of calculating the ESR, the normal range for males is 8 to 10 mm in 1 h; the normal range for females is 0 to 15 mm in 1 h. In the Westergren method, the normal range for males is 0 to 13 mm in 1 h; the normal range for females is 0 to 20 mm in 1 h.
   **B.** *YES.* A serum TSH test is useful in diagnosing either hyper- or hypothyroid conditions. The TSH ranges indicating euthyroid, hypothyroid, and hyperthyroid states vary depending on the type of laboratory methods used. Low TSH levels suggest hyperthyroid states, and marked improvements in the sensitivity of the TSH assay by radioimmunologic techniques make it possible to diagnose hyperthyroidism solely on the basis of the absence of detectable TSH. On the other hand, hypothyroid states are indicated when the TSH is elevated.

C. *YES.* A free $T_4$ index is useful in confirming either hypo- or hyperthyroid states. A low free $T_4$ and an increased TSH are essentially diagnostic of primary hypothyroidism, even in the absence of a palpable thyroid gland. On the other hand, an elevated free $T_4$ and low TSH indicate a hyperthyroid state.

D. *NO.* The free $T_4$ is a better measure of thyroid function than the total $T_4$, which is affected by changes in thyroid-binding globulin independent of thyroid function.

E. *NO.* Although total $T_3$ is often routinely ordered as part of a battery of thyroid function tests, the assay is expensive to perform and the results correlate poorly with thyroid status, as they are affected by such events as a fall in peripheral conversion of $T_4$ to $T_3$, which is common in the elderly and in nonthyroid illness. Measurement of $T_3$ is not necessary unless the patient is clinically thyrotoxic, and $T_3$ toxicosis is uncommon.

F. *NO.* A RAIU test is an unnecessary expense to diagnose subacute thyroiditis with a patient profile of neck pain following an apparent viral illness, an elevated $T_4$, a low TSH level, and an elevated ESR level. Nor is an RAIU necessary to confirm the diagnosis of Graves' disease if the patient has ophthalmopathy, clinical hyperthyroidism, and a diffusely enlarged thyroid gland. In the absence of clear clinical indicators, however, an RAIU does help differentiate causes of hyperthyroidism related to overproduction (i.e., Graves' disease, a multinodular goiter, or a hot nodule) from those related to excessive release but not production (i.e., subacute thyroiditis, postpartum thyroiditis, or silent thyroiditis), as well as excessive thyroid hormone ingestion. In these three types of thyroiditis, the RAIU test will be low, whereas in Graves' disease, multinodular goiter, and a hot nodule, the RAIU is elevated. A diagnosis of subacute thyroiditis is reinforced with a low RAIU in the presence of an elevated ESR.

**QUESTION 5.** Which one of the following diseases is most likely, considering Theresa's symptoms, her laboratory results, and her tender, asymmetrically enlarged thyroid gland?

A. *NO.* Primary myxedema is advanced and/or undiagnosed hypothyroidism. The clinical picture of florid myxedema includes dull, expressionless facies; slow movements; periorbital puffiness; sparse, coarse hair; macroglossia; and cool, pale, coarse skin. The most characteristic clinical finding in advanced hypothyroidism is the delayed relaxation phase of deep tendon reflexes. Theresa did not present with this constellation of symptoms. Primary myxedema is not to be confused with pretibial myxedema, which is a dermopathy of the legs affecting some Graves' disease patients.

B. *NO.* Hashimoto's thyroiditis is a chronic form of thyroiditis characterized as an inflammatory disorder with progressive destruction of the thyroid gland. An autoimmune condition, it is the leading cause of multinodular goiter in the United States. During the onset of Hashimoto's thyroiditis, patients are commonly euthyroid, although hyperthyroidism is also common in the early stages of the disease. As the disease progresses and the gland is further damaged, hypothyroidism results from the glandular damage and the thyroid's inability to manufacture thyroid hormones. Unlike Theresa, patients with Hashimoto's thyroiditis typically have a slightly elevated TSH.

C. *NO.* Graves' disease often presents with ophthalmopathy, pretibial myxedema (nonpitting edema; erythematous, mildly scaly plaques limited to the skin of the ankles and pretibial area), and a diffusely enlarged thyroid gland. Like subacute thyroiditis, Graves' disease patients usually have decreased TSH levels and elevated free $T_4$ levels. However, in addition to Theresa's lacking the classic symptoms of Graves' disease, the fact that her symptoms began after a viral respiratory illness strongly suggests a diagnosis of subacute thyroiditis. The occurrence of Graves' disease in former President Bush and his wife have raised an interest in the possibility of environmental precipitants such as an infectious agent.

D. *YES.* Theresa's presentation is typical of subacute thyroiditis, which includes symptoms following an apparent viral illness, pain in the thyroid area with radiation to the ears or jaw, malaise, and low-grade fever. On physical examination, a tender, enlarged thyroid is characteristic. Acute hemorrhage into a thyroid nodule can also cause a painful thyroid. Patients with subacute thyroiditis are initially hyperthyroid and may present with symptoms similar to Graves' disease, with the exception of exophthalmos and pretibial myxedema. Following the hyperthyroid state, as the subacute thyroiditis progresses, patients may become mildly hypothyroid. Therefore, symptoms representing each state may be present in the same patient and confound the clinical picture. However, Theresa's symptoms in addition to her elevated free $T_4$ and low TSH levels lead to a diagnosis of subacute thyroiditis.

**QUESTION 6.** What is the standard treatment for Theresa's condition?

A. *YES.* Subacute thyroiditis is a self-limiting illness; thus, treatment is aimed at relieving symptoms. Aspirin or nonsteroidal anti-inflammatory medications are usually very effective in relieving the neck, muscle, and joint pains.

B. *NO.* However, if Theresa's symptoms were not controlled with ibuprofen, prednisone 20 to 40 mg in divided doses might be prescribed. The side effects of suppressing normal adrenal function and normal immune response and inflammation make this a much less desirable treatment than aspirin and nonsteroidal anti-inflammatory medications. Complete recovery is expected within approximately 2 to 6 months.

C. *NO.* Beta-adrenergic blockers such as propranolol or atenolol, as well as calcium channel blockers, are useful medications in the treatment of tachycardia and palpitations of hyperthyroidism. However, Theresa had no symptoms that would warrant such treatment.

D. *NO.* Iodine in the form of Lugol's solution or SSKI solution is used in the treatment of thyroid storm (a life-threatening complication of thyrotoxicosis) and for preparation of patients for surgery.

E. *NO.* Antithyroid drugs (ATDs) belong to a group of compounds known as thionamides. They act by inhibiting thyroid peroxidase and therefore block iodine organification and thyroid hormone synthesis. The two ATDs available in the United States are propylthiouracil (PTU) and methimazole (Tapazole). As Theresa's subacute thyroiditis is self-limiting and not true hyperthyroidism, such medications would not be prescribed in her case.

F. *NO.* Synthetic preparations of levothyroxine sodium ($L$-$T_4$) or natural thyroid hormones, such as desiccated thyroid preparations, are prescribed for patients with hypothyroidism and must be taken indefinitely.

## REFERENCES

Braham, R. L., Lemberg, L. A., Pong, P., Rucker, L. M., Stulman, J. K. (1997). Endocrinology and metabolic disorders. In L. Rucker (ed.), *Essentials of Adult Ambulatory Care, 540.* Baltimore: Williams & Wilkins.

Goroll, A. H. (1995). Approach to the patient with hyperthyroidism. In A. H. Goroll, L. A. May, A. G. Mulley (eds.), *Primary Care Medicine: Office Evaluation and Management of the Adult Patient, 565–578.* Philadelphia: J. B. Lippincott.

Kasper, P. (1996). Thyroid disorders. In R. R. Rubin, C. Voss, D. J. Derksen, A. Gateley, R. W. Quenzer (eds.), *Medicine: A Primary Care Approach, 290–294.* Philadelphia: W. B. Saunders.

Mudge-Grout, C. L. (1992). *Immunologic Disorders.* Chicago: Mosby.

Ridgeway, E. C. (1994). Endocrinology. In R. Schrier (ed.), *The Internal Medicine Casebook: Real Patients, Real Answers, 67–121.* Boston: Little, Brown.

Traub, S. L. (1996). Endocrine disorders. In S. L. Traub (ed.), *Basic Skills in Interpreting Laboratory Data, 245–280.* Bethesda, MD: American Society of Health-System Pharmacists.

Uphold, C., Graham, M. (1993). *Clinical Guidelines in Family Practice.* Gainesville, FL: Barmarrae Books.

Wallach, J. (1996). *Interpretation of Diagnostic Tests.* Boston: Little, Brown.

# VI

# MIDDLE
# ADULT

# Introduction

*Arlene Miller*

The midlife years, from approximately ages 45 to 65, are marked by significant psychological and physical changes. Personality in adulthood is influenced by the ability to interpret past experiences from an adult cognitive and emotional stance. Midlife provides potential opportunities for greater psychological autonomy, self-actualization, and self-evaluation. Life goals are reassessed in terms of time left to live, and no longer seem limitless. This is a time marked by a sense of increased freedom, use of more mature strategies for dealing with life's complexities, and some relaxation of polarized gender roles. Generativity vs. stagnation continues to be important throughout adulthood. In spite of the emphasis in the popular literature on midlife crises, most adults adjust to and accept the challenges encountered during this period of life.

Developmental tasks in midlife include psychological adaptation to predictable transitional events or normative crises, such as having children leave home and the disability or death of parents. They can also include events for which little psychological or behavioral preparation exists. Nonnormative crises that may have particular implications during midlife include the unexpected death of a spouse, job loss, or early retirement. Immigration to a new country during midlife poses particular difficulties, as older age and female gender are highly correlated with acculturative stress. Developing enjoyable community, social, physical and solitary leisure time activities during midlife supports success in retirement and later years.

Symptoms of normal physiologic aging experienced most frequently in midlife include joint pains, backaches, fatigue, and sleep disorders. Cognitively, memory changes begin to occur, manifested most commonly as mild forgetfulness and decreased word retrieval. Visual changes are common after age 40, and include decreased accommodation of the lens to near objects. Hearing tends to decline after age 50. Menopause creates many physiological changes, but is experienced without psychological crisis for the majority of women. Psychological symptoms, including depressed mood and anxiety, appear to be more strongly related to extenuating social circumstances than to changes in hormonal balance.

Increased risk of heart disease and cancer for men and women during midlife necessitates the initiation or continuation of several routine screening tests. Screening for hypertension and diabetes, both of which have increased incidence during midlife compared to early adulthood, should be continued annually. Rectal examinations for men and Papanicolaou testing for women should also be continued. Total blood cholesterol screening should be instituted for women after age 45, when the protective effects of estrogen are diminished. Sigmoidoscopy and tests for fecal occult blood should be done regularly after age 50 in men and women. Mammograms with clinical breast examinations should be obtained yearly by women after age 50.

Other routine health promotion and education activities include screening and counseling for stress management, smoking cessation, substance abuse, and dental health. Initiation of regular physical activity programs is important, particularly for sedentary adults. Diets that emphasize grains, fruits, and vegetables and limit fat and cholesterol have been shown to decrease the incidence of cancer and heart disease. Assuring adequate calcium intake is important to reduce the development of osteoporosis, which can occur in both men and women in later life. Although there are still controversies regarding the benefits and risks associated with hormone replacement therapy (HRT), it is commonly prescribed to relieve vasomotor and vaginal symptoms of menopause. Reasons for long-term use of HRT include prevention of cardiovascular disease and osteoporosis.

The case studies in this part include health promotion visits that address the prevention and screening needs of midlife men and women, as well as health problems that are commonly seen in primary care settings. Evaluation of breast masses is important and has particular implications for African American women. Back pain is a common problem for employed adults, and anxiety is a presenting problem that is often inadequately managed by primary care providers. Finally, as individuals age, their health is often maintained in the context of chronic diseases such as hypertension and diabetes.

## REFERENCES

Berry, J. W., Kim, U., Minde, T., Mok, D. (1987). Comparative studies of acculturative stress. *International Migration Review 21*, 491–511.

Erikson, E. H. (1982). *The Life Cycle Completed*. New York: Norton.

Fogel, C. I., Woods, N. F. (1995). Midlife women's health. In C. I. Fogel, N. F. Woods (eds.), *Women's Health Care: A Comprehensive Handbook*, 79–100. Thousand Oaks, CA: Sage.

Hoyer, W. J., Rybash, J. M. (1994). Characterizing adult cognitive development. *Journal of Adult Development 1*, 7–12.

Matthews, K., Wing, R., Kuller, L., Meilahn, E., Kelsey, S. (1990). Influences of natural menopause on psychological characteristics and symptoms of middle-aged healthy women. *J Consult Clin Psychol 58*, 345–351.

Miller, A., Wilbur, J., McDevitt, J. (1997). Health promotion: The perimenopausal to mature years (45–64). In K. Allen, J. Phillips (eds.), *Women's Health Across the Lifespan: A Comprehensive Perspective*, 55–71. Philadelphia: J. B. Lippincott.

Murray, R. B., Zentner, J. P. (1997). *Nursing Assessment and Health Promotion: Strategies through the Life Span*, 6th ed. Stamford, CT: Appleton & Lange.

U.S. Preventive Services Task Force. (1996). *Guide to Clinical Preventive Services*, 2nd ed. Baltimore: Williams & Wilkins.

Wilbur, J., Miller, A., Montgomery, A. (1995). The influence of demographic characteristics, menopausal status, and symptoms on women's attitudes toward menopause. *Women Health, 23*(3), 19–39.

# 26

# Health Promotion: Midlife Woman

*JoEllen Wilbur*
*Arlene Miller*

Sylvia C., a 50-year-old Caucasian woman, was last seen 1 year ago for a routine well-woman examination including a Papanicolaou (Pap) smear. Her record indicates that she is married, has two adolescent children, and has been working in a secretarial position for the past 15 years. She had a normal mammogram when she was 48 years old. At the time of her last visit, her Pap smear was normal and she had a high-density lipoprotein (HDL) of 69, low-density lipoprotein (LDL) of 98, and a total cholesterol level of 180. Her weight at that time was 165 lb, and her height was 5 ft 5 in.

## CHIEF COMPLAINT

"During the past few months, I have occasionally felt hot and clammy over my face and chest."

## HISTORY OF PRESENT HEALTH

Mrs. C. feels she is generally in good health, but perhaps "out of shape." During the last several months she has periodically felt a sensation of warmth and flushing over her upper chest and neck. It lasts for a minute or so, and then she feels clammy. This occurs several times a week. Her last menstrual period was 6 weeks ago. Although she usually does not keep track of her menses, she has noticed that the time between periods has increased from about every 4 weeks to every 6 to 8 weeks during the past year. Recently the flow has appeared darker and lasts only 1 to 2 days. She denies spotting between menses and dyspareunia. She has successfully used a diaphragm since her last pregnancy 15 years ago, but admits to recently using it sporadically. She expresses much concern about hormone replacement (HRT) therapy and cancer. Mrs. C. has no regular exercise routine. She drinks two to three cups of coffee in the morning and one can of diet cola in the afternoon. She drinks two to three glasses of wine during weekends. She denies smoking. Her 75-year-old mother had a myocardial infarction and triple bypass heart surgery when she was 70 years old. Her maternal grandmother had breast cancer at the age of 72 years.

## PHYSICAL FINDINGS

| | |
|---|---|
| Vital signs: | Blood pressure 124/80 right arm sitting, 120/76 right arm lying, 126/80 left arm lying; height 5 ft 5 in (165 cm); weight 175 lb (79.54 kg); body mass index (BMI) 29. |
| Skin: | No lesions, moles, or excessive perspiration. |
| Breasts: | Symmetric, without retraction, discharge, or lesions. |
| External genitalia: | No infestations, lesions, swelling, or redness. Urethra, Bartholin's and Skene's glands intact. |
| Vagina: | Walls pale, smooth, without lesions, odor, or discharge. |
| Cervix: | Pink, no lesions or discharge. No cervical motion tenderness. Pap smear taken. |
| Uterus: | Midline without enlargement, masses, or tenderness. |
| Adnexae: | No enlargement or tenderness. |
| Rectum: | No hemorrhoids, fissures, or lesions. Rectal walls intact without masses or tenderness. |

## ASSESSMENT

Mrs. C. is a sedentary midlife woman with hot flashes and weight gain.

QUESTION 1. Which of the following screening tests should be requested at this visit? (Select all that apply.)
A. Mammogram
B. Serum follicle-stimulating hormone (FSH) and estradiol levels
C. Fecal occult blood test (FOBT)
D. Lipid profile
E. Bone density screening

QUESTION 2. What information will help Mrs. C. make a decision regarding HRT? (Select all that apply.)
A. In order to gain any benefit for the prevention of osteoporosis, HRT must be started shortly after the cessation of menstruation.
B. Her family history of breast cancer is a contraindication to HRT.
C. Her family history of cardiovascular disease is a strong indicator for using HRT.
D. HRT should include both estrogen and progestin.
E. To obtain relief from hot flashes, she needs to consider long-term use of HRT.

QUESTION 3. Which of the following nutritional information should be provided? (Select all that apply.)
A. She should consume a diet that has approximately 1500 mg of calcium per day.
B. The calcium supplement with the highest percentage of elemental calcium is calcium gluconate.
C. There is little that can be done from a dietary perspective to alleviate or prevent her hot flashes.
D. A dietary goal should be to limit fat intake.

QUESTION 4. What information should you provide regarding sexuality? (Select all that apply.)
A. Birth control should continue until 1 year after her last menstrual period (LMP).
B. Vaginal dryness and discomfort during intercourse are inevitable if she does not take HRT.
C. Sexual interest will decrease substantially with aging.
D. Physical changes may require her to alter her sexual activity as she ages.

QUESTION 5. Which of the following information should be shared with her about starting an exercise program? (Select all that apply.)
A. One must engage in at least 30 min of continuous moderate-intensity activity five or six days of the week to obtain cardiovascular benefits.
B. The components of an exercise prescription include frequency, intensity, duration, and mode of activity.
C. Her exercise program should include both aerobic conditioning and weight training.
D. Adherence to an exercise program will be enhanced if she participates in a group program.
E. Because of her age and medical history, she should have an aerobic fitness test prior to starting an exercise program.

QUESTION 6. What information should be shared with her regarding weight gain? (Select all that apply.)
A. Weight gain is inevitable during and following menopause.
B. Her BMI is acceptable for her age.
C. The advantage of added weight is that it places her at less risk for osteoporosis.
D. If she loses weight, her hot flashes will probably intensify.

## ANSWERS

QUESTION 1. Which of the following screening tests should be ordered at this visit?
A. *YES.* There is general agreement among the American Cancer Society, the U.S. Preventive Services Task Force, and the Canadian Task Force on Periodic Examination that a mammogram should be done every 1

to 2 years after age 40, and yearly after age 50. Since her last examination was 2 years ago, it is time for another mammogram.

B. *NO.* Screening for FSH and estradiol is expensive and may be difficult to interpret, since serum levels fluctuate during the perimenopausal period. A high serum FSH level may be useful to diagnose premature menopause or to differentiate between pregnancy and menopausal amenorrhea, but it is not used routinely to identify the onset of normal perimenopausal symptoms. Results of these tests would not influence the management of this woman's health care.

C. *YES.* She is at average risk for colorectal cancer. Although there has been some controversy regarding the best strategy for screening individuals at average risk, there is now general agreement that a digital rectal examination should be included yearly in the periodic health examination, with annual stool testing after the age of 50. The American College of Physicians also recommends a screening sigmoidoscopy in adults at average risk at age 50 and every 3 to 5 years thereafter. Factors that would place one at high risk include colorectal cancer in a first-degree family member; familial polyposis coli; personal history of endometrial, ovarian, or breast cancer; ulcerative colitis; and prior colon cancer.

D. *NO.* The National Cholesterol Education Program of the National Heart, Lung, and Blood Institute recommends that total blood cholesterol and HDL cholesterol should be measured at least once every 5 years in adults with a desirable blood cholesterol (<200 mg/dL). Her cholesterol and HDL were both in the desirable range 1 year ago, so screening is not warranted at this time.

E. *NO.* There are no recommendations for routine screening for bone density with any of the currently available methods. Also, there are no guidelines regarding intervals for screening and subsequent treatment. Although one indication for screening, recommended by the National Osteoporosis Foundation, is for women who want to make a decision regarding estrogen replacement, it is not mandatory.

**QUESTION 2.** What information will help her make a decision regarding HRT?

A. *NO.* If she is worried about having osteoporosis later in life, the decision to begin HRT does not have to be made immediately after the cessation of menstruation in order to gain benefits. In the past, women were told that they had to begin therapy within 3 to 5 years of natural menopause to prevent bone loss, but recent evidence suggests that starting HRT 5 or more years after the cessation of menstruation provides protective effects. The effect of estrogen on bone mass continues throughout the course of HRT administration, and positive effect has been shown up to 75 years of age.

B. *NO.* The relationship between the use of estrogen and the risk of breast cancer is not clear. Although there is some evidence suggesting that among women with a family history of breast cancer, those who have used estrogen replacement have a higher risk for breast cancer than those women who have not, family history of breast cancer is not included in either the absolute or relative contraindications to estrogen use. Research to date has been contradictory. For example, a meta-analysis of the results of 16 studies indicated that the risk of breast cancer did not increase until after more than 5 years of estrogen use.

C. *YES.* Her family history of heart disease may be a factor to consider in deciding to use hormone therapy. The results of the Postmenopausal Estrogen/Progestin Interventions (PEPI) showed that triglyceride levels increased significantly, LDL was reduced, and HDL was elevated in all formulations tested. The effect on cardiovascular morbidity and mortality has not been determined yet.

D. *YES.* Since this women has not had a hysterectomy, she would need a regimen that included both estrogen and progestin. The use of unopposed estrogen increases the risk for endometrial cancer. This risk appears to be eliminated with the addition of a progestin. Cyclic use of progestins will result in withdrawal bleeding. The newer regimens of estrogen and progestin given continuously or on a 3-month sequential regimen eliminate monthly withdrawal bleeding.

E. *NO.* Relief of hot flashes is the most common reason women give for starting HRT. For this purpose alone, 2 to 5 years of therapy may be adequate.

**QUESTION 3.** Which of the following nutritional information should be provided?

A. *YES.* Calcium is important in the prevention of osteoporosis. The recommended intake of calcium from puberty to age 25 and for postmenopausal women taking estrogen is 1200 mg. For postmenopausal women not on HRT, the recommendation is 1500 mg of calcium daily. This woman is approaching menopause, so it is appropriate to recommend that she take 1500 mg of calcium daily, through either dietary intake or supplement.

B. *NO.* She needs to be advised that there is a difference between total calcium and the amount of elemental calcium contained in a tablet. It is the total number of milligrams of elemental calcium that is important. The percentage of elemental calcium in calcium gluconate is only 9.3 percent. Calcium carbonate has the highest percentage (40 percent).

C. *YES.* Dietary strategies for women experiencing hot flashes are found in the literature, although there is little confirmatory research as yet. Some data suggest avoiding spices, sugar, hot drinks, wine, and caffeine, as they have been implicated as triggers for hot flashes. She may want to track these or other foods or drinks that seem to precipitate hot flashes. Phytoestrogens are naturally occurring compounds in plants that produce estrogenic effects. They are found in a diverse variety of plant products, with the highest concentrations being found in legumes such as soy, cereals, and linseed (flaxseed) oil. Evidence from other countries suggests that these products may have an impact on menopausal symptoms and may have protective effects against cancer and heart disease. Additional research is necessary before specific recommendations can be made.

D. *YES.* Menopause equalizes the risk for cardiovascular disease for men and women. Thus, limiting fat intake is even more important at midlife than in the earlier stages of a woman's life. The best strategy for controlling weight is reduction of dietary fat intake to no more than 30 percent of calories. She should increase the amounts of whole grain foods and cereals, vegetables and fruits, and complex carbohydrates and fiber in her diet.

**Question 4.** What information should be provided regarding sexuality?
A. *YES.* The general recommendation is for women to continue to use contraception for 1 year after the last menstrual period. Although there is a sharp decrease in fertility starting around age 40, as long as women are menstruating, they are potentially fertile. Among women who do become pregnant in midlife, the incidence of miscarriages is higher than for women in their twenties and thirties.
B. *NO.* Sexually active women have less vaginal atrophy and report fewer vaginal symptoms than women who are not sexually active, and regular sexual stimulation and intercourse seem to overcome the effects of decreased estrogens on the vagina. If needed, vaginal creams with or without estrogens may be helpful.
C. *NO.* Sexual interest can continue throughout life.
D. *YES.* Sexual behaviors may need to be modified, such as allowing adequate time for stimulation, using alternative positions during coitus, using water-soluble lubricants, and identifying alternative forms of sexual activity.

**Question 5.** Which of the following information should be shared with her about starting an exercise program?
A. *NO.* For people who cannot set aside 30 min on most days of the week for moderate-intensity activity, recent studies suggest that gains in cardiorespiratory fitness may be obtained when physical activity occurs in several short sessions (e.g., 10 min at a time).
B. *YES.* An exercise prescription includes mode or type of aerobic activity, intensity, duration, and frequency. She needs to identify an activity that she enjoys and that is suitable to her lifestyle. Moderate-intensity effort is recommended to avoid injuries and increase adherence. The recommended duration is 20 to 30 min at a frequency of three to four times a week.
C. *YES.* Aerobic conditioning improves cardiorespiratory endurance and reduces the risk of cardiovascular disease. Weight training improves muscle strength and bone density.
D. *NO.* Women's leisure time is often fragmented and depends on the priorities of others. There is some research that suggests that women's adherence to an exercise program is higher if the time and location are flexible. Group programs usually do not provide a great deal of flexibility.
E. *NO.* Women who are 50 years of age or younger, have no symptoms or signs suggestive of cardiopulmonary disease, and have no more than one major coronary risk factor do not need exercise testing prior

to participation in moderate intensity exercise. Risk factors include a family history of myocardial infarction or sudden death before 55 years in the father or 65 years in the mother or other first-degree relatives, current cigarette smoking, hypertension, hypercholesterolemia, diabetes mellitus, and sedentary lifestyle/ physical inactivity. She has only one risk factor (sedentary lifestyle), so exercise testing is not recommended.

**QUESTION 6.** What information should be shared with her regarding weight gain?

**A.** *NO.* There is an increasing prevalence of overweight in women with each decade of life until 59 years of age, but a natural menopause has not been specifically found to affect body weight.

**B.** *NO.* The desirable BMI for women 45 to 54 years of age is 22 to 27. She is in the overweight range for BMI.

**C.** *YES.* Heavier women have a reduced risk for osteoporosis. The constant weight borne by the skeletal system helps maintain bone density.

**D.** *NO.* The research to date on body weight and hot flashes is not conclusive. Higher endogenous estrogen associated with obesity suggests that heavier women may have fewer hot flashes than thin women. Several studies contradict this theory, however. One study found that thin women who smoke have more of a problem with hot flashes.

## REFERENCES

Fogel, C., Woods, N. (1995). Midlife women's health. In C. Fogel, N. Woods (eds.), *Women's Health Care,* 79–110. Thousand Oaks, CA: Sage.

Knight, D. C., Eden, J. A. (1995). Phytoestrogens—a short review. *Maturitas 22,* 167–175.

Miller, A., Wilbur, J., McDevitt, J. (1997). Health promotion: The perimenopausal to mature years (45–64). In K. Allen, J. Phillips (eds.), *Women's Health across the Lifespan,* 55–71. Philadelphia: J. B. Lippincott.

Murray, R., Zentner, J. (1997). Assessment and health promotion for the middle-aged person. In R. Murray, J. Zentner (eds.), *Health Assessment and Promotion Strategies through the Life Span* 6th ed., 637–992. Stamford, CT: Appleton & Lange.

Woolf, S. H., Jonas, S., Lawrence, R. S. (1996). *Health Promotion and Disease Prevention in Clinical Practice.* Baltimore: Willliams & Wilkins.

# 27

# Health Promotion: Midlife Man

*Susan A. Fontana*
*Marie L. Talashek*

Richard M. is a 52-year-old African American man and a regular patient who presents to the clinic because he needs a history and physical for job certification as a school bus driver. Review of his record reveals that he was last seen 1½ years ago for a routine checkup. He is a nonsmoker and has never been hospitalized. A chemistry screen, including a lipid panel, was done at his last visit. Results were normal, and the lipid panel revealed below-average risk for heart disease. A prostate-specific antigen (PSA) test was ordered at the patient's request because his father died of prostate cancer. The level was 2.0 ng/mL; the upper limit of normal is 4.0 ng/mL.

## CHIEF COMPLAINT

"I need another checkup, since it's been 2 years. Also, please fill out this health evaluation form from my employer."

## PAST MEDICAL HISTORY

Mr. M. is not taking any medications. Other significant family history is that his mother and brother have hypertension. He follows no regular exercise pattern or diet plan. He sleeps 7 to 8 h nightly without difficulty. He lives with his wife of 30 years and two daughters who attend city colleges.

QUESTION 1. Preventive care includes screening for potential problems. The utility of the screening is based on which of the following criteria? (Select all that apply.)
  A. The condition must have a significant effect on the quality of life.
  B. The condition must have a significant effect on the quantity of life.
  C. Acceptable methods of treatment must be available.

D. The incidence of the condition must be high enough to justify the cost of screening.
E. The condition can be detected in the asymptomatic period by tests that are acceptable to patients at a reasonable cost.

QUESTION 2. The frequency of age-related screening depends on which of the following? (Select all that apply.)
A. The sensitivity of the screening test
B. The rate of progression of the disease
C. The person's risk status
D. The discomfort of the examination

## OBJECTIVE DATA

| | |
|---|---|
| Vital signs: | Blood pressure, right arm sitting 140/92, left arm sitting 142/94; pulse 88, sinus rhythm; respiration 18 breaths/min; height 5 ft 9 in; weight 195 lb. |
| General: | Overweight, middle-aged male in no distress; appears relaxed and pleasant without obvious deformities. |
| Skin: | Warm and moist. Hair thick. Nails pink. |
| Head: | Normocephalic, nontender. |
| Eyes: | Extraocular movements intact, conjunctivae pink; pupils equal, round, reactive to light and accommodation; funduscopic benign. |
| Ear, nose, | Tympanic membranes intact. Turbinates pink without throat: discharge. Throat not injected. |
| Mouth: | Membranes pink without lesions. Teeth in good repair. |
| Neck: | Thyroid not palpable. No regional nodes tender or palpable. |
| Breast/axillae: | No masses or nodes palpable. |
| Lungs: | Clear to auscultation and percussion. No adventitious sounds. |
| Heart: | Point of maximum impulse at fifth intercostal space at midclavicular line. $S_1$ and $S_2$ without $S_3$, $S_4$, or murmurs. No peripheral edema. |
| Abdomen: | Protuberant. Active bowel sounds, without bruits. No masses, organs, hernias, or inguinal nodes palpable. |
| Musculo-skeletal: | Joints nontender, not swollen. Back no deformities or tenderness. |
| Neurologic: | Cranial nerves II to XII intact. Deep tendon reflexes 2+. Sensory and motor intact. |
| Genital: | Penis circumcised without lesions. No scrotal masses. |
| Rectal: | External hemorrhoids noted. No intrarectal masses. Stool brown, hemoccult negative. Prostate nontender, symmetrical, not enlarged. |

QUESTION 3. Based on the history and physical examination, which of the following screening tests are recommended. (Select all that apply.)
A. Repeat lipid panel
B. Home fecal occult blood test (FOBT)

   C. Sigmoidoscopy
   D. Thyroid screening using TSH
   E. Repeat of PSA at this visit

## ASSESSMENT

QUESTION 4. Which of the following is an appropriate assessment? (Select all that apply.)
   A. Increased risk for prostate cancer
   B. Essential hypertension
   C. Ten pounds above ideal body weight
   D. Lack of a regular exercise pattern

## PLAN

QUESTION 5. What should be included in an exercise prescription for a person over age 50? (Select all that apply.)
   A. Aerobic or cardiovascular endurance activities
   B. Strengthening or resistance activities
   C. Improving flexibility
   D. Treatment of uncontrolled conditions
   E. An exercise stress test

QUESTION 6. Which of the following dietary recommendations for weight control are appropriate for Mr. M.? (Select all that apply.)
   A. Setting high goals.
   B. Daily self-monitoring.
   C. Follow-up at every visit.
   D. Avoid acknowledging a lack of progress.

## ANSWERS

QUESTION 1. Preventive care includes screening for potential problems. The utility of the screening is based on which of the following criteria.
   A. *YES.* A condition having a significant effect on the quality of life is one of six explicit evidence-based criteria for recommending a preventive procedure.
   B. *YES.* A condition having a significant effect on the quantity of life is another explicit evidence-based criterion for recommending a preventive procedure.
   C. *YES.* Acceptable methods of treatment must be available if a preventive procedure is recommended.
   D. *YES.* If the condition is rare or has a low incidence, the cost of screening large numbers of people would be prohibitive.
   E. *YES.* It is necessary for a test to be acceptable and affordable. In addition, treatment during the asymptomatic phase must yield a therapeutic result superior to that obtained by delaying treatment until symptoms appear.

**QUESTION 2.** The frequency of age-related screening depends on which of the following?

   **A.** YES. If the sensitivity of the test (proportion of persons who correctly test positive when screened) is poor, then the test will miss cases and the number of false positives will be high.

   **B.** *YES.* The rate of progression of the disease is important in determining whether early detection truly improves outcome. Early detection should lead to the implementation of clinical interventions that can prevent or delay progression of the disorder.

   **C.** *NO.* A person's risk status supersedes criteria for age-related screening. For example, if there is a family history of coronary artery disease earlier, more frequent screening may be called for.

   **D.** *NO.* Though discomfort may be a barrier to the acceptability to patients of a screening test, it does not preclude recommendation.

**QUESTION 3.** Based on the history and physical examination, which of the following screening tests are recommended?

   **A.** *NO.* Current recommendations are to repeat the lipid panel every 5 years if it is within the acceptable reference range (less than 200 mg/dL).

   **B.** *YES.* An annual FOBT is recommended for persons age 50 years and older. Although a single FOBT can be performed in the examation room as part of the digital rectal examination, it is less accurate than home testing. Home testing involves the patient's collecting two specimens from each of three separate consecutive stool samples using three FOBT cards.

   **C.** *YES.* Most health professional groups or organizations recommend that all persons over age 50 receive sigmoidoscopy screening every 3 to 5 years.

   **D.** *NO.* The American Thyroid Association recommends screening adults who are asymptomatic with a strong family history of thyroid disease, persons over age 60 years, postpartum women, patients with hypercholesterolemia or a prior history of thyroid disease, and patients with autoimmune disease. Mr. M. meets none of these criteria.

   **E.** *YES.* Prostate-specific antigen testing is recommended yearly for all men over 50 years old by the American Cancer Society. Mr. M. has a family history and a desire to be screened for prostate cancer. However, there continues to be a great deal of controversy over this recommendation because of the lack of evidence that early detection and treatment of prostate cancer lowers morbidity or mortality. In addition, the treatment of prostate cancer can produce complications (impotence, incontinence) that seriously affect the quality of life.

**QUESTION 4.** Which of the following is an appropriate assessment?

   **A.** *YES.* The incidence of prostate cancer in African American males is 50 percent higher than in Caucasians. Family history is also a risk factor.

   **B.** *NO.* Although the patient's blood pressure is elevated at today's visit and the family history is significant for this condition, there is no previous personal history of elevated blood pressure. Further confirmation of a sustained elevation at another one to two visits is needed before this diagnosis can be established.

C. NO. Ideal body weight (I.W.) can be estimated using tables for population norms. Another method for estimating I.W. for men is to start with 106 lb for the first 5 feet of height and add 6 lb for every additional inch. Using this method, Mr. M.'s I.W. is 160 pounds. Regardless of body frame, he is approximately 35 pounds or 22 percent over his I.W.

D. YES. The patient does not report any regular physical activity.

QUESTION 5. What should be included in an exercise prescription for a person over age 50?

A. YES. A balanced exercise prescription for most people includes some aerobic and some strengthening activities. Exercise programs for older persons are not very different from those for younger persons. Examples of aerobic exercise include walking, hiking, swimming, bicycling, and stair climbing.

B. YES. Most experts agree that to improve strength substantially, the exerciser needs to train a muscle to more than 70 percent of the maximum force the muscle can generate. Each group of contractions or repetitions performed until the muscle is fatigued is called a "set." Two to five sets per exercise session are recommended.

C. YES. Flexibility exercises are important to reduce the risk of injuring muscles and tendons. Injuries can be prevented by warming up with slow movements and walking before lifting weights or performing endurance activities.

D. YES. An exercise prescription must address the patient's overall health status. Therefore, chronic conditions must be considered and any uncontrolled conditions treated prior to undertaking an exercise program.

E. NO. Most authorities believe that treadmill testing is necessary only for those beginning a vigorous program or for those planning a moderate program who have symptoms of or known cardiovascular, pulmonary, or metabolic disease. Some would add to that list persons with two or more cardiac risk factors. The American College of Sports Medicine recommends an exercise stress test for all men and women older than 60 prior to initiating an aerobic exercise program.

QUESTION 6. Which of the following dietary recommendations for weight control are appropriate for Mr. M.?

A. NO. Setting high weight loss goals often leads to failure and makes persons want to give up. Nutritional goals should be realistic, measurable, and achievable with reasonable effort. It is important for the patient to experience success and to make progress. Goals are typically related to calorie or fat intake, or to weight. A common goal is to keep protein consumption to 10 to 20 percent and carbohydrate consumption to 50 to 60 percent of total calories. For fat consumption, the goal is to keep it to no more than 30 percent of total calories. Weight loss of approximately 2 lb a week has been demonstrated to be safe and effective for long-term management.

B.  *YES.* Self-monitoring is typically done daily and involves having patients record the variables that they are trying to change, e.g., calorie intake or grams of fat consumed.
C.  *YES.* Follow-up is critical because it presents the opportunity to facilitate success and provide feedback. It is important to recognize and reinforce successful behavior when it occurs.
D.  *NO.* Addressing lack of progress is helpful to patients. In order to overcome barriers, the clinician must acknowledge problems and explore them with the patient. Common barriers include long hours at work, stress at home, misunderstanding nutritional guidelines, poor motivation, and a lack of family support.

## REFERENCES

Brawer, M. K. (1995). How to use prostate-specific antigen in the early detection or screening for prostatic carcinoma. *Cancer Journal for Clinicians 45*(3), 148–164.

Fiatarone, M. A., O'Brien, K., Rich, B. S. (1996). Exercise: RX for healthier old age. *Patient Care, 30*(16), 145–158.

Snelling, A. M. (1997). A concise guide to nutrition counseling. *Patient Care 31*(8) 47–53.

U.S. Preventive Services Task Force. (1996). *Guide to Clinical Preventive Services,* 2d ed. Baltimore: Williams & Wilkins.

Woolf, S. H., Jonas, S., Lawrence, R. S. (eds.). (1996). *Health Promotion and Disease Prevention in Clinical Practice.* Baltimore: Williams & Wilkins.

# 28

# Breast Mass

*Janice M. Phillips*
*Arlene Miller*

Yvonne B., a 45-year-old African American woman, presents at the HMO complaining of a lump in her left breast. Ms. B. initially discovered the lump approximately 4 months ago. The clinic nurse notes that Ms. B. is extremely anxious and concerned about the possibility of breast cancer, because her mother was diagnosed with it at age 47 and died at age 50.

## CHIEF COMPLAINT

"I have a lump in my left breast, found about 4 months ago."

## HISTORY OF PRESENT ILLNESS

Ms. B. was last seen in the clinic a year ago, when she had a normal physical examination. She was instructed to return within a year for her annual physical. She did not have a screening mammogram at that time. Ms. B. recalls being told a long time ago she had very lumpy breasts. She does not do breast self-examinations (BSEs) routinely, but found the breast lump unexpectedly during a shower.

QUESTION 1. What additional data are required for Ms. B.'s history of present illness? (Select all that apply.)
  A. Previous breast biopsy
  B. Mammography history
  C. History of pain in the left breast
  D. Last chest x-ray

QUESTION 2. What information should be included to complete an initial history to identify risk factors for breast cancer? (Select all that apply.)
  A. Previous personal history of breast cancer
  B. Number of pregnancies and age at first birth
  C. Use of exogenous estrogen

**D.** Additional maternal and paternal family history of breast cancer

**E.** Weight changes over time

## PAST MEDICAL HISTORY

Ms. B. has no known history of any diseases, illnesses, or allergies and is currently taking no medicines. She complains of occasional sinus problems relieved by over-the-counter sinus medicine. Review of systems reveals the following additional information:

| | |
|---|---|
| General: | Denies recent illness, increase or decrease in weight, or change in eating patterns. Denies history of fever, sweats, fatigue, or malaise. |
| Skin: | Denies lesions, color changes, petechiae, pruritis, or rash; overall skin turgor good. |
| Respiratory/ cardiovascular: | No history of cough, upper respiratory infection, dyspnea, or cardiovascular problems. |
| Gastrointestinal: | Reports normal bowel habits. |
| Genitourinary: | Denies problems with urination, burning, frequency, or vaginal discharge. Last menstrual period 3 weeks ago. Gravida 1 Para 1 at age 25 years; using condoms for birth control method now; has used oral contraceptive pills in the past for a total of 6 years. Denies estrogen use at this time. Last Papanicolaou smear 6 months ago. All other systems are within normal limits. |

## PHYSICAL FINDINGS

| | |
|---|---|
| Vital signs: | Temperature 36.6°C (98.6°F), pulse 92, respirations 20, blood pressure 110/70. |
| General: | Well-developed adult female; weight 146 lb, height: 5 ft, 1 in. |
| Skin: | Slight facial acne lower borders of face, otherwise clear skin with overall good skin turgor. No evidence of lesions, color changes, petechiae, pruritis, or rash. |
| Respiratory: | Lungs clear to auscultation and percussion. |
| Cardiovascular: | Point of maximum impulse at fifth intercostal space, $S_1$, $S_2$, $S_2 > S_1$ at the base, no $S_3$, $S_4$, or murmurs. Extremities symmetrically warm, no evidence of edema or clubbing, peripheral pulses equal bilaterally. |
| Breast: | 1-cm, nonmobile, nontender, firm mass in the upper inner quadrant of the left breast. No bloody or other nipple discharge, no nipple retraction, skin dimpling, ulceration, or redness. No palpable mass or nipple discharge in the right breast. There is swelling and tenderness of the left axillary lymph nodes. |
| Gastrointestinal: | Abdomen round, soft, slightly protruded; bowel sounds in all four quadrants. No organ enlargement; no palpable masses or tenderness. |

Genitourinary:    External genitalia nontender, without lesions, inflammation, or discharge. Cervix nulliparous, pink; uterus nonpregnant size, no masses or tenderness.

Neuromuscular:    Alert and oriented ×3, good mobility of all extremities.

## ASSESSMENT

Breast mass in the left breast.

**QUESTION 3.** Based on the history and physical examination, which of the following diagnoses is most likely?
A. Breast cancer
B. Fibrocystic breast condition
C. Fibroadenoma
D. Gynecomastia

## PLAN

A work-up for suspicious breast mass is initiated. The plan includes a diagnostic mammogram.

**QUESTION 4.** Which of the following is the best diagnostic tool for effectively distinguishing between a benign and a cancerous lesion?
A. Screening mammogram
B. Ultrasonography
C. Biopsy
D. Clinical breast examination

**QUESTION 5.** Which of the following statement(s) is/are true regarding breast cancer in African American women? (Select all that apply.)
A. The increase in reported breast cancer rates for African American women is due solely to advances in breast cancer screening.
B. The American Cancer Society provides specific recommendations for breast cancer detection in African American women.
C. African American women are less likely than Caucasian women to obtain treatment for breast cancer at an early stage, when the potential for cure is greatest.
D. The single most important risk factor for the development of breast cancer is race.

## ANSWERS

**QUESTION 1.** What additional data are required to complete Ms. B.'s history?
A. *YES.* Biopsy history should be ascertained. Benign proliferative breast disease, particularly a diagnosis of atypical hyperplasia confirmed by biopsy, is associated with an increased risk of breast cancer.
B. *YES.* Mammography history, location, findings, and follow-up recommendations should be ascertained. Previous mammography findings should be compared with those of a current mammogram. Screening of women between ages 40 to 49 is not universally recommended. The

decision to provide mammography screening for women under the age of 50 may be influenced by health care setting policy, provider beliefs and practices, patient request, and patient risk factors, such as family history and previous breast findings. Although this debate is of concern for all women, it is of particular concern for African American women. African American women under the age of 45 years have a higher incidence of breast cancer than Caucasian women.

C. YES. Presence and onset of pain in the breast should be ascertained. One of the most important physical symptoms of breast cancer is a painless mass, although breast pain may be present with advanced disease. Approximately 10 percent of women present with breast pain and no mass.

D. *NO.* Chest x-rays are not done routinely at age 45, and would not be expected to contribute to the history.

**QUESTION 2.** What information should be included in the initial history to identify risk factors for breast cancer?

A. *YES.* A personal history of breast cancer, invasive and in situ cancers, increases the lifetime risk of developing breast cancer in the unaffected breast.

B. *YES.* Late age at first live birth and few pregnancies may increase a woman's risk of breast cancer because of the prolonged exposure to hormones, particularly estrogen. Researchers postulate that hormones may promote cell division in breast tissue and increase the risk of mutations.

C. *YES.* Although the relationship between exogenous hormones [estrogen replacement therapy (ERT), or oral contraceptive pills (OCP)] and the development of breast cancer is controversial, a detailed history should include this information. Oral contraceptive pills may explain the diagnosis of breast cancer at young ages and long-term use of ERT may also increase risk. However, research in this area is currently under way.

D. *YES.* Family history of breast cancer is one of the established risk factors for the development of breast cancer, particularly if a first-degree relative (mother, daughter, and/or sister) has a history of breast cancer. An assessment of family history should include age at onset and history of bilateral breast cancer. Genetically influenced breast cancers occur at younger ages and are more likely to be bilateral. Contrary to popular belief, paternal family history of breast cancer has also been linked to the development of breast cancer and needs to be assessed.

E. *YES.* A detailed history should include weight and height measurements. While studies examining the relationship between obesity and breast cancer have been difficult because of measurement issues, obesity, especially in postmenopausal women, has been linked to the development of breast cancer. Of all risk factors, body weight is perhaps the most modifiable. Breast cancer appears to be related to a combination of factors, rather than one single factor. However, while a variety of factors have been associated with the development of breast cancer, these factors have failed to identify approximately 70 to 80 percent of all breast cancer cases. Thus, all women should be considered at risk.

**Question 3.** Based on the history and physical examination, which of the following diagnoses is most likely?
  **A.** *YES.* Breast cancer is the most likely diagnosis, given the family history of breast cancer. The patient's mother was diagnosed with breast cancer in her forties. In addition, a painless, nonmobile mass is characteristic of breast cancer (see Table 28–1 and Fig. 28–1*B*).
  **B.** *NO.* Fibrocystic breast condition is not as likely to be the diagnosis as cancer in this case. Fibrocystic breast condition is characterized by bilateral, multiple painful and somewhat mobile lesions. These symptoms increase during the menstrual cycle (see Fig. 28–1*A*).
  **C.** *NO.* Fibroadenomas are benign breast lesions associated with fibrocystic disease. Fibroadenomas are generally found in women between age 15 and 35 and are characterized by solitary, unilateral fibrous and glandular tissue (see Fig. 28–1*C*).
  **D.** *NO.* Gynecomastia is the enlargement of male breast tissue. Contributing factors include hormonal influences of leukemia, drugs or cirrhosis.

TABLE 28-1   Differentiating Breast Lumps

|  | Fibroadenoma | Benign Breast Disease | Cancer |
|---|---|---|---|
| Likely age | 15–30, can occur up to 55 | 30–55, decreases after menopause | 30–80, risk increases after 50 |
| Shape | Round, lobular | Round, lobular | irregular, star-shaped |
| Consistency | Usually firm, rubbery | Firm to soft, rubbery | Firm to stony hard |
| Demarcation | Well demarcated, clear margin | Well demarcated | Poorly defined |
| Number | Usually single | Usually multiple, may be single | Single |
| Mobility | Very mobile, slippery | Mobile | Fixed |
| Tenderness | Usually none | Tender, usually increases before menses, may be noncyclic | Usually none, can be tender |
| Skin retraction | None | None | Usually |
| Pattern of growth | Grows quickly and constantly | Site may increase or decrease rapidly | Grows constantly |
| Risk to health | None, they are benign—must diagnose by biopsy | Benign although general lumpiness may mask other cancerous lump | Serious, needs early treatment |

Source: Jarvis, C. (1996). *Physical Examination and Health Assessment,* 2nd ed. Philadelphia, PA: W. B. Saunders. With permission.

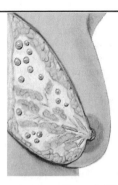
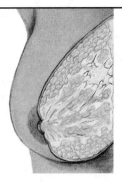

## Benign Breast Disease (Formerly Fibrocystic Breast Disease)

Multiple tender masses. Fibrocystic disease is no longer a useful term because it covers too many entities. Actually, six diagnostic categories exist, based on symptoms and physical findings (Love, 1990b):

- Swelling and tenderness (cyclic discomfort)
- Mastalgia (severe pain, both cyclic and noncyclic)
- Nodularity (significant lumpiness, both cyclic and noncyclic)
- Dominant lumps (including cysts and fibroadenomas)
- Nipple discharge (including intraductal papilloma and duct ectasia)
- Infections and inflammations (including subareolar abscess, lactational mastitis, breast abscess, and Mondor's disease)

About 50% of all women have some form of benign breast disease. Nodularity occurs bilaterally; regular, firm nodules that are mobile, well demarcated, and feel rubbery, like small water balloons. Pain may be dull, heavy, and cyclic or just before menses as nodules enlarge. Some women have nodularity but no pain, and vice versa. Cysts are discrete, fluid-filled sacs. Dominant lumps and nipple discharge must be investigated carefully and may need biopsy to rule out cancer. Nodularity itself is not premalignant, but may produce difficulty in detecting other cancerous lumps.

## Cancer

Solitary unilateral nontender mass. Single focus in one area, although it may be interspersed with other nodules. Solid, hard, dense, and fixed to underlying tissues or skin as cancer becomes invasive. Borders are irregular and poorly delineated. Grows constantly. Often painless, although the person may have pain. Most common in upper outer quadrant. Usually found in women 30 to 80 years of age; increased risk in ages 40 to 44 and in women older than 50 years. As cancer advances, signs include firm or hard irregular axillary nodes; skin dimpling; nipple retraction, elevation, and discharge.

*A*                                    *B*

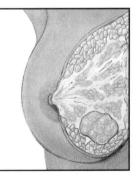

## Fibroadenoma

Solitary nontender mass. A category of benign breast disease that deserves mention due to its frequency and characteristic appearance. Solid, firm, rubbery, and elastic. Round, oval or lobulated; 1 to 5 cm. Freely movable, slippery; fingers slide it easily through tissue. Most common between 15 and 30 years of age, but can occur up to age 55 years. Grows quickly and constantly. Benign, although it must be diagnosed by biopsy.

*C*

FIGURE 28-1.   Breast lump. *A.* Benign breast disease. *B.* Cancer. *C.* Fibroadenoma. (See Color Plate 6*A*–*C*.) Carolyn Jarvis (1996). *Physical Examination and Health Assessment,* 2nd ed. Philadelphia, PA: W. B. Saunders. With permission.

**QUESTION 4.** Which of the following is the *best* diagnostic tool for effectively distinguishing between a benign and a cancerous lesion?

**A.** *NO.* A screening mammogram is a mammogram done to detect suspicious lesions in asymptomatic individuals; it cannot provide reliable results in distinguishing a benign from a malignant lesion. Because Ms. B. presents with symptoms, a diagnostic mammogram, which includes a variety of views with an emphasis on the suspicious area, should be ordered, and a comparison should be made with previous mammograms if available.

**B.** *NO.* Ultrasonography is frequently used to distinguish between a fluid-filled cyst and a solid mass. Ultrasonography may be used in women with dense breast tissue as an adjunct to mammography. Like the mammogram, the ultrasound cannot provide reliable results in distinguishing a benign from a malignant lesion.

**C.** *YES.* The biopsy, generally performed after a mammogram and perhaps after ultrasound, is the only tool that can distinguish a benign lesion from a malignant lesion. While a diagnosis of cancer may be suspected as a result of both physical and mammography findings, a tissue sample by means of a biopsy is essential for confirmation.

**D.** *NO.* A clinical breast examination is an important part of a general physical examination. The American Cancer Society recommends a clinical breast examination annually after age 40. A small percentage of lesions are not visible on mammography but are palpable on examination. The accuracy of a clinical breast examination is dependent upon provider skill and experience. A clinical breast examination cannot provide reliable results in distinguishing a benign from a malignant lesion.

**QUESTION 5.** Which of the following statement(s) is/are true regarding breast cancer in African American women?

**A.** *NO.* While the increases in breast cancer incidence have been largely due to the increased use of screening methods, especially mammography, other factors have also been related to this trend. Researchers also speculate that delayed childbearing, an aging population, and environmental factors may contribute to the increased rates. However, part of this increase in cancer incidence is due to the detection of asymptomatic cancers in both African American women and Caucasian women.

**B.** *NO.* There are no specific guidelines for African American women. Generally, the National Cancer Institute (NCI) and the American Cancer Society (ACS) screening guidelines are targeted toward all asymptomatic women. Currently, the ACS recommends the following:

> Age 20–39, monthly BSE, clinical breast examination every 3 years
> Age 40–49 monthly BSE, annual clinical breast exam, annual mammography, as well as a baseline mammogram by age 40
> Age 50+, monthly BSE, annual clinical breast examination, annual mammography

These guidelines apply to all women regardless of ethnicity. In 1997, the ACS changed its mammography guidelines for women age 40 to

49 to annually, rather than every 1 to 2 years. This change may be viewed favorably because of the higher incidence of breast cancer among African American women under age 50.

C. *YES.* While breast cancer is the second leading cause of cancer death for all American women, it is the leading cause of cancer death among African American women. In numerous studies, when compared with their Caucasian counterparts, African American women were less likely to present with breast cancers at an early stage, when the potential for cure was greatest. Recent statistics revealed that the relative 5-year survival rate for African American women was 69 percent compared to 84 percent for Caucasians, primarily because of the late stage at diagnosis. Breast cancer mortality is distributed disproportionately among the socioeconomically disadvantaged, many of whom are African American women. These and other findings highlight the tremendous need for promoting early detection among this population.

D. *NO.* Overall, the risk of developing breast cancer is influenced by a variety of factors for both African American women and Caucasian women. Both groups of women are at risk for developing breast cancer as they age. The risk of developing breast cancer increases with age, particularly after the age of 50.

## REFERENCES

American Cancer Society. (1996). *Breast Cancer Facts and Figures—1996.* Atlanta: Author.

Barkauskas, V. H., Stoltenberg-Allen, K., Baumann, L. C., Darling-Fisher, C. (1994). *Health and Physical Assessment.* St. Louis: Mosby.

Dow, K. H. (ed.). (1996). *Contemporary Issues in Breast Cancer.* Boston: Jones and Bartlett Publishers.

Harris, J. R. Morrow, M., Lippman, M. E., Hellman, C. (1996). *Diseases of the Breast.* Philadelphia: Lippincott-Raven.

Hogstel, M. O., Keen-Payne, R. (1996). *Practical Guide to Health Assessment throughout the Lifespan.* Philadelphia: F. A. Davis.

McCorkle, R., Grant, M., Frank-Stromborg, M., Baird, S. (1997). *Cancer Nursing: A Comprehensive Textbook.* Philadelphia: W. B. Saunders Company.

Wellis, L. A. (1996). *Modern Breast and Pelvic Examination.* New York: National Council on Women's Health, Inc.

# 29

# Acute Sinusitis

*Marilyn Scott*
*Marie Lindsey*

Maria M. is a 46-year-old Latina who is employed as a grocery store manager and resides in a suburban setting. She is being seen today for an acute care visit. She was last seen 6 months ago for her well-woman care. Her physical examination at that time was normal, and she was taking no medications.

## CHIEF COMPLAINT
"I've had a cold for the past week, and it's getting worse."

## HISTORY OF PRESENT ILLNESS
Initially, the cold began with rhinorrhea and occasional cough. Since last night, she has had a headache, facial pain that increases with bending, thick, white nasal discharge, decreased appetite, and a fever. She has tried over-the-counter cold remedies with no improvement.

## PAST MEDICAL HISTORY
No known allergies, no history of major illnesses, asthma, frequent colds, sinus infections, hospitalizations, or surgeries.

## PHYSICAL FINDINGS
Vital signs: Temperature 37.4°C (100°F), pulse 84, respiration 22, blood pressure 128/70.

General
appearance: Appears ill and tired.

Head/neck: Tenderness with percussion over the maxillary sinuses; bilateral lymphadenopathy.

Eyes: Watery.

Ears: Tympanic membranes pearly gray, landmarks visualized.

Nose: Edema and erythema of turbinates with mucopurulent rhinorrhea.

Oropharynx: Mucous membranes pink, moist, no tonsillar edema or exudate; mucopurulent postnasal drip; halitosis present.

QUESTION 1. What diagnostic tests are appropriate at this time?
   A. Plain sinus radiography
   B. Computed tomography (CT) scan
   C. Transillumination
   D. Sinus puncture and aspiration
   E. Nasal endoscopy

## ASSESSMENT

QUESTION 2. What is the likely diagnosis?
   A. Acute sinusitis
   B. Allergic rhinitis
   C. Upper respiratory infection (URI)
   D. Chronic sinusitis

QUESTION 3. Most children and adults with acute sinusitis are infected with which of the following organisms?
   A. *Streptococcus pneumoniae, Haemophilus influenzae,* or *Moraxella catarrhalis*
   B. Group A or C beta-hemolytic streptococci, *Streptococcus viridans*, peptostreptococci, or *Eikenella corrodens*
   C. *Staphylococcus aureus*
   D. Rhinovirus

QUESTION 4. Which sinuses are most likely infected in Ms. M.?
   A. Ethmoid
   B. Maxillary
   C. Frontal
   D. Sphenoid

## PLAN

QUESTION 5. In addition to an analgesic with an antipyretic effect, which of the following classifications of medication would be considered in the treatment plan? (Select all that apply.)
   A. Antibiotic
   B. Oral decongestant
   C. Antihistamine
   D. Intranasal steroid
   E. Mucoevacuant

QUESTION 6. Besides medications, what other recommendations could be included in the treatment plan? (Select all that apply.)
   A. Warm, moist soaks over the maxillary sinus
   B. Steam inhalation, vaporizer/humidifier, saline nasal spray, increased oral fluids
   C. Eating yogurt
   D. Smoking cessation, adequate rest, and balanced nutrition

**QUESTION 7.** Which of the following antibiotics should be used as first line treatment? (Select all that apply.)
  A. Amoxicillin 500 mg, 1 tablet orally t.i.d. for 10 to 14 days
  B. Trimethoprim and sulfamethoxazole (160/800 mg),1 tablet orally b.i.d. for 10 to 14 days
  C. Amoxicillin with clavulanate potassium 500/125 mg, 1 tablet orally t.i.d. for 10 to 14 days
  D. Clarithromycin 500 mg, 1 tablet orally b.i.d. for 10 to 14 days

**QUESTION 8.** When should referral to a specialist be considered? (Select all that apply.)
  A. Treatment failure after two courses of appropriate antibiotics
  B. More than three episodes in a year
  C. Immunocompromised host
  D. Deterioration of patient's condition

## ANSWERS

**QUESTION 1.** What diagnostic tests are appropriate at this time?
  A. *NO.* Plain sinus radiographs are of questionable value because not all sinuses are visualized. There is no consensus on how standard radiography should be used by primary care providers in the initial clinical evaluation of acute sinusitis. Many experts believe that imaging is an unwarranted expense when a high clinical suspicion for sinusitis exists and the patient has not been previously treated.
  B. *NO.* Although a CT scan has increased sensitivity over plain films, it should be reserved for patients in whom maximal medical therapy has failed. Some 85 percent of patients with colds have abnormalities on CT scan that resolve spontaneously in 2 weeks. If a scan done while the patient is symptomatic is absolutely benign, the symptoms are not the result of sinusitis.
  C. *YES.* Transillumination of the frontal and maxillary sinuses is a noninvasive procedure that may be helpful in diagnosing disease in adolescents and adults. In children less than 10 years of age, the increased thickness of both the soft tissue and the bony vaults limits the clinical usefulness of transillumination. However, as with any transillumination, practice is necessary and accuracy is controversial. Transillumination results are reported as opaque (no light transmission), dull (reduced light transmission), or normal (light transmission typical of a normal subject).
  D. *NO.* Although the "gold standard" for diagnosis is sinus aspiration and culture, it is appropriate only for patients with complications or refractory sinusitis.
  E. *NO.* Nasal endoscopy is reserved for recurrent acute or chronic sinusitis.

**QUESTION 2.** What is the likely diagnosis?
  A. *YES.* Five independent predictors of sinusitis are maxillary toothache, abnormal transillumination, poor response to decongestants, and a history or examination finding of purulent nasal discharge. If all five clinical

predictors are present, there is a 92 percent probability of sinusitis. However, research has also found that the provider's overall clinical impression was superior to any single historical or physical finding. The most common clinical scenario is the presence of signs and symptoms of a URI extending beyond the typical 7 to 10 days, or symptoms that are more severe than usual. Although headache and facial pain can be seen in patients with a URI or allergic rhinitis, these tend to be more of a pressure sensation and less severe than those encountered in acute sinusitis. Populations at increased risk for sinusitis include those who have recently recovered from diabetic acidosis, those who have been intubated or had a nasogastric tube, those who are HIV positive, and those who have asthma.

**B.** *NO.* Allergic rhinitis is characterized by an itchy and runny nose; paroxysmal sneezing; thin, watery nasal discharge; nasal obstruction; and nasal congestion.

**C.** *NO.* Although Ms. M.'s present symptoms follow an apparent URI, her present symptoms indicate that she is suffering from a subsequent acute sinus infection.

**D.** *NO.* Chronic sinusitis is defined as sinus inflammation lasting more than 8 to 12 weeks or lasting longer than 4 weeks after medical therapy, as seen by radiographic imaging. Chronic sinusitis differs from acute sinusitis in that chronic sinusitis has nasal congestion and discharge as its major symptoms. Pain and headache are usually absent or mild, and fever is not typical.

**QUESTION 3.** Most children and adults with acute sinusitis are infected with which of the following organisms?

**A.** *YES.* In sinusitis that progresses to acute infection, the most common pathogens are *Streptococcus pneumoniae, Haemophilus influenzae,* and *Moraxella catarrhalis.* In one study, *S. pneumoniae* was the organism in 20 to 35 percent of the cases, *H. influenzae* in 6 to 26 percent, and *M. catarrhalis* in 2 to 19 percent. In patients with acute sinusitis, 75 percent of the cultures obtained by antral puncture contained either *H. influenzae* or *S. pneumoniae.*

**B.** *NO.* In a recent study, group A or C beta-hemolytic streptococci, *S viridans,* peptostreptococci, and *Eikenella corrodens* did not account for any of the cases of sinusitis.

**C.** *NO. Staphylococcus aureus* accounted for only 0 to 8 of the cases of sinusitis in a recent study.

**D.** *NO.* While rhinoviruses are responsible for many URIs, they are rarely implicated in the development of sinusitis.

**QUESTION 4.** Which sinuses are most likely infected in Ms. M.?

**A.** *NO.* Pain or pressure that is felt at the inner canthus, tenderness at the medial edge of the eye over the lacrimal fossa, and headache that is periorbital or temporal suggest that the probable site of infection is the ethmoid sinus. Coughing, straining, and the supine position typically exacerbate the pain; raising the head upright improves the pain.

   **B.** *YES.* Pain that is periorbital, is felt over one cheekbone or is like a toothache, tenderness that is evoked over the maxillary sinus, and headache that is temporal suggest that the probable site of infection is the maxillary sinus. Purulent secretions are seen most often in the middle meatus. The head in the upright position exacerbates the pain, whereas the supine position improves pain. The maxillary sinus is the sinus most frequently infected in adults.

   **C.** *NO.* If pain is evoked over the frontal sinus or by pressing up against the floor of the frontal sinus, and the headache is severe and frontal, the probable site of infection is the frontal sinus. The supine position exacerbates pain, whereas the head in the upright position improves the pain.

   **D.** *NO.* If the headache has multiple foci or is occipital plus frontal, temporal, retroorbital, or at the vertex, the probable site of infection is the sphenoid sinus. The supine position, bending forward, or Valsalva effort exacerbates pain, whereas the upright position improves pain.

**QUESTION 5.** In addition to an analgesic with an antipyretic effect, which of the following classifications of medication would be considered in the treatment plan? (Select all that apply.)

   **A.** *YES.* Antibiotics are the conventional baseline therapy for acute sinusitis. However, very recent studies indicate that acute maxillary sinusitis appears to have a good prognosis whether or not it is treated with antibiotics. Although more of the antibiotic group improved than of the placebo group, most of the differences were not significant. However, side effects (rash or gastrointestinal symptoms) were significantly more common with the antibiotic used in the study (amoxicillin).

   **B.** *YES.* Oral decongestants are baseline therapy for acute sinusitis. Blockage of the sinus ostia appears to initiate the cycle of events leading to sinusitis, and decongestants may help to maintain ostial patency. The sequence of sinusitis is inflammation of the nasal mucosa, leading to occlusion of the sinus ostia leading to obstruction of mucus outflow, leading to sinusitis. Pseudoephedrine and phenylpropanolamine are the oral decongestants usually chosen. These alpha-adrenergic receptor agonists reduce nasal blood flow and may maintain ostial patency through a decongestant effect deep within the ostiomeatal complex. When taken at recommended doses in patients with stable hypertension, oral agents do not cause clinically significant changes in blood pressure. If insomnia occurs, the medication should be taken only in the morning. Nasal decongestants, such as oxymetazoline hydrochloride 0.05%, can also be used. However, use should be limited to no more than 3 days, as rebound congestion can occur with longer usage.

   **C.** *NO.* Allergy, long believed to be an initiating factor, is now considered to be relatively unimportant as a cause of sinusitis. Therefore, antihistamines are rarely indicated, unless the patient's history strongly suggests an underlying allergic component. Furthermore, the use of antihistamines should also be avoided because their drying effect may thicken secretions and worsen outflow obstruction.

D. *NO.* Intranasal steroids reduce inflammation and edema, but are indicated for use with allergic rhinitis, not with sinusitis, as they can take up to 3 weeks before becoming effective. Oral steroids are not indicated.

E. *YES.* Mucoevacuants may also help maintain ostial patency. The most frequently used is guaifenesin, which comes in capsules, tablet, liquid, and syrup forms. For adults and children over 12 years, dose recommendation is 100 to 400 mg q 4 h, not to exceed 2.4 g/day; children 6 to 12 years: 100 to 200 mg q 4 h, not to exceed 1.2 g/day; and children 2 to 6 years: 50 to 100 mg q 4 h, not to exceed 600 mg/day. If nausea occurs, the dose should be decreased.

**QUESTION 6.** Besides medications, what other recommendations could be included in the treatment plan?

A. *YES.* Warm, moist soaks over the maxillary sinus help to liquefy and mobilize mucus.

B. *YES.* Steam inhalation, a vaporizer/humidifier, saline nasal spray, and increased oral fluids also help to liquefy and mobilize mucus.

C. *YES.* Daily ingestion of yogurt with active cultures or acidophilus may help prevent some of the diarrheal effects of certain antibiotics and may also decrease the incidence or severity of yeast infections.

D. *YES.* Smoking cessation, rest, and nutrition contribute as both primary and secondary prevention.

**QUESTION 7.** Which of the following antibiotics should be used as first-line treatment?

A. *NO.* In the past, amoxillicin was considered the first-line agent for sinusitis due to its broad spectrum of coverage and its low cost. However, because of the proliferation of beta-lactamase-producing organisms throughout many communities, amoxicillin as a single-agent therapy is no longer recommended as the drug of choice.

B. *YES.* Trimethoprim and sulfamethoxazole (Bactrim DS, Septra DS) continue to be an effective first-line treatment for sinusitis. They are the only inexpensive antibiotics that offer a fairly high rate of cure for beta-lactamase-producing *H. influenzae.*

C. *YES.* Amoxicillin with potassium clavulanate (Augmentin) is now considered the first-line treatment of sinusitis because of its effectiveness against beta-lactamase-producing organisms, which seem to be prevalent throughout many communities. However, a common side effect of Augmentin is gastrointestinal upset; therefore, it is recommended that it be taken with food. Furthermore, it is more expensive than amoxicillin preparations without clavulanate.

D. *NO.* Clarithromycin (Biaxin) is too expensive for initial treatment, but would be appropriate to treat sinusitis that is unresponsive to first-line therapy. It is indicated for patients with a history of severe penicillin allergy.

**QUESTION 8.** When should referral to a specialist be considered?

A. *YES.* Treatment failure after two courses of appropriate antibiotics may indicate an underlying disorder. Referral to an otolaryngologist for further evaluation would be appropriate at that time. On the other hand, evidence that the sinusitis is from a dental source should initiate a prompt referral to a provider who performs root canal or drainage of periapical abscesses.

B. *YES.* Chronic sinusitis that is unresponsive to medical treatment and recurrent acute sinusitis can be a result of abnormalities of the osteomeatal complex. Referral to an otolaryngologist for evaluation with possible endoscopic sinus surgery may be indicated to restore sinus drainage.

C. *YES.* The clinical presentation of sinusitis in immunocompromised patients, particularly those with severe leukopenia, may be subtle, making an early diagnosis difficult and increasing the likelihood of a fulminant and fatal course. Because of these risks and because fungal origins may be suspected, the immunocompromised patient should be referred to an otolaryngologist earlier in the treatment course.

D. *YES.* Clinical deterioration of a patient suggests the presence of possible complications of sinusitis: subdural empyema, frontal lobe abscess, intrahemispheric abscess, cavernous and superior sagittal sinus thrombosis, orbital cellulitis, and osteomyelitis. Such complications warrant surgical intervention by an otolaryngologist. Symptoms can include fever, malaise, frontal headache, change in mental status, vomiting, or severe facial swelling.

## REFERENCES

Chow, J. M. (1995). The diagnosis and management of sinusitis. *Comp Ther 21*(2), 74–79.

Ferguson, B. J. (1995). Acute and chronic sinusitis. *Postgrad Med 97*(5), 45–57.

Haugen, J. R., Ramlo, J. H. (1993). Serious complications of acute sinusitis. *Postgrad Med 93*(1), 115–125.

Lewis, C. M. (1994). Protocol for acute and chronic sinusitis. *College Health 42*, 237–239.

Mickelson, S. A., Benninger, M. S. (1996). The nose and paranasal sinuses. In J. Noble (ed.), *Textbook of Primary Care Medicine*, 2d ed., 425–444. St. Louis: Mosby.

Sanford, J. P., Gilbert, D. N., Moellering, R. C., Sande, M. A. (1997). *The Sanford Guide to Antimicrobial Therapy*. Vienna, VA: Antimicrobial Therapy, Inc.

Schwartz, R. (1994). The diagnosis and management of sinusitis. *Nurse Pract 19*(12), 58–63.

Simon, H. (1995). Approach to the patient with sinusitis. In A. Goroll, L. May, A. Mulley, Jr. (eds.), *Primary Care Medicine*. Philadelphia: J. B. Lippincott, 1004–1007.

Williams, J. W., Simel, D. L. (1993). Does this patient have sinusitis? *JAMA 270*, 1242–1246.

Williams, J. W., Simel, D. L., Roberts, L., Samsa, G. P. (1992). Clinical evaluation for sinusitis. *Ann Intern Med 117*, 705–709.

Wilson, J. (1994). Current approaches to sinusitis. *Practitioner 238*, 467–472.

# 30

# Back Pain

*Sharon E. Muran*
*Marie Lindsey*

Ms. C. is a 42-year-old African American female. She works 40 h a week as a geriatric staff nurse. She is employed in a large urban hospital that has recently experienced staff reduction. She uses mass transportation and walks several blocks to reach her job. Ms. C. is a single parent with two active children, ages 4 and 8. This is her first visit to this clinic.

## CHIEF COMPLAINT

"I've had low back pain for 1 week and it just doesn't get any better."

## HISTORY OF PRESENT ILLNESS

Ms. C.'s back pain began 1 week ago following an unaided transfer of an elderly, frail man from his bed to a wheelchair. She feels a constant aching pain across her lower back and down into her buttocks. The pain is always present when sitting, but worsens with bending. She has continued to work and keep up with her daily activities, but came in today because "the pain is not improving."

QUESTION 1. To complete the history of present illness (HPI), additional inquiry would include which of the following? (Select all that apply.)
    A. Nature and onset of pain
    B. Aggravating and alleviating factors of pain
    C. Previous history of back problems
    D. Occupational history and work environment

**QUESTION 2.** A pertinent review of systems would include which of the following? (Select all that apply.)
A. Constitutional symptoms of weight loss, chills, and fever
B. Bladder/bowel problems or paresthesias
C. History of cancer
D. History of depression

## PAST MEDICAL HISTORY

Ms. C. has no known allergies and no history of major illnesses, surgeries, fractures, injuries, or previous back problems.

## PHYSICAL FINDINGS

| | |
|---|---|
| Vital signs: | Temperature 36.6°C (98.6°F), pulse 78, regular; respirations 18; blood pressure 120/76; height 5 ft 4 in; weight 190 lb. |
| General: | African American female; appears most comfortable standing for interview. |
| Back: | Cervical spine, thoracic spine, and lumbosacral (LS) spine symmetrical, no atrophy; erect posture, normal lordotic curve.Cervical spine range of motion (ROM) within normal limits. Thoracic and LS spine ROM indicates normal extension; flexion produces pain at 70° at the level of L4-L5.L-S spine tender at L4-L5 extending bilaterally to paravertebral muscles. No point of maximum tenderness (PMT). No sciatic notch sensitivity.No cervical or thoracic pain on palpation. No costovertebral angle tenderness. |
| Lower extremities: | Full ROM of knees and ankles and feet, no atrophy noted. Thigh and calf circumferences equal bilaterally. Muscle strength: Full extension of quadriceps, normal dorsiflexion and plantar flexion of great toes and feet. |
| Neurological: | Deep tendon reflexes within normal limits. Cutaneous sensation of anterior thigh, lateral calf, and lower lateral foot intact bilaterally. Straight leg raising (SLR) produces pain at 75° bilaterally at L4-L5 with radiation to buttocks (see Fig. 30-1); no increase of pain on dorsiflexion or internal rotation of feet. No crossover pain; sitting knee extension negative (see Fig. 30-2). Able to squat and rise, normal heel walking and toe walking bilaterally. |

**QUESTION 3.** Which of the following best describes Ms. C.'s SLR test findings? (Select all that apply.)
A. Her SLR testing is negative for nerve root compression.
B. The sitting knee extension test does not relate to her SLR test results.
C. The results of having her walk on her toes and heels indicate nerve root compression.
D. Her negative results on crossover testing contributes to ruling out nerve root compression.

QUESTION **4.** Which of the following should be obtained to establish a diagnosis? (Select all that apply.)

A. Plain x-ray of the LS spine.
B. Complete blood count (CBC), erythrocyte sedimentation rate (ESR), and urinalysis (UA).
C. Further diagnostic testing is not indicated with symptoms of less than 4 weeks' duration.
D. Computed tomography (CT) or magnetic resonance imaging (MRI).

(1) Ask the patient to lie as straight as possible on a table in the supine position.

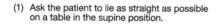

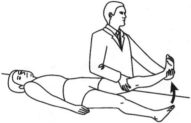

(2) With one hand placed above the knee of the leg being examined, exert enough firm pressure to keep the knee fully extended. Ask the patient to relax.

(3) With the other hand cupped under the heel, slowly raise the straight limb. Tell the patient, "If this bothers you, let me know, and I will stop."

4) Monitor for any movement of the pelvis before complaints are elicited. True sciatic tension should elicit complaints before the hamstrings are stretched enough to move the pelvis.

(5) Estimate the degree of leg elevation that elicits complaint from the patient. Then determine the most distal area of discomfort: back, hip, thigh, knee, or below the knee.

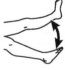

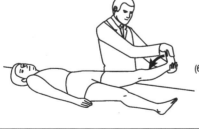

(6) While holding the leg at the limit of straight leg raising, dorsiflex the ankle. Note whether this aggravates the pain. Internal rotation of the limb can also increase the tension on the sciatic nerve roots.

FIGURE 30-1.   Instructions for the straight leg raising (SLR) test. U.S. Department of Health and Human Services. *Acute Low Back Problems in Adults: Assessment and Treatment.* AHCPR Publication No. 0643, December 1994.

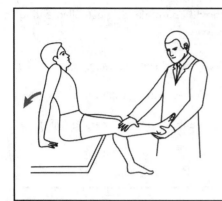

With the patient sitting on a table, both hip and knees flexed at 90 degrees, slowly extend the knee as if evaluating the patella or bottom of the foot. This maneuver stretches nerve roots as much as a moderate degree of supine SLR.

FIGURE 30-2.   Instructions for sitting knee extension test. U.S. Department of Health and Human Services. *Acute Low Back Problems in Adults: Assessment and Treatment.* AHCPR Publication No. 0643, December 1994.

## ASSESSMENT

QUESTION 5. Which one of the following is the appropriate diagnosis? (Select all that apply.)
  A. Sciatica with nerve root compression
  B. Infection of the LS spine
  C. Vertebral fracture
  D. Cauda equina syndrome
  E. Lumbosacral strain

## PLAN

QUESTION 6. Which of the following elements of a short-term treatment plan would be appropriate? (Select all that apply.)
  A. Bed rest—supine position for 4 days
  B. Ice or heat for pain relief
  C. As pain abates, isometric tightening exercises of abdominal and gluteal muscles
  D. Over-the-counter (OTC) nonsteroidal anti-inflammatory drugs (NSAIDs), in the absence of ulcer or aspirin intolerance
  E. Follow-up in 7 to 10 days for moderate to severe pain; referral in 4 weeks for evaluation of persistent pain

QUESTION 7. Which of the following should be discussed with Ms. C. regarding her employment? (Select all that apply.)
  A. It is important that she report the injury/problem to the employer.
  B. The employer should be contacted about Mrs. C.'s returning to work with restrictions.
  C. A copy of Ms. C.'s job description should be sent to the clinic to be included in the patient record.
  D. Ms. C. should seek Workers' Compensation indemnity benefits if time off is required.

QUESTION **8.** In future appointments, counseling should include which of the following? (Select all that apply.)
A. Preventive exercises
B. Avoiding heavy lifting
C. Instruction in proper lifting and body mechanics
D. Weight reduction

## ANSWERS

QUESTION **1.** To complete the history of present illness, additional inquiry would include which of the following?
A. *YES.* The nature and mode of onset of pain are important clinical clues to the diagnosis of back problems. Sudden pain is an indicator of severity and is more likely to be associated with rupture or acute pressure on a disk. Gradual pain is more likely related to repetitive stress and soft tissue trauma. Constant unremitting pain, especially night pain or pain unrelieved by bed rest, indicates the need to rule out cancer. A sense of pressure associated with pain is suspicious for nerve root irritation. The extent, location, and distribution of radiating pain are subjective symptoms that should be objectively quantified by tests of sensation and range of motion (ROM). Sciatica, a sharp or burning pain radiating down the posterior or lateral aspect of the leg to the ankle or foot, is the symptomatic hallmark of clinically significant disk herniation. Therefore, radiating pain is often related to sciatica and various other neuromusculoskeletal diagnoses of varying severity, whereas nonradiating pain may be limited to injury of soft tissue.
B. *YES.* Identifying aggravating and alleviating factors is important in back pain. In terms of position changes, mechanical pain is relieved when supine, whereas pain that is worse at night or unimproved with bed rest indicates the need to rule out infection or tumor. Pain or spasm associated with coughing, sneezing, or straining suggest nerve root compression. Movement that results in pain can help localize the cause of the pain. Weather changes related to increased pain and stiffness are associated with arthritic conditions. Medication use and response is an important, but not strong, diagnostic indicator, since most musculoskeletal pain will be relieved to some degree with anti-inflammatory drugs (NSAIDs) regardless of whether the cause is arthritic, soft tissue strain or trauma, or disk-related. However, the degree of response to medications is a better indicator of the severity of the condition.
C. *YES.* A history of previous back problems is a key part of the HPI, since the risk for reinjury is great, particularly in the first 6 months after an injury. Repeated episodes of self-diagnosis and treatment must also be considered, since they are suggestive of chronicity. Identifying activities associated with previous episodes will aid in detecting problems associated with poor body mechanics and repetitive trauma. For example, pain that is worsened by standing, walking, or other activities that cause spinal extension is characteristic of spinal stenosis.
D. *YES.* The occupational history and work environment are very important to the HPI. Previous back injuries and problems reported at

work need to be carefully investigated, since the physical demands of the job, the patient's capacity to perform them, the patient's perceptions of the job, and attitudes about the work environment help to identify psychological and social factors that have been found to be significant in the recovery from back problems and in their recurrence.

**QUESTION 2.** A pertinent review of systems would include which of the following?

A. *YES.* Although back pain resulting from infection is rare, it is an important cause to detect. The constitutional symptoms of weight loss, chills, and fever suggest infection, and have special meaning in the intravenous drug user, diabetic, or immune-suppressed patient. Common sources of infection include urinary tract infection, skin abscess, and an indwelling catheter.

B. *YES.* A herniated intervertebral disk with resulting nerve root compression may present with the following: sciatica, paresthesias, dysesthesias, hypoesthesias, anesthesias, paresis, sphincter problems, pelvic pain, painful sex, and impotence. Compression of the lower portion of the nerve roots inferior to the spinal cord proper, known as cauda equina syndrome, is a rare *surgical emergency* whose signs include central back pain associated with weakness of the leg muscles, impotence, urinary frequency, urinary retention (sometimes with overflow), incontinence, loss of sphincter tone, and saddle anesthesia (reduction in sensation over the buttocks, upper posterior thighs, and perineum). Cauda equina syndrome requires immediate referral to an orthopedist or neurosurgeon.

C. *YES.* The most common spinal tumor is *metastatic carcinoma*, which often presents with waist-level or midback pain of insidious onset, gradually increasing in severity and aggravated by activity. About 80 percent of patients with spinal tumors are older than 50 years of age. Although only 30 percent of patients with spinal tumors give a history of previous cancer, those who do have a high probability of spinal metastasis. Breast, lung, prostate, gastrointestinal, and genitourinary neoplasms often metastasize to the spine. A history of prior malignancy and insidious increase in midback pain that is not relieved by lying down is highly predictive of metastatic tumor.

D. *YES.* Patients with depression may present complaining of chronic low back pain. Often there is a history of previous back problems or onset at the time of a minor injury, with depression amplifying the presentation and prolonging the clinical course. Characteristically, the intensity of complaints and degree of disability are much greater than the minor limitations found on examination.

**QUESTION 3.** Which of the following best describes Ms. C.'s SLR test findings?

A. *YES.* Ms. C.'s SLR test of 75° is negative for nerve root compression because a positive SLR test requires a sharp, burning, sciatic pain to be produced when raising the leg between 30 and 60°.

B. *NO.* A sitting knee extension test does relate to an SLR test in that a *positive* sitting knee extension test is an affirmation of a *positive* SLR.

Conversely, as Ms. C.'s knee extension test was *negative*, it is an affirmation of her *negative* SLR test. The sitting knee extension is usually done following the supine SLR and is often used to rule out symptom amplification or malingering.

C. *NO.* That Ms. C. was able to perform toe and heel walking bilaterally indicates that she does *not* have nerve root compression. Compression radiculopathy of the S1 root by L5-S1 disk herniation is associated with weakness of plantar flexion, best demonstrated by the patient's having difficulty walking on his or her toes. Dorsiflexion weakness is associated with L5 radiculopathy from L4-L5 disk herniation, and is demonstrated by the patient's having difficulty walking on his or her heels.

D. *YES.* Crossover or contralateral pain on the SLR test does contribute to the differential diagnosis of nerve root compression and is an even stronger indication than pain on the affected side. Ms. C.'s physical examination was negative for crossover pain, further supporting the premise that she does not have nerve root compression.

QUESTION 4. Which of the following should be obtained to establish a diagnosis?

A. *NO.* X-rays of the LS spine are not indicated in the absence of a history or signs of a fracture.

B. *NO.* Complete blood count, ESR, and UA would be useful at this stage only when signs of infection or tumor are present.

C. *YES.* In the absence of indicators of serious illness, further diagnostic testing is not indicated in symptoms of less than 4 weeks' duration. The majority of these cases actually respond with no treatment, and testing at this point is not clinically useful.

D. *NO.* Expensive tests such as a CT scan or an MRI are not indicated, since there are no signs of cauda equina syndrome or other conditions of an emergency nature. In fact, an MRI at this time might actually obscure the diagnosis. Reviews of adults who have had an MRI indicate that as many as 30 percent with positive readings had no clinical disease and were asymptomatic at the time the test was taken.

QUESTION 5. Which one of the following is the appropriate diagnosis?

A. *NO.* The absence of pain radiation to the lower extremities, a negative SLR, and normal sensory distribution indicate that there is no evidence of sciatica with nerve root compression.

B. *NO.* Infection of the LS spine is ruled out by the absence of fatigue, chills, and fever.

C. *NO.* The absence of trauma, absence of a PMT, and a history negative for cancer or autoimmune problems rule out fracture of the LS spine.

D. *NO.* Cauda equina syndrome is ruled out by the negative history of genitourinary and bowel complaints, sciatica, saddle anesthesia, and weakness of the leg muscles, and by the absence of significant physical examination findings.

E. *YES.* Lumbosacral strain is the accurate diagnosis based upon negative review of systems and physical examination.

QUESTION 6. Which of the following elements of a short-term treatment plan would be appropriate?

A. *NO*. Bed rest is not indicated in the absence of severe pain or herniated disk. If it were indicated, it should be limited to no more than 2 days; studies indicate that bed rest beyond 2 days actually contributes to atrophy and deconditioning. Work and activities of daily living (ADLs) should be adjusted for short-term avoidance of lifting of weights greater than 20 lb; and repeated bending, twisting, and reaching; and prolonged sitting.

B. *YES*. Immediately following the onset of pain, ice is the most efficacious, but given the time elapsed since the onset of pain (1 week), either ice or heat may be helpful in relieving pain. The choice is the patient's, since this is primarily a comfort measure.

C. *YES*. Isometric tightening exercises of abdominal and gluteal muscles are the first step in the introduction of exercise therapy, as they help to maintain muscle strength. The exercises should begin as soon as intense pain decreases, and can be practiced even by those on bed rest.

D. *YES*. Over-the-counter NSAIDs are the hallmark medication for musculoskeletal pain and have been found to be very efficacious. In cases of severe pain, the following other NSAIDs may be ordered: naproxen (Naprosyn) 500 mg initially, followed by 250 mg every 6 to 8 h, or piroxicam (Feldene) 20 mg every day. For those suffering intense pain, Tylenol #3 (1 to 2 tablets) four times a day may be prescribed for a short time (i.e., 1 to 2 days) and/or used at bedtime to aid with sleep. Research is inconclusive as to the benefits of muscle relaxants, but if the patient has muscle spasms, the following may be used: cyclobenzaprine hydrochloride (Flexeril) 10 mg every day to three times a day; methocarbanol (Robaxin) two tablets, 750 mg each, four times a day, then 750 to 1000 mg four times a day. This may be most beneficial at bedtime. All medications must be closely monitored and restricted to short-term use. Tylenol #3 and muscle relaxants are not appropriate for use in the operation of machinery or in the workplace.

E. *YES*. Follow-up is clearly indicated so that progress may be monitored, complications detected, and rehabilitation intensified as appropriate. Follow-up on a 7- to 10-day frequency is usual for moderate to severe pain. If pain remains unchanged 4 weeks following onset, the patient should be referred for additional evaluation.

QUESTION 7. Which of the following should be discussed with Ms. C. regarding her employment?

A. *YES*. Reporting the injury/problem to the employer provides the employee with access to the benefits afforded by Workers' Compensation. Reporting should occur immediately after a work-related injury or illness to ensure coverage for medical costs and lost time.

B. *YES*. A key element in recovery from a back injury is the avoidance of disability. Maintenance of ADLs, including work, is actually an important part of therapy. It is the provider's responsibility to actively participate in and help to guide the return to work process from a safety and health perspective. The patient should be advised of his or her part in the process and encouraged to ask the employer about returning to work with restrictions.

C. *YES.* A job description is essential in assessing the potential for safe return to work. The job description will help determine whether the patient should return to work in a restricted or transitional duty position. It should be objectively quantified with respect to the physical demands of the essential functions of the job. The provider's responsibility is to identify what the patient can safely do and how long the employee is anticipated to require restrictions. This information must be clearly communicated to the employee and provided in writing to the employer. The employer makes the determination about his or her ability to accommodate the employee in a restricted or transitional duty position.

D. *YES.* Assuming that the injury is truly work-related, if time off from work is medically indicated, the employee should notify the employer, submit the written order for time off to the employer, and complete the necessary forms to receive payment for lost time (e.g., indemnity).

**QUESTION 8.** In future appointments, counseling should include which one of the following?

A. *YES.* Preventive exercises, especially aerobic conditioning such as walking and swimming, help to avoid debilitation. These exercises produce no more stress than an equal amount of time spent sitting and can be gradually increased to 20 to 30 min daily within the first 2 weeks. Patients should be counseled that symptoms may seem somewhat more apparent when exercise is first begun and that the exercise routine may be modified to accommodate the patient. Conditioning exercises for trunk muscles do help in regaining activity tolerance, but are more mechanically stressful than aerobic exercises. Therefore, such exercises should not begin until 3 to 4 weeks have elapsed from the onset of injury.

B. *NO.* Given this diagnosis and the anticipated uncomplicated recovery, there is no indication that the patient will not be able to return to heavy lifting as required by her job. Actually, in regard to the risk for reinjury, the amount of weight is less of an issue than the manner in which it is lifted, as well as the frequency of the tasks. Guidelines for unassisted lifting are as given in Table 30-1.

C. *YES.* Instruction in proper lifting and body mechanics is essential in the prevention of reinjury. Workplaces have become very involved in this area, especially for high-risk jobs such as staff nursing. It is not unusual for an employee who has suffered a work-related back injury to be required to attend a back prevention program prior to clearance for return to full duty. The patient should be counseled to inquire about the availability of these programs.

D. *YES.* Obesity places stress on the supportive muscles of the abdomen and back. Weight reduction counseling is indicated to assist the patient in the prevention of future back injuries.

TABLE 30-1   Guidelines for Sitting and Unassisted Lifting

| | Symptoms | | | |
|---|---|---|---|---|
| | Severe | Moderate | Mild | None |
| Men | 20 lb | 20 lb | 60 lb | 80 lb |
| Women | 20 lb | 20 lb | 35 lb | 60 lb |

SOURCE: Bigos, S., Bowyer, O., Braen, G., et al. (1994). Acute Low Back Problems in Adults: Clinical Practice Guidelines, Quick Reference Guide for Clinicians, No. 14. AHCPR Publication No. 95-0643. Rockville, MD: Agency for Health Care Policy and Research, Public Health Service, Department of Health and Human Services.

## REFERENCES

Bigos, S., Bowyer, O., Braen, G., et al. (1994). *Acute Low Back Problems in Adults: Clinical Practice Guideline No.14.* AHCPR Publication No. 95-0642. Rockville, MD: Agency for Health Care Policy and Research, Public Health Service, Department of Health and Human Services.

Bigos, S., Bowyer, O., Braen, G., et al. (1994). *Acute Low Back Problems in Adults: Clinical Practice Guidelines, Quick Reference Guide for Clinicians, No.14.* AHCPR Publication No. 95-0643. Rockville, MD: Agency for Health Care Policy and Research, Public Health Service, Department of Health and Human Services.

Boyd, R. J. (1995). Evaluation of back pain. In A. H. Goroll, L. A. May, A. G. Mulley, (eds.), *Primary Care Medicine: Office Evaluation and Management of the Adult Patient,* 742–751. Philadelphia: J. B. Lippincott.

Foreman, L. (1997). Orthopaedics: Back pain. In L. Rucker, (ed.), *Essentials of Adult Ambulatory Care,* 539–545. Baltimore: Williams & Wilkins.

Hefferman, J. J. (1996). Low back. In J. Noble (ed.), *Textbook of Primary Care Medicine,* 1026–1040. St. Louis: Mosby.

Seller, R. H. (1996). *Differential Diagnosis of Common Complaints.* Philadelphia: W. B. Saunders.

Uphold, C. R., Graham, M. V. (1993). *Clinical Guidelines in Family Practice.* Gainesville, FL: Barmarrae Books.

# 31

# Anxiety

*Laina M. Gerace*
*Arlene Miller*

Doris J., a 53-year-old Caucasian woman, presents to her urban HMO with vague complaints of insomnia, restlessness, and fatigue. Mrs. J. has been widowed for 2 years. Mrs. J.'s daughter accompanies her and describes her mother as "more worried than usual."

## CHIEF COMPLAINT

"I've been worried and tired and have had trouble relaxing and sleeping through the night for the past 6 months."

## HISTORY OF PRESENT ILLNESS

Mrs. J.'s symptoms began about 6 months ago, soon after she sold the family home of 20 years and moved to the city to be closer to her daughter and grandchildren. Her history reveals no recent illnesses or history of serious or chronic illnesses. She has gone for regular checkups and is on postmenopausal hormone-replacement therapy. Mrs. J. states that she was "alcohol dependent" when she was in her 40s, but that she "has been in recovery" and has been abstinent for over 10 years with no relapses.

QUESTION 1. Which of the following would help to complete the history of present illness (HPI) regarding Mrs. J.'s vague complaints of fatigue and restlessness? (Select all that apply.)
  A. Additional somatic symptoms
  B. Heat or cold intolerance
  C. Weight loss or gain
  D. Last menstrual period

QUESTION 2. Which of the following information about Mrs. J.'s complaint of insomnia would be helpful? (Select all that apply.)
A. Caffeine consumption patterns
B. Diurnal sleep pattern
C. Onset, middle, or terminal insomnia
D. Snoring and frequent awakenings

QUESTION 3. What additional health history is needed to complete the HPI? (Select all that apply.)
A. Previous treatment for psychiatric disorders
B. Description of the onset and nature of her "worrying"
C. Previous response to stressful situations
D. Adjustment to the loss of her husband

## ADDITIONAL HISTORY

Appetite normal, no weight loss or gain, able to carry out household work and care for grandchildren. Able to enjoy activities and friendships.
Substance abuse: Daughter corroborates that Mrs. J. is alcohol- and drug-free and has been abstinent for over 10 years.
Nature and onset of "worrying": Mrs. J.'s worries center on routine circumstances, such as household chores (what if the washing machine breaks down?), her grandchildren (what if they get hurt?), and her social life (what if her friends don't like her anymore?). These worries are pervasive and are distressful to Mrs. J. because they preoccupy her and interfere with her ability to fall and stay asleep.
Cognitive functioning: No memory problems, concentration impaired.

## PHYSICAL FINDINGS

General:     Face appears strained and tired. No psychomotor agitation noted.
Vital signs:  All are normal, except pulse is 90, which is higher than her usual pulse rate of 76.

Laboratory tests, including complete blood count, urinalysis, gamma-glutamyltransferase (GGT), and thyroid function tests, are normal.

QUESTION 4. Based on the objective data above, which is the appropriate diagnosis?
A. Major depression
B. Primary sleep disorder
C. Obsessive-compulsive disorder
D. Somatization disorder
E. Generalized anxiety disorder

## PLAN

QUESTION 5. Which prescription medications may be appropriate for Mrs. J.? (Select all that apply.)
A. Alprazolam
B. Buspirone

C. Imipramine
D. Haloperidol

QUESTION **6.** Which interventions are appropriate for Mrs. J.? (Select all that apply.)
A. Relaxation training.
B. Cognitive behavioral therapy.
C. Evaluate for cardiac problems.
D. Explain that anxiety is "all in your head."

## ANSWERS

QUESTION **1.** Which of the following would help to complete the HPI regarding Mrs. J.'s vague complaints of fatigue and restlessness?
A. *YES.* Complaints of seemingly unrelated somatic symptoms, such as muscle tension, dry mouth, nausea, urinary frequency, headaches, and difficulty swallowing may indicate an anxiety-related disorder.
B. *YES.* While less likely, Mrs. J.'s complaints could indicate a thyroid dysfunction. Cold intolerance and fatigue may occur in hypothyroidism, heat intolerance and restlessness may occur in hyperthyroidism.
C. *YES.* Weight loss or gain can occur in psychiatric disorders, especially depression, as well as in thyroid dysfunction.
D. *NO.* Mrs. J. has been followed for postmenopausal hormone-replacement therapy; therefore, this information is not needed to evaluate her current complaints. It would be appropriate to question her about compliance with hormonal therapy.

QUESTION **2.** Which of the following information about Mrs. J.'s complaint of insomnia would be helpful?
A. *YES.* Caffeine-containing beverages such as coffee and colas can cause "wired" or anxious symptoms. Their stimulating effects interfere with induction of sleep and may reduce REM sleep, causing the person to not feel restored after sleep. Other drugs associated with insomnia include bronchodilators, alcohol, some antidepressant medications, and thyroid medications.
B. *YES.* Diurnal sleep pattern refers to daytime sleeping in addition to nighttime sleeping. Mrs. J.'s sleeping pattern could be due to her moving to a new environment; however, as people age, they tend to awaken more frequently during the night and make up for the lack of sleep by napping more during the day. Furthermore, some women have sleep changes as part of menopausal changes, although hormone-replacement therapy may ameliorate this problem.
C. *YES.* Sleep problems are typical in both anxiety disorders and depression. Anxiety disorders are usually associated with difficulty falling asleep, whereas depression is more often associated with a pattern of middle-of-the-night or early-morning awakenings.
D. *YES.* Breathing-related sleep disorders are often accompanied by heavy snoring and frequent awakenings. Sleep apnea is usually caused by obstruction of the upper airway. The soft palatal tissue and muscles of

the upper airway collapse during sleep. Obesity can contribute to this blockage, as can alcohol and sleeping pills. Patients stop breathing for 30 s to 2 min many times a night. Oxygen saturation decreases significantly during these periods, causing the person to gasp and awaken to resume breathing. The person will be exhausted during the day.

**QUESTION 3.** What additional health history is needed to complete the HPI?
- **A.** *YES.* History of treatment for previous psychiatric disorders would shed light on whether or not Mrs. J. is predisposed to anxiety or depression, since many of these disorders are characterized by relapses.
- **B.** *YES.* Worrying is found in a variety of anxiety-related disorders, but the nature of the worrying varies. Panic disorders are characterized by worries about having another attack; obsessive-compulsive disorders, by concern about germs, money, and/or contamination; hypochondriasis, by preoccupation with illnesses; depression, by ruminations of inadequacy. Generalized anxiety disorders are characterized by pervasive apprehensive expectation and worry about routine life events, such as daily activities, job and family responsibilities, and social events.
- **C.** *YES.* Because Mrs. J. has made a recent major life change by selling her home and moving to an urban area, data about how she normally handles stressful events would be useful. Anxiety-related disorders and depression can be triggered by stressful events.
- **D.** *YES.* Mrs. J. has been widowed for 2 years. Normal grieving lasts up to 2 years. Data about how she is adjusting to widowhood would be helpful in evaluating her symptoms.

**QUESTION 4.** Based on the objective data above, which is the appropriate diagnosis?
- **A.** *NO.* While major depression needs to be considered, the above data do not support that diagnosis. Mrs. J. has experienced no changes in weight and is able to carry out daily activities. Her insomnia seems to be due to excessive worrying about daily events, a symptom more characteristic of generalized anxiety disorder.
- **B.** *NO.* While Mrs. J. has insomnia, it appears to be secondary to symptoms of anxiety. A diagnosis of primary insomnia is not given if the symptoms are due to a mental disorder, a medical condition, or substance use or abuse.
- **C.** *NO.* While Mrs. J.'s worrying preoccupies her, it does not fit the description of obsessive-compulsive disorder. Obsessions are persistent, recurrent thoughts or images that cause marked anxiety or distress. These thoughts are not simply excessive worries about real-life problems, but are more intrusive in nature. For example, the person may be plagued by thoughts and images of something gruesome.
- **D.** *NO.* Somatization disorder is characterized by physical symptoms that cannot be fully explained by medical findings or known physiology. Somatic symptoms in generalized anxiety disorder tend to reflect central nervous system tension. In someone with somatization disorder, if there are medical problems, complaints about symptoms are

beyond what would be expected in the condition. Typical symptoms of somatization disorder include clusters of complaints such as vomiting, difficulty swallowing, muscle and limb pains, weakness, dizziness, vague internal pains, burning sensations, dysmenorrhea, and shortness of breath. Mrs. J.'s symptoms do not follow this pattern.

**E.** *YES*. Mrs. J.'s symptoms are typical of generalized anxiety disorder and fit the DSM-IV criteria for this disorder. Criteria include excessive anxiety and worry about a number of daily events or activities, occurring more days than not for at least 6 months, and at least three of the following symptoms: restlessness or feeling keyed up, fatigue, impaired concentration, irritability, muscle tension, sleep disturbance. Mrs. J.'s symptoms do not seem to be due to any physical condition or substance abuse problems. Further, Mrs. J.'s daughter characterizes Mrs. J. as "more worried than usual," indicating that Mrs. J. tends to be an anxious person. About half of adults who seek treatment for generalized anxiety disorder report that symptoms of anxiety started before 20 years of age. Overall lifetime prevalence of this disorder is about 5 percent (3 to 4 percent in men; 6 to 7 percent in women). Usually these patients present in primary care settings, and often the diagnosis is overlooked.

**QUESTION 5.** Which prescription medications may be appropriate for Mrs. J.?

**A.** *NO*. Alprazolam is a benzodiazepine. Benzodiazepines are not appropriate for Mrs. J. because of her history of alcoholism, as these agents are cross-addicting with alcohol. If Mrs. J.'s anxiety was overwhelming to the point of jeopardizing her health and safety, she might be offered a brief course of alprazolam with an explanation about the addiction potential, given her history. Benzodiazepines are, however, appropriate for treatment of generalized anxiety disorders in those patients who are not at risk for addiction. Care must be taken because tolerance and withdrawal can occur. Dosages should be monitored and tapered before discontinuing.

**B.** *YES*. Buspirone, an azapirone with serotonergic inhibitory effects, is an approved medication for generalized anxiety disorder and is superior to benzodiazepines in several ways. Buspirone targets the symptoms of worry, apprehension, irritability, difficulty concentrating, cognitive slowing, and indecision, rather than creating a tranquilizing effect. Buspirone is a safe medication that has no euphoriant effects or withdrawal syndrome. It does not tend to cause muscle relaxation, fatigue, or sedation, and it does not interact with alcohol. Efficacy generally lags behind that of benzodiazepines, and patients need to be advised of its slow onset. Sometimes people who have been treated with benzodiazepines find it difficult to accept buspirone because the effects are not immediate. Patient education is essential.

**C.** *YES*. While not the first medication of choice, imipramine is a tricyclic antidepressant that has shown effectiveness in treating anxiety disorders, especially panic disorder and agoraphobia. Imipramine alleviates symptoms of anxiety, interpersonal sensitivity, paranoia, and depression. When given before bedtime, it also enhances sleep. Disadvantages include unpleasant side effects such as drowsiness, dizziness, dry mouth, and constipation. Tricyclics do interact with alcohol, but Mrs. J. has been abstinent for over 10 years.

**D.** *NO.* Haloperidol is a neuroleptic (antipsychotic) medication used to treat acute and chronic psychosis, Tourette's syndrome, and (in children) severe behavior problems. This would be an inappropriate medication choice for Mrs. J., since her symptoms are clearly not psychotic.

**QUESTION 6.** Which interventions are appropriate for Mrs. J.?

**A.** *YES.* Relaxation training can be effective in the treatment of generalized anxiety disorder, although it has not been shown to be as effective as cognitive behavioral approaches. Relaxation training is more effective than nondirective therapy. The relaxation training should be specific to anxiety control.

**B.** *YES.* Cognitive behavioral therapy focuses on bringing the worry process itself under the patient's control and incorporates problem-solving strategies to address sources of anxiety. Cognitive behavioral therapy has been shown to be effective in most anxiety disorders; however, patients must do homework and be amenable to cognitive strategies. Some dependent persons prefer to "take a pill" rather than invest in the self-discipline needed to successfully engage in cognitive therapy.

**C.** *YES.* Because Mrs. J.'s pulse is elevated and cardiac problems are associated with anxiety disorders, it would be wise to evaluate for potential heart problems such as atrial fibrillation or mitral valve prolapse (usually associated with panic attacks).

**D.** *NO.* Anxiety disorders are considered medical conditions, and any attitudes that threaten the patient's self-esteem and sense of integrity should be avoided. Acceptance of the patient's symptoms and providing adequate treatment decreases unnecessary diagnostic work-ups and increases the patient's quality of life.

## REFERENCES

Barlow, D. H., Lehman, C. L. (1996). Advances in the psychosocial treatment of anxiety disorders: Implications for national health care. *Arch Gen Psychiatry* 53(8), 727–735.

Bell, J. A. (1996). Generalized anxiety disorder. In J. L. Jacobson, A. M. Jacobson (eds.), 88–91. *Psychiatric Secrets*. Philadelphia: Hanley & Belfus.

Goldberg, R. J. (1995). Diagnostic dilemmas presented by patients with anxiety and depression. *Am J Med, 98*(3), 278–284.

Kelter, N. L., Folks, D. G. (1997). Psychotropic Drugs. St. Louis: Mosby.

Maxmen, J. S., Ward, N. G. (1995). *Essential Psychopathology and Its Treatment*. New York: W.W. Norton.

Pi, E. H., Gross, L. S., Nagy, R. M. (1994). Biochemical factors in anxiety and related disorders. In B. B. Wolman, G. Stricker (eds.), *Anxiety and Related Disorders*. New York: J. Wiley.

# 32

# Diabetes

*Terese M. Bertucci*
*Marie Lindsey*

Mrs. Adeline M., a 55-year-old Caucasian patient, has an appointment today at her suburban health center. She was last seen 6 months ago for her yearly physical. At that time, her physical examination was normal, but she was approximately 20 lb overweight. Routine tests, including a complete blood count (CBC), fasting blood sugar (FBS), lipid profile, blood urea nitrogen (BUN), creatinine, liver function tests, Papanicolaou (Pap) smear, and mammogram were normal. She was referred to a dietician and asked to start brisk walking to tolerance and increase gradually; however, she has not been following the diet or exercise program. She has been otherwise healthy and takes no medication. She has come to the health center today because she is not feeling well.

## CHIEF COMPLAINT

"I've been urinating more for the past several weeks, especially this past week, and I've been really tired for several weeks, too."

## HISTORY OF PRESENT ILLNESS

Mrs. M. states she had been waking up once during the night to urinate for several weeks. This past week the frequency has increased to two to three times a night, and she has also needed to urinate more frequently during the day. She has been very thirsty, but feels she is urinating more than she is drinking. She has been feeling hungrier than usual and seems more tired, especially after meals. Yesterday she felt so tired after lunch that she took a nap at her desk at work. She has been trying to get at least 8 h of sleep per night, but it doesn't seem to help.

QUESTION 1. Information on which of the following should be elicited to complete the history of present illness regarding Mrs. M.'s urinary symptoms? (Select all that apply.)
   A. Urinary urgency or dysuria
   B. Vaginal discharge
   C. Fever
   D. Back pain

QUESTION 2. Which of the following information would help complete the HPI for Mrs. M.'s symptoms of fatigue? (Select all that apply.)
   A. Weight history (gain or loss)
   B. Shortness of breath
   C. Hearing loss
   D. Sleep patterns

QUESTION 3. If diabetes mellitus is suspected, additional history should include which of the following? (Select all that apply.)
   A. Family history
   B. Gestational history
   C. Smoking history
   D. Diet history

## PHYSICAL FINDINGS

General:     Middle-aged, overweight, white female in no acute distress.
Vital signs: Temperature 36.5°C (97.8°F), pulse 80, respirations 20, blood pressure, 122/84, weight: 165 lb (74.9 kg)—a weight loss of 10 lb since last visit, height: 67 in. (170 cm), body mass index: 26. Urine dipstrick: glucose 3+; negative for white blood cells (WBCs), red blood cells (RBCs), ketones, and nitrites. Postprandial fingerstick for glucose: 344 mg/dL.
Eyes:        Pupils equal, round, reactive to light: extraocular movements intact. Funduscopic: disk margins sharp, no exudates, vessels normal.
Heart:       Apical pulse 80, regular rate and rhythm; no murmurs; no $S_3$, no $S_4$.
Lungs:       Clear to auscultation, anteriorly and posteriorly. No costovertebral angle (CVA) tenderness bilaterally.
Abdomen:     Normal bowel sounds in all four quadrants; no tenderness, no masses, no organomegaly.

QUESTION 4. Which of the following should also be included in the examination? (Select all that apply.)
   A. Thyroid examination
   B. Gross hearing test
   C. Breast examination
   D. Oral examination
   E. Skin examination

Mrs. M. was instructed to obtain a fasting glucose the next morning, which was 215 mg/dL.

## ASSESSMENT

**QUESTION 5.** Which one of the following is the most likely diagnosis for Mrs. M.?
A. Hypothyroidism
B. Pyelonephritis
C. New-onset diabetes mellitus type 2
D. New-onset diabetes mellitus type 1

## PLAN

**QUESTION 6.** Which one of the following would be the initial treatment of choice for Mrs. M.?
A. Diet and exercise only
B. Glyburide (Micronase) 10 mg b.i.d.
C. Metformin (Glucophage) 500 mg with breakfast
D. 70/30 insulin 35 units ½ h before breakfast and 25 units ½ h before dinner
E. Trimethoprim and sulfamethoxazole (Bactrim DS) b.i.d. × 7 days

**QUESTION 7.** In addition to the fasting glucose, what other tests should have been ordered when Mrs. M. returned the next day? (Select all that apply.)
A. Hb $A_{1c}$
B. A blood chemistry panel that includes electrolytes, and cholesterol
C. Urinalysis
D. Thyroid function tests
E. Electrocardiogram (ECG)

**QUESTION 8.** Which would be appropriate in the management plan at this point? (Select all that apply.)
A. Nutritional therapy
B. Sliding scale for insulin adjustment
C. Recommendations for appropriate physical activity
D. Reinforcement regarding the importance of regular follow-up

**QUESTION 9.** What additional information would this patient require regarding her disease? (Select all that apply.)
A. Basic pathophysiology
B. Signs and symptoms of high and low blood glucose and what to do
C. Information regarding her medication
D. Information regarding self-monitoring of blood glucose
E. Breast self-examination

## ANSWERS

**QUESTION 1.** Information about which of the following should be elicited to complete the HPI regarding Mrs. M.'s urinary symptoms?
A. *YES.* Symptoms of urgency and dysuria along with frequent voiding, usually of small amounts of urine, would point to a urinary tract infection (UTI). Frequent voiding of large amounts of urine, or polyuria, is associated with poorly controlled diabetes. However, as diabetics are more prone to UTIs, these two conditions may coexist.

B.  *YES.* Vaginal infections can also cause urinary symptoms, so this needs to be ruled out as the cause of the patient's urinary symptoms.
C.  *YES.* Since fever is often present with UTIs, a history of fever needs to be elicited to help rule out infection as the cause of the patient's symptoms.
D.  *YES.* Flank pain, referred to in common terms as "back" pain, is often present with pyelonephritis. This should be asked of any patient with urinary tract symptoms.

QUESTION 2. Which of the following information would help complete the HPI for Mrs. M.'s symptoms of fatigue?
A.  *YES.* Fatigue associated with weight loss, polyuria, polydipsia, and polyphagia are classic symptoms of diabetes mellitus. Fatigue associated with weight loss and/or anorexia may indicate depression or carcinoma. Symptoms of fatigue associated with significant weight gain may indicate hypothyroidism.
B.  *YES.* Symptoms of fatigue associated with shortness of breath may indicate congestive heart failure or anemia.
C.  *NO.* Hearing loss is not associated with fatigue.
D.  YES. Fatigue may be the result of inadequate sleep as a result of nocturia, depression, or metabolic disorders, such as thyroid disease or diabetes mellitus.

QUESTION 3. If diabetes mellitus is suspected, additional history should include which of the following?
A.  *YES.* Diabetes is more prevalent in patients with a family history of diabetes.
B.  *YES.* Patients with gestational diabetes are at increased risk for developing diabetes mellitus later in life.
C.  *YES.* Smoking increases the risk for atherosclerosis in patients with diabetes. If the patient smokes, smoking cessation counseling needs to be part of the treatment plan.
D.  *YES.* Since nutrition therapy is a cornerstone of diabetes management, a diet history is essential. Changes in Mrs. M.'s current diet could make a significant difference in the management of her diabetes.

QUESTION 4. Which of the following should also be included in the examination?
A.  *YES.* Since Mrs M. is complaining of feeling tired, a thyroid examination can rule out an enlarged thyroid or nodules. Fatigue can be a symptom of hypothyroidism.
B.  *NO.* A gross hearing test is unnecessary if the patient is not complaining of hearing loss or ear pain.
C.  *NO.* A breast examination is not necessary, as Mrs. M. had a complete physical examination and a normal mammogram 6 months ago.
D.  *YES.* An oral examination will help to determine if the patient is dehydrated as a result of her polyuria and will rule out gingivitis or other oral infections that sometimes accompany uncontrolled diabetes.
E.  *YES.* A skin examination will help to determine if the patient is hydrated. Also, dry itchy skin can be a symptom of hyperglycemia.

**Question 5.** Which one of the following is the most likely diagnosis for Mrs. M.?

A. *NO*. A definitive diagnosis of hypothyroidism cannot be made until the results of a thyroid function test are obtained; however, Mrs. M.'s constellation of symptoms really points to another diagnosis. If thyroid disease was the most likely suspected reason for Mrs. M.'s fatigue, then the appropriate tests would be a TSH and $T_4$.

B. *NO*. Without fever, pyuria, or CVA tenderness, pyelonephritis is an unlikely diagnosis.

C. *YES*. Mrs. M. presents with the classic symptoms of diabetes: polyuria, polydipsia, and unexplained weight loss. The urine dipstick of 3+ glucose and the fasting plasma glucose (FPG) of 215 mg/dL confirm the diagnosis. An FPG of $\geq$ 126 mg/dL or casual (random) plasma glucose of $\geq$ 180 mg/dL is diagnostic of diabetes.

D. *NO*. Although type 1 diabetes can occur at any age, the fact that this patient is middle-aged, overweight, and not ketotic with such a high blood glucose rules out type 1 diabetes.

**Question 6.** Which one of the following would be the initial treatment of choice for Mrs. M.?

A. *NO*. Although diet and exercise should be instituted, the degree to which Mrs. M.'s blood sugar is elevated and the fact that she is so symptomatic warrant pharmacologic intervention. As her diabetes comes more under control, it may be possible to discontinue medication.

B. *NO*. Micronase is an appropriate treatment for a new type 2 diabetic, but not at the dose listed, which is the maximum dose. Micronase should be started at 2.5 to 5.0 mg once daily.

C. *YES*. Glucophage, one of the newer diabetes medications, is a good choice for this patient at the starting dose of 500 mg daily. It needs to be taken with food to decrease gastrointestinal side effects. One of the side effects of this drug is a decrease in appetite which may help Mrs. M. with weight loss. Use of Glucophage should be avoided in patients with renal dysfunction, liver dysfunction, history of alcohol abuse, acute or chronic metabolic acidosis, disease states that can increase tissue hypoxia/renal insufficiency, and pregnancy. The patient's history and normal blood chemistries performed 6 months ago suggest no contraindications for Mrs. M.

D. *NO*. The insulin dosage listed in this answer is too high. A new-onset type 2 diabetic with a moderately high glucose who is not ketotic is usually started on one of the new oral hypoglycemic agents such as Glucophage. Recently, however, some experts have recommended that new type 2 diabetics start on insulin when plasma glucose levels are over 300, beginning with a low dose of an intermediate insulin such as NPH, using 5 units 30 min before breakfast and increasing by 5 units based on the FPG response.

E. *NO*. Since the patient is not febrile and has no CVA tenderness or pyuria, there is no need to start an antibiotic.

**QUESTION 7.** In addition to the fasting glucose, what other tests should have been ordered when Mrs. M. returned the next day?

**A.** *YES.* A baseline Hb $A_{1c}$ (also called glycated or glycosylated hemoglobin or glycohemoglobin) should be obtained. It should be rechecked quarterly in uncontrolled diabetics and one to two times per year in well-controlled patients. A Hb $A_{1c}$ level reflects the state of an individual's glycemia in the preceding 2 to 3 months (see Table 32-1).

**B.** *YES.* While it is unlikely that Mrs. M.'s chemistries would show a significant change from the values of 6 months ago, a new baseline should be obtained. In particular, Mrs. M.'s creatinine should be monitored for renal dysfunction. Glucophage should not be continued if the patient's creatinine is above 1.5 mg/dL. Lipids should also be checked to assess additional cardiovascular risk, as elevations in lipids, particularly triglycerides, are common in diabetes (see Table 32-1).

**C.** *YES.* A complete urinalysis should be done yearly in all diabetics to assess for protein, particularly in this patient with her predominant urinary symptoms. An office dipstick alone is not sufficient because reagent strips are subject to possible errors from alterations in urine concentration. A positive test by reagent strip must be confirmed by more specific testing.

**D.** *NO.* Thyroid function tests should not be done in a patient with type 2 diabetes unless specific symptoms of thyroid disease are present. However, in type 1 diabetes, assessment of thyroid function is appropriate. Both thyroid disease and type 1 diabetes mellitus are considered autoimmune disorders. Having one can predispose an individual to other autoimmune disorders. Coexistence of more than one disorder can also occur.

**E.** *YES.* The American Diabetes Association (ADA) recommends baseline ECGs on all newly diagnosed diabetics because of the additional cardiovascular risk incurred with the disease.

TABLE 32-1   Guidelines for Diabetes Care 1

| Assessment | Frequency | Goal | Action Required[a] |
|---|---|---|---|
| Glycated Hgb | Every 6 months if | | |
| Hb $A_{1c}$ | ≤ action required level: | ≤ 7% | >8% |
| other | every 3 months if greater | ≤1% above upper limit of normal | >2% above upper limit of normal |
| LDL-C | Yearly or more often | | |
| CAD absent | as necessary | ≤ 130 mg/dL | >160 mg/dL |
| CAD present | | ≤100 mg/dL | >130 mg/dL |
| TG | Yearly or more often | ≤200 mg/dL | >400 mg/dL |

[a]If target level exceeded for 1 yr, action (depending on individual patient circumstances) may indicate enhanced diabetes self-management education, comanagement with a diabetes team, referral to an endocrinologist, change in pharmacologic therapy, initiation of or increased SMBG, or more frequent contact with patient.

SOURCE: American Diabetes Association: Clinical Practice Recommendations 1997. *Diabetes Care* 20(suppl 1), 1997.

TABLE 32-2   Guidelines for Diabetes Care 2

| Assessment | Frequency |
|---|---|
| Renal profile | Yearly or more often as necessary<br>• Dipstick for proteinuria<br>— if positive and confirmed, ACE inhibitor unless contraindicated; serum creatinine as appropriate<br>— if negative, evaluation for microalbuminuria; if positive and confirmed, ACE inhibitor unless contraindicated |
| Blood pressure | Minimum every 6 months (or more often as necessary) as long as target level of ≤130/85 mmHg met; if target level exceeded for 1 year, action (depending on individual patient circumstances) may include change in pharmacologic therapy or referral as appropriate |
| Office visit | Minimum every 6 months as long as all action required levels not exceeded and all target levels met; otherwise a contact at least every 3 months |

SOURCE: American Diabetes Association: Clinical Practice Recommendations 1997. *Diabetes Care* *20*(suppl 1), 1997.

QUESTION **8.** Which would be appropriate in the management plan at this point? (See Tables 32-2 and 32-3.)

A. *YES.* Since nutritional therapy is a cornerstone of diabetes management, at least some basic guidelines would be appropriate at this visit. The patient should be scheduled for further diet counseling in the near future, preferably with a registered dietician.

B. *NO.* Since the patient is not starting on insulin, this is not an issue. In addition, a sliding scale would be inappropriate for a newly diagnosed diabetic.

C. *YES.* Mrs. M. should be encouraged to begin a regular aerobic exercise program. Exercise has been found to increase insulin sensitivity, thus improving glycemic control. Furthermore, exercise enhances cardiovascular conditioning. The ADA recommends that all diabetics over 35 have an exercise stress ECG to uncover silent ischemic heart disease prior to embarking on an exercise program.

TABLE 32-3   Guidelines for Diabetes Care 3

| Assessment | Frequency |
|---|---|
| Eye exam | Yearly dilated funduscopic exam in all patients with diabetes except those with type I within 5 years of diagnosis |
| Foot exams | Minimum every 6 months or more often as necessary |
| Weight | Minimum every 6 months |
| Smoking | Yearly; if current smoker, counseling or referral for cessation |

SOURCE: American Diabetes Association: Clinical Practice Recommendations 1997. *Diabetes Care* *20*(suppl 1),1997.

**D.** *YES.* Regular follow-up is essential for optimum management. As a newly diagnosed diabetic, Mrs. M. will have a great deal to learn about comanaging her illness with her health care provider. Regular follow-up is also necessary to address Mrs. M.'s questions and provide emotional support, as anxiety is often high at this time.

**QUESTION 9.** What additional information would this patient require regarding her disease (see Tables 32-2 and 32-3)?

**A.** *YES.* Patients frequently want to know how they got their disease and what it means. A discussion of basic pathophysiology is appropriate at the initial diagnosis.

**B.** *YES.* Mrs. M. needs to be aware of how well her blood sugar is controlled. A measure of control is the presence or absence of symptoms of hyperglycemia and hypoglycemia; thus, this information and the appropriate interventions should be reviewed with her. Though Glucophage alone infrequently causes hypoglycemia, the patient should know the signs and symptoms and what to do. Written information should also be given to the patient to review at home.

**C.** *YES.* Since Mrs. M. is starting on a new medication, she should be instructed on how it works, when to take it, and the side effects in terms she can understand. Glucophage needs to be taken with food to minimize gastrointestinal side effects. The symptoms of lactic acidosis, a rare side effect of Glucophage if prescribed appropriately, should be reviewed briefly and the patient instructed to call immediately if symptoms develop. Onset of symptoms can be subtle and can include malaise, unusual muscle or stomach pain, lightheadedness, respiratory distress, irregular or slow heartbeat, hypothermia, or hypotension.

**D.** *YES.* Monitoring of blood glucose is a vital component of diabetes care. Results from blood glucose monitoring are used to adjust medication, diet, and exercise in order to maintain blood glucose levels as close to normal as safely possible. Research has shown that diabetics who maintain tight control of blood glucose levels are less likely to experience the complications of neuropathy, nephropathy, and retinopathy. The frequency of glucose testing for type 2 diabetics should be individualized, with frequency decreasing as blood glucose goals are maintained. Many blood glucose machine companies offer substantial rebates for their products. They are available at pharmacies, clinics, or individual health care facilities. The patient should be offered this information and can return with a machine at a future visit for teaching. Urine glucose testing may be considered *only* if the patient is unwilling or unable to perform blood glucose testing, as urine testing is less accurate than testing the blood for glucose levels.

**E.** *NO.* Although Mrs. M. should understand the basics of breast selfexamination, such information is not related to a diagnosis of diabetes. Careful follow-up of her diabetes will reveal how she is adapting to her newly diagnosed disease. Once it is clear that she understands diabetes control, other self-care information can be incorporated into health maintenance discussion.

# REFERENCES

American Diabetes Association. (1997). Diabetes and exercise (position statement). *Diabetes Care 20*(Suppl.1), S51.

American Diabetes Association. (1997). Guide to diagnosis and classification of diabetes mellitus and other categories of glucose intolerance (position statement). *Diabetes Care 20*(Suppl.1), S21–S23.

American Diabetes Association. (1997, June). *Highlights from the Report of the Expert Committee on the Diagnosis and Classification of Diabetes Mellitus.*

American Diabetes Association. (1997). Standards of medical care for patients with diabetes mellitus (position statement). *Diabetes Care 20*(Suppl. 1), S5–S13.

American Diabetes Association. (1997). Tests of glycemia in diabetes (position statement). *Diabetes Care 20*(Suppl.1), S18–S20.

Burr, R. E. (1996). Endocrine syndromes. In J. Nobel (ed.), *Textbook of Primary Care Medicine*, 566–573. St. Louis: Mosby.

Chipkin, S. R., Gottlieb, P. A., Bogorad, D. D., Parker, F. (1996). Diabetes mellitus. In J. Noble (ed.), *Textbook of Primary Care Medicine*, 476–497. St. Louis: Mosby.

Lebovitz, H. (1994). *Therapy for Diabetes Mellitus and Related Disorders*, 2d ed. Alexandria, VA: American Diabetes Association.

Physicians' Desk Reference. (1997). Montvale, NJ: Medical Economics Company.

White, J. R. (1997). The pharmacologic management of patients with type II diabetes mellitus in the era of new oral agents and insulin analogs. *Diabetes Spectrum 9,* 227–233.

# 33

# Hypertension

*Marie Lindsey*
*Marie L. Talashek*

Joe D., a 46-year-old African American male, is a supervisor for a large utility company located in the suburb where he lives. Mr. D.'s visits to health care providers have been sporadic over the years. However, he decided to have his blood pressure checked at work when the occupational health nurse offered to do so. His blood pressure reading was 160/104 on that day. At the nurse's urging, Mr. D. sought care at a private practice in his town a week later. He had a complete physical examination at that time, and his blood pressure was still 160/104. He was given advice on lifestyle modifications and advised to return in one month (see Table 33-1).

**TABLE 33-1** Recommendations for Follow-up Based on Initial Blood Pressure Measurements for Adults

| Initial Blood Pressure, mmHg[a] | | Follow-up Recommended[b] |
|---|---|---|
| Systolic | Diastolic | |
| <130 | <85 | Recheck in 2 years |
| 130–139 | 85–89 | Recheck in 1 year[c] |
| 140–159 | 90–99 | Confirm within 2 months[c] |
| 160–179 | 100–109 | Evaluate or refer to source of care within 1 month |
| ≥180 | ≥110 | Evaluate or refer to source of care immediately within 1 week depending on clinical situation |

[a]If systolic and diastolic categories are different, follow recommendations for shorter time follow-up (e.g., 160/86 mmHg should be evaluated or referred to source of care within 1 month).
[b]Modify the scheduling of follow-up according to reliable information about past blood pressure measurements, other cardiovascular risk factors, or target organ disease.
[c]Provide advice about lifestyle modifications.

Source: The Sixth Report of the Joint National Committee on Prevention, Detection, Evaluation, and Treatment of High Blood Pressure (1997). NIH Publication. Washington, D.C.

## CHIEF COMPLAINT

"I'm here for a blood pressure check because it was still high last month."

## HISTORY OF PRESENT ILLNESS

Mr. D. has always considered himself to be in good health, as he has no chronic diseases and takes no medications. He denied headaches, blurred vision, chest pain, shortness of breath, or pedal edema.

**QUESTION 1.** What additional data should be obtained to rule out secondary causes of hypertension in patients with an elevated blood pressure? (Select all that apply.)
    **A.** Urinary symptoms
    **B.** Muscle cramps or weakness
    **C.** Palpitations or excessive perspiration
    **D.** Dietary intake
    **E.** Over-the-counter medications

**QUESTION 2.** Which of the following must be explored in Mr. D.'s. history to identify the risk factors for hypertension? (Select all that apply.)
    **A.** Family history
    **B.** Patient history
    **C.** Lifestyle behaviors
    **D.** Psychosocial and environmental factors

## MEDICAL HISTORY

Mr. D. has smoked one pack of cigarettes a day for 30 years. He drinks five to six beers on Fridays and Saturdays, but denies using street drugs. His job is very sedentary, and he never exercises. A 24-h diet recall reveals an intake of high-fat, high-sodium foods.

## FAMILY HISTORY

Father died at age 60 of a heart attack. Mother, age 70, had a stroke 5 years ago. Sister, age 52, is being treated for hypertension.

## SOCIAL HISTORY

Mr. D. has been married for 25 years and has three daughters, ages 22, 19, and 15, all of whom live at home. As is the case for most of his friends, his job has gotten harder over the years as a result of downsizing. In an area once covered by three supervisors, he is the only one remaining. As a result, what was previously an 8-h workday is now 10 to 12 h. He has not had a raise in five years.

**QUESTION 3.** Which of the following should be included in the physical examination for a person with an elevated blood pressure? (Select all that apply.)
    **A.** Cardiovascular examination
    **B.** Measurement of height, weight, and waist circumference

C. Eye examination
D. Neck examination
E. Abdominal examination

## PHYSICAL EXAMINATION

Vital signs:      Temperature 98.4°F; pulse 84, regular rate and rhythm; respirations 20.
Blood pressures:  160/104 left arm sitting; 162/108 right arm sitting; 160/100 right arm standing.
Height/weight:    5 ft. 10 in. (177.8 cm), 195 lb (88.5 kg).
Funduscopic:      Some arteriovenous (A-V) nicking bilaterally; no hemorrhages, exudates, or papilledema.
Neck:             No jugular venous distention, carotid bruits. Thyroid without nodules or enlargement.
Heart:            Apical impulse at the fifth intercostal space at the mid-clavicular line; $S_1 > S_2$ at apex, no $S_3$ or $S_4$, clicks, or murmurs.
Thorax:           Lungs clear. No costovertebral angle tenderness.
Abdomen:          No bruits, masses, or organomegaly.
Extremities:      Peripheral pulses all 2+ bilaterally. No edema or calf tenderness. Deep tendon reflexes all 2+ bilaterally.

QUESTION 4. Which of the following laboratory tests should be included in the evaluation of all hypertensive patients? (Select all that apply.)
A. Urinalysis
B. Blood glucose
C. Cholesterol level
D. Other blood chemistries
E. Electrocardiography

## ASSESSMENT

QUESTION 5. In light of Mr. D.'s blood pressure readings and physical examination, how would his hypertension be staged?
A. Stage 1
B. Stage 2
C. Stage 2 with target organ disease
D. Stage 3
E. Stage 3 with target organ disease

## PLAN

QUESTION 6. Which of the following nonpharmacologic therapies are important for Mr. D. to follow? (Select all that apply.)
A. Weight reduction
B. Alcohol intake reduction
C. Smoking cessation

D. Dietary changes
E. Hypnotherapy

QUESTION 7. Which of the following classes of medications would be appropriate for Mr. D.? (Select all that apply.)
A. Tranquilizers
B. Beta blockers
C. Diuretics
D. Angiotensin-converting enzyme (ACE) inhibitors
E. Calcium channel blockers (CCBs)
F. Angiotensin II receptor blockers (ARB)

QUESTION 8. If after 3 weeks of continuing nonpharmacologic measures and initiation of pharmacologic measures, Mr. D.'s blood pressure is not below 140/90, what further treatment options would be instituted? (Select all that apply.)
A. Increase the dose of his diuretic
B. Add an $alpha_1$-receptor blocker or alpha-beta blocker.
C. Add a centrally acting $alpha_a$-agonist, a peripheral acting adrenergic antagonist, or a direct vasodilator.
D. Add a CCB.

## ANSWERS

QUESTION 1. What additional data should be obtained to rule out secondary hypertension in patients with an elevated blood pressure?
A. *YES.* There are several secondary causes of hypertension that have urinary symptoms. Polyuria may be present in renal parenchymal disease or primary aldosteronism. Hematuria or flank pain may be presentations of renal vascular disease.
B. *YES.* In addition to polyuria and polydipsia, muscle cramps or muscle weakness may also be symptoms of aldosteronism. Leg claudication may be a symptom of coarctation of the aorta. Patients presenting with muscle weakness associated with fatigue, impotence, amenorrhea, capillary fragility, edema, excess hair growth, truncal adiposity, and purplish striae of the skin should be evaluated for Cushing's syndrome.
C. *YES.* Palpitations, tachycardia, excessive perspiration, severe headaches, and weight loss are all symptoms of pheochromocytoma.
D. *YES.* Sodium intake can contribute to an elevated blood pressure. Furthermore, hypertensive patients should also be asked about excessive consumption of licorice, as it contains glycyrrhetinic acid, which produces a mineralocorticoid-like activity.
E. *YES.* Many over-the-counter medications, and herbal preparations such as pseudoephederine, phenylpropanolamine, and nonsteroidal anti-inflammatory agents, can contribute to an elevated blood pressure. Of course, many commonly recommended prescription medications also can affect the blood pressure, such as oral contraceptives, steroids, bronchodilators, amphetamines and other sympathomimetic drugs, and thyroid hormone.

**QUESTION 2.** Which of the following must be explored in Mr. D.'s. history to identify the risk factors for hypertension?

  A. *YES.* Information should be obtained regarding a family history of high blood pressure, premature coronary heart disease, stroke, diabetes mellitus, and dyslipidemia, and renal disease.

  B. *YES.* The patient's personal history should be explored for evidence of coronary heart disease (CHD), heart failure, cerebrovascular, peripheral vascular, or renal disease; diabetes; dyslipidemia; gout; or sexual dysfunction.

  C. *YES.* Several different lifestyle behaviors must be examined, including history of weight gain; smoking or other tobacco use; intake of sodium, alcohol, saturated fats, and caffeine; and lack of regular exercise.

  D. *YES.* Psychosocial and environmental factors may influence blood pressure control, such as family situation, employment status and working conditions, and educational level.

**QUESTION 3.** Which of the following should be included in the physical examination for a person with an elevated blood pressure?

  A. *YES.* A thorough cardiovascular examination must be performed, including assessing the heart for increased rate, increased size, precordial heave, clicks, murmurs, arrhythmias, and third and fourth heart sounds. Furthermore, the extremities should be examined for diminished or absent peripheral arterial pulsations, bruits, and edema. Two or more blood pressure measurements separated by 2 min with the patient either supine or seated and after standing for at least 2 min should be done. The blood pressure should be verified in the contralateral arm; if the values are different, the higher value should be recorded.

  B. *YES.* Measurement of height and weight is important to determine if the patient is overweight. A body mass index (BMI) equal to or greater than 27 is correlated with increased blood pressure. The BMI is calculated by dividing weight in kilograms by height in meters squared. Waist circumference is used to estimate excess visceral or abdominal fat, which has been associated with risk for hypertension. Specifically a waist circumference of equal to or greater than 39 inches for men and equal to or greater than 34 inches for women has been associated with risk for dyslipidemia, diabetes, and coronary heart disease mortality in addition to hypertension.

  C. *YES.* A funduscopic examination (with pupil dilatation if necessary) is necessary to determine the presence of arteriolar narrowing, arteriovenous nicking, hemorrhages, exudates, or papilledema, all of which suggest target organ damage.

  D. *YES.* The neck should be examined for carotid bruits and distended veins, as well as for an enlarged or nodular thyroid, which would suggest thyroid disease as a possible secondary cause for the hypertension.

  E. *YES.* The abdomen should be examined for bruits, enlarged kidneys, masses, and abnormal pulsations.

**QUESTION 4.** Which of the following laboratory tests should be included in the evaluation of all hypertensive patients?

A. *YES.* A urinalysis should be done to assess for renal disease.
B. *YES.* A fasting blood glucose should be obtained to determine the presence of diabetes, which would greatly add to the risk for cardiovascular disease.
C. *YES.* It is important to obtain a total cholesterol and high-density lipoprotein (HDL) to further assess the patient's risk for cardiovascular disease. Low-density lipoprotein (LDL), and fasting triglycerides are optional tests.
D. *YES.* Other blood chemistries, specifically potassium, sodium, and creatinine, should be performed. Blood calcium and uric acid levels are optional tests. While not definitive, there is some evidence that adequate levels of potassium and calcium are required for blood pressure control. Furthermore, a low potassium level might influence a provider's choice of pharmacological treatment, as would an elevated uric acid level. Elevated creatinine levels indicate renal disease.
E. *YES.* Electrocardiography is helpful in determining left ventricular hypertrophy (evidence of target organ damage) as well as concomitant coronary disease.

**QUESTION 5.** In light of Mr. D.'s blood pressure readings and physical examination, how would his hypertension be staged? (See Table 33-2.)

A. *NO.* Stage 1 (previously called mild) hypertension is reserved for systolic blood pressures of 140 to 159 and diastolic blood pressures of 90 to 99.

**TABLE 33-2   Classification of Blood Pressure for Adults Age 18 and Older[a]**

| Category | Systolic, mmHg | | Diastolic, mmHg |
|---|---|---|---|
| Optimal[b] | <120 | and | <80 |
| Normal | <130 | and | <85 |
| High-normal | 130–139 | or | 85–89 |
| Hypertension[c] | | | |
| Stage 1 | 140–159 | or | 90–99 |
| Stage 2 | 160–179 | or | 100–109 |
| Stage 3 | ≥180 | or | ≥110 |

[a]Not taking antihypertensive drugs and not acutely ill. When systolic blood pressures fall into different categories, the higher category should be selected to classify the individual's blood pressure status. For example, 160/92 mmHg should be classified as stage 2 hypertension, and 174/120 mmHg should be classified as stage 3 hypertension. Isolated systolic hypertension is defined as SBP of 140 mmHg or greater and DBP below 90 mmHg and staged appropriately (e.g., 170/82 mmHg is defined as stage 2 isolated systolic hypertension). In addition to classifying stages of hypertension on the basis of average blood pressure levels, clinicians should specify presence or absence of target organ disease and additional risk factors.
[b]Optional blood pressure with respect to cardiovascular risk is below 120/80 mmHg. However, unusually low readings should be evaluated for clinical significance.
[c]Based on the average of two or more readings taken at each of two or more visits after an initial screening.

SOURCE: The Sixth Report of the Joint National Committee on Prevention, Detection, Evaluation, and Treatment of High Blood Pressure (1997). NIH Publication. Washington, D.C.

Mr. D.'s blood pressures are too high for a stage 1 hypertension diagnosis. It must be noted that in Joint National Committee VI, even 140/90 is too high for diabetic patients; instead, their maximum acceptable blood pressure (above which treatment should be instituted) is 130/84.

B. *NO*. It is true that Mr. D.'s blood pressures are within the stage 2 (previously called moderate) hypertension range: systolic blood pressures of 160 to 179 and diastolic blood pressures of 100 to 109. However, the A-V nicking noted in the funduscopic examination is evidence of target organ damage. Therefore, his full diagnosis should be stage 2 hypertension with target organ disease (A-V nicking). This specificity is necessary for risk classification and management.

C. *YES*. In light of Mr. D.'s blood pressure readings and the presence of funduscopic A-V nicking, his full diagnosis would be stage 2 hypertension with target organ disease (A-V nicking).

D. *NO*. Stage 3 (previously called severe) is reserved for systolic blood pressures equal to or greater than 180 and diastolic blood pressures equal to or greater than 110.

E. *NO*. Mr. D. does have evidence of target organ damage, but his blood pressures are under the criteria set for stage 2 hypertension.

QUESTION 6. Which of the following nonpharmacologic therapies are important for Mr. D. to follow? (See Table 33-3.)

A. *YES*. At 5 ft 10 in and 195 lb, Mr. D. is overweight. His body mass index (BMI) of 28.5 was calculated by dividing his weight in kilograms (88.5) by the square of his height in meters ($5.83^2 = 3.16$). Excess body weight is correlated closely with increased blood pressure. Weight reduction enhances antihypertensive agents and can significantly reduce concomitant cardiovascular risk factors. Therefore, Mr. D. should be encouraged to lose weight through caloric restriction, with a focus on limiting foods that are high in cholesterol and saturated fats, and through increased caloric expenditure by regular physical activity. Often a reduction in blood pressure occurs early during a weight loss program, with as small a weight loss as 10 lb.

B. *YES*. Hypertensive male patients should be encouraged to limit their daily alcohol intake to no more than 1 oz of ethanol (2 oz of 100 proof whiskey, 10 oz of wine, or 24 oz of beer). Hypertensive female patients should limit their daily alcohol intake to half of the recommended amount for males. Mr. D.'s reported alcohol intake of five to six beers on Fridays and Saturdays is typical of many Americans whose alcohol consumption is limited to the weekends. Even though his weekly average of 10 to 12 beers seems within the moderate range, consumption of five to six beers in one day is not acceptable. In addition, he may be underreporting his weekly intake. He should be encouraged to decrease his alcohol intake, since doing so is an inexpensive, safe measure that is likely to contribute to a reduction in blood pressure. If Mr. D. has difficulty reducing his alcohol intake, he should be evaluated and treated for alcohol dependence.

C. *YES*. Nicotine is a vasoconstrictor, and smoking a cigarette causes a significant rise in blood pressure. Current recommendations state

TABLE 33-3   Risk Stratification and Treatment[a]

| Blood Pressure Stages, mmHg | Risk Group A (No Risk Factors; No TOD/CCD)[b] | Risk Group B (At Least 1 Risk Factor, Not Including Diabetes; No TOD/CCD) | Risk Group C (TOD/CCD and/or Diabetes, with or without Other Risk Factors) |
|---|---|---|---|
| High-normal (130–139/85–89) | Lifestyle modification | Lifestyle modification | Drug therapy[c] |
| Stage 1 (140–159/90–99) | Lifestyle modification (up to 12 months) | Lifestyle modification[d] (up to 6 months) | Drug therapy |
| Stages 2 and 3 (≥160/≥100) | Drug therapy | Drug therapy | Drug therapy |

For example, a patient with diabetes and a blood pressure of 142/94 mmHg plus left ventricular hypertrophy should be classified as having stage 1 hypertension with target organ disease (left ventricular hypertrophy) and with another major risk factor (diabetes). This patient would be categorized as **stage 1, risk group C,** and recommended for immediate initiation of pharmacologic treatment.

[a]Lifestyle modification should be adjunctive therapy for all patients recommended for pharmacologic therapy.
[b]TOD/CCD indicates target organ disease/clinical cardiovascular disease.
[c]For those with heart failure, renal insufficiency, or diabetes.
[d]For patients with multiple risk factors, clinicians should consider drugs as initial therapy plus lifestyle modifications.
SOURCE: The Sixth Report of the Joint National Committee on Prevention, Detection, Evaluation, and Treatment of High Blood Pressure (1997). NIH Publication. Washington, D.C.

that blood pressure readings should be taken no less than 30 min after a patient smokes a cigarette. Smoking is also a major risk factor for cardiovascular disease (CVD); furthermore, those who continue to smoke may not receive the full degree of protection against CVD from antihypertensive therapy. Therefore, tobacco avoidance is essential. Mr. D. should receive repetitive messages to quit smoking by attending smoking cessation meetings and/or using a nicotine patch or chewing gum.

D. *YES.* Increased lipid levels pose significant risk for CVD, and fat intake is strongly correlated to increased lipid levels. Therefore, in addition to the overall caloric restriction to achieve weight loss, Mr. D. should be counseled to limit his fat intake to no more than 30 percent of his daily caloric intake (with saturated fat contributing no more than 10 percent of total calories). Furthermore, Mr. D. should limit his sodium intake to no more than 2300 mg per day. Finally, it is recommended that all hypertensive patients maintain an adequate intake of dietary potassium, calcium, and magnesium.

E. *NO.* Although positive effects on blood pressure may be achieved by stress reduction techniques, there is no evidence that hypnotherapy is a preferred modality to control stress and/or that its use would positively affect a patient's blood pressure in any other way.

**QUESTION 7.** Which of the following classes of medications would be appropriate for Mr. D.? (See Fig. 33.1.)

   **A.** *NO.* Although stress can be a factor in hypertension and Mr. D.'s history reveals some job-related stress, there is no evidence that Mr. D. is suffering from an anxiety disorder requiring a tranquilizer. Mr. D.'s ethnic background and family history are major contributing factors in his developing the disease. Furthermore, hypertensive patients must be treated with medications that will have a direct, positive effect on the other cardiovascular components of their disease.

   **B.** *NO.* Although beta blockers are one of the two preferred first-line medications recommended for hypertension, monotherapy using beta blockers is less effective in African Americans. However, in the general population, beta blockers, as well as diuretics, have been shown to reduce cardiovascular morbidity and mortality in controlled clinical trials.

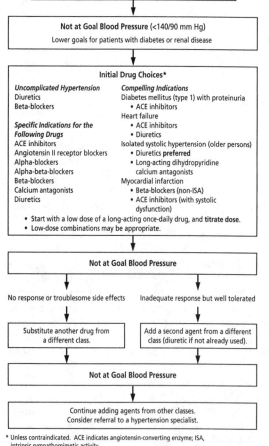

FIGURE 33-1.  Algorithm for the treatment of hypertension. (From *The Sixth Report of the Joint National Committee on Prevention, Detection, Evaluation, and Treatment of High Blood Pressure (1997).* NIH Publication. Washington, D.C.)

Alternative medications such as alpha blockers, alpha-beta blockers, calcium channel blockers (CCB), and ACE inhibitors are equally effective in reducing blood pressure, but diuretics and beta blockers continue to be most recommended as the first-line agents because more long-term data exist regarding their efficacy in reducing morbidity and mortality than with the newer medications. However, there are a few compelling indications (unless contraindicated) in which the new agents are recommended as first-line agents: ACE inhibitors for patients with diabetes mellitus (type 1) with proteinuria; ACE inhibitors and/or diuretics for patients with heart failure; diuretics (preferred) or the calcium channel blocker dihydropyridine for older patients with isolated systolic hypertension; beta blockers (without intrinsic sympathetic activity) for patients with myocardial infarction, or ACE inhibitors for patients with myocardial infarction and systolic dysfunction.

C. *YES.* Diuretics, the other recommended first-line medication (in addition to beta blockers), have been proven in controlled trials to reduce hypertensive morbidity and mortality in African Americans. Thus, diuretics should be the agent of first choice in the absence of other conditions that prohibit their use. Often a low dose of a diuretic (the equivalent of 12.5 mg hydrochlorothiazide) is sufficient to reduce the blood pressure. Patient may select the time of day to take their diuretic that is most convenient in terms of adapting to the diuresis. The common side effects of diuretics are hypokalemia, hyponatremia, gout related to hyperuricemia, impaired glucose tolerance, and small increases in LDL cholesterol and triglyceride levels. However, these side effects are less common with lower doses. Furthermore, in nonedematous patients taking thiazide diuretics, restriction of sodium intake (1.5 to 2 g of elemental sodium, the equivalent of 4 to 6 g of salt) will decrease the risk of hypokalemia in most patients. However, because ventricular ectopy may be precipitated by hypokalemia, patients should have potassium levels assessed at 3 to 4 weeks after initial therapy, and if their level is greater than 3.5 milliequivalents per liter, then twice yearly. Another potential side effect is impotence; however, starting at a low dose reduces its risk. Nonetheless, at subsequent visits, it would be important to assess the medication's effect on Mr. D.'s sexual functioning, so that alternative therapy could be instituted if necessary.

D. *NO.* Monotherapy using ACE inhibitors is less effective in controlling the blood pressures of African Americans. Furthermore, long-term data regarding ACE inhibitors' efficacy in reducing morbidity and mortality in the general population are lacking.

E. *NO.* While calcium channel blockers have been demonstrated to effectively control the blood pressure of hypertensive African Americans, they are not recommended as first-line agents. Diuretics are also very effective in African Americans and have the benefit of more long-term data regarding their efficacy in reducing morbidity and mortality than do CCBs. Furthermore, recent research has revealed life-threatening risks with some CCBs. Immediate-release nifedipine has precipitated ischemic events and in large doses may increase coronary mortality in patients who have had a myocardial infarction. Therefore, this agent should be used only with great caution if at all. There have been inconsistent reports regarding adverse health effects of short-acting or immediate-release formulations of nifedipine, diltiazem hydrochloride, and vera-pamil hydrochloride. Randomized controlled trials are now in progress with long-acting types and formulations of calcium antagonists approved for treatment of hypertension.

F.  NO. Angiotensin II receptor blockers is the newest class of anti-hypertensive agents. The mechanism of action is to block uptake of angiotensin II at the receptor site, whereas ACE inhibitors block the conversion of angiotensin I to angiotensin II in the lungs. One rationale for the development of ARBs is that angiotensin II is produced in loca-tions other than the AI to AII conversion in the lungs. Their other reputed benefit is to provide the efficacy of blood pressure control typical of ACE inhibitors, but without the common ACE-inhibitor side effect of cough. However, early data suggest that ARBs lack the efficacy in African American populations that has been noted with ACE inhibitors.

QUESTION 8. If after 3 weeks of continuing nonpharmacologic measures and initiation of pharmacologic measures, Mr. D.'s blood pressure is not below 140/90, what further treatment options would be instituted?

A.  YES. If Mr. D. was started at the equivalent of 12.5 mg of hydrochloro-thiazide, increasing the dose to 25 mg is a possible second step.

B.  YES. Although beta blockers are less effective in African Americans, alpha$_1$-receptor blockers or alpha-beta blockers are as effective in African Americans as in Caucasian patients. Furthermore, the greater rate of severe hypertension in African Americans often requires that they receive multidrug therapy. Therefore, adding a low dose of one of these agents to his current dose of diuretic has the advantage of lower-ing the blood pressure even further with minimal side effects.

C.  NO. Although, centrally acting alpha agonists, peripheral acting adrener-gic antagonists, and direct vasodilators are effective in controlling the blood pressure, they have many side effects. If the decision is to add a second agent at this time, it would be better to add either an alpha$_1$-receptor blocker, alpha-beta blocker, or a CCB and maintain Mr. D.'s same dose of diuretic.

D.  YES. As CCBs are very effective in controlling the blood pressures of African Americans, adding one of these agents in a low dose would be a logical second step in his treatment.

## REFERENCES

Barker, L., Burton, J., Zieve, P. (eds.). (1995). *Principles of Ambulatory Medicine,* 4th ed. Philadelphia: Williams & Wilkins.

Edwards, W. L. (1997, September). *Cardiovascular Update.* Symposium conducted at the meeting of Nurse Practitioner Associates for Continuing Education, Chicago, IL.

Green, H. L., Hoffman, R. M., Ingelfinger, J. A. (1996). In J. Noble (ed.), *Textbook of Primary Care Medicine,* 2d ed., 170–198. St. Louis: Mosby.

*The Sixth Report of the Joint National Committee on Prevention, Detection, Evaluation, and Treatment of High Blood Pressure (1997).* NIH Publication. Washington, DC: National Heart Lung and Blood Institute, U.S. Department of Health and Human Services.

# VII

## OLDER ADULT

# Introduction

*Arlene Miller*

As a result of increased longevity, older adulthood is divided into the "young-old" (approximately 65 to 85) and "frail-old" (over 85) periods. Health status, however, cannot be predicted from chronological age. Although men and women in the United States can expect to live an average of 15 to 19 years after age 65, there are wide variations in physical and psychological quality of life.

Older adults may express generativity vs. stagnation issues as they engage in transmitting their expertise to younger family members or their communities. Erikson's final developmental crisis, ego integrity vs. despair, is successfully resolved by coming to terms with one's own life decisions or achievements, dealing with loneliness, and ultimately accepting one's own mortality. The increased interiority or introspection that comes during later life does not eliminate the need for continued social participation, however. Developmental tasks of later life include adjusting to changes in physical performance and health. New roles for older adults may include becoming a grandparent or a caregiver to one's spouse. Other changes result from becoming retired or widowed, and from the role reversal that occurs as parents become increasingly dependent on their mature children. An average 7-year difference in life expectancy for women compared to men means that many older women must live alone and perform tasks and responsibilities previously allocated to their husbands.

Although one's ability to adjust to environmental challenges may decrease with age, some degree of autonomy, adaptability, and resilience is still present and can be a measure of successful aging. Mental health reflects the ability to cope with the inevitable disappointments, losses, and conflicts that are beyond one's control. Studies of older adults indicate that being healthy and participating in health promotion activities depends on the ability to make choices and take responsibility for one's actions, in spite of the presence of significant chronic illnesses. Relatively little is known, however, about the patterns of healthy lifestyle practices in older adults, how they differ from those of midlife and younger adults, and how sociocultural characteristics influence choices and behaviors. Values and expectations of successful aging vary across cohorts and cultures.

Neurological changes associated with the normal aging process include slower nerve impulse transmission and decline in the integration of sensory and motor function. Slower response time, stiffness, and slower voluntary movements have implications for physical activity as well as driving. Sensory decline in vision, hearing, taste, and smell has implications for both safety and nutrition. Changes in sleep quality, including insomnia, are common problems for older adults. Systemic changes throughout the body have implications for increased incidence of cardiovascular, kidney, and gastrointestinal diseases. Older adults may be highly susceptible to medication effects and drug interactions. Drug dosages must be prescribed and monitored carefully. Osteoporosis increases the risk of fractures of all types, with accompanying disability, morbidity, and mortality. In addition, osteoarthritis of the knee is one of the top five conditions accounting for physical disability in noninstitutionalized elderly women and men. The leading causes of death for older people are heart disease, cancer, cardiovascular accident, pneumonia/influenza, and chronic obstructive lung disease.

In general, the recommendations for annual or biannual screening for blood pressure, fecal occult blood screen/sigmoidoscopy, mammogram/clinical breast examination, Papanicolaou smear, and questioning concerning alcohol use continue throughout adulthood. Additionally, screening for vision and hearing impairment should be included in primary care visits. People with risk factors should be screened for skin cancer and counseled regarding excessive sun exposure and use of protective clothing. Counseling for substance and tobacco use, dental health, exercise, and diet should be included in primary care visits. In particular, many older people do not consume enough water, fiber, calcium, B vitamins, and other minerals, and should be advised to limit fat and cholesterol while maintaining adequate caloric intake. Counseling on injury prevention should include discussion of fall prevention, seat belt use, smoke detectors, and CPR training for household members. Assessing functional status is important, and health providers should be alert to changes in performing activities of daily life. Brief tests such as the mini-mental status examination may be useful for assessing cognition, but there is insufficient evidence to recommend routine screening for dementia in asymptomatic elderly persons. Older adults should receive pneumococcal vaccine, tetanus-diphtheria boosters every 10 years, and an annual influenza vaccine injection. Older adults who are at risk for tuberculosis (TB), including those with chronic medical conditions, those with TB contacts, immigrants, and alcoholics, should have an annual purified protein derivative (PPD) test. In addition, hepatitis A vaccine and a PPD test are recommended for institutionalized persons.

The case studies in this chapter address common presenting problems relating to the gastrointestinal, pulmonary, and urinary systems. In addition, although some cognitive decline in older adults is inevitable, a case study regarding differentiation between dementia and depression, both of which may be precipitated by a wide range of factors, is included.

# REFERENCES

Davis, L., Maryland, M. (1996). Health promotion: The mature years. In K. Allen, J. Phillips (eds.), *Women's Health across the Lifespan: A Comprehensive Perspective*, 90–101. Philadelphia: J.B. Lippincott.

German, P. S. (1994). The meaning of prevention for older people: Changing common perceptions. *Generations: The Journal of the Western Gerontological Society 18*(1), 28–32.

Guccione, A. A., Felson, D. T., Anderson, J. J., Anthony, J. M., Zhang, Y., Wilson, P. W., Kelly-Hayes, M., Wolf, P. A., Kreger, B. E., Kannel, W. B. (1994). The effects of specific medical conditions on the functional limitations of elders in the Framingham Study. *Am J Public Health 84*, 351–358.

Miller, A.M., Iris, M. (1997). *Health Promotion Attitudes and Strategies in Older Adults.* Manuscript submitted for publication.

Mold, J. W. (1993). Nutritional assessment and dietary recommendations. In J. Yoshikawa (ed.), *Ambulatory Geriatric Care*, 175–186. St. Louis: Mosby.

Murray, R. B., Zentner, J. P. (1996). *Nursing Assessment and Health Promotion: Strategies through the Life Span*, 6th ed. Norwalk, CT: Appleton & Lange.

National Center for Health Statistics. (1992). *Healthy People 2000: National Health Promotion and Disease Prevention Objectives.* DHHS Publication No. PHS 91-50213. Washington, DC: U.S. Department of Health and Human Services, Public Health Services.

Walsh, J. (1993). Successful aging. In J. Yoshikawa (ed.), *Ambulatory Geriatric Care*, 168–174. St. Louis: Mosby.

Wrightsman, L. (1994). *Adult Personality Development: Theories and Concepts.* Thousand Oaks, CA: Sage.

# 34

# Gastroenteritis

*Diane Graybill Pineda*
*Lorrita Verhey*

Mr. B., a 74-year-old male, drove himself to the clinic today. He was seen approximately 1 month ago for routine management of hypertension, which was diagnosed 12 years ago. His blood pressure has been well controlled with Monopril 10 mg daily, which he took this morning. He lives alone since his wife's sudden death 6 months ago from a massive cardiovascular accident. He has one daughter who lives out of state, with whom he corresponds by E-mail on a regular basis.

## CHIEF COMPLAINT

"I feel so weak and tired because I've been vomiting and had diarrhea for two days."

## HISTORY OF PRESENT ILLNESS

Two nights ago, Mr. B. prepared and ate a medium-well steak, baked potato, and carrots, visited briefly with some neighbors, and went to bed. He was awakened by abdominal cramping followed by several episodes of explosive watery diarrhea. Yesterday he vomited bile and was unable to tolerate liquids. He vomited several times during the day; the last episode was approximately 8 h ago. Today he is tolerating sips of room temperature lemon-lime soda. His vomiting and diarrhea have subsided. He had a vague generalized headache and felt feverish yesterday, but didn't take his temperature. The headache is gone, but he feels lightheaded now. His urine is darker today, and he has voided smaller amounts than usual the last few days.

## FAMILY HISTORY

Mr. B.'s older brother, John, had a colostomy for colon cancer at age 75. Mr. B. is his main support.

## PAST MEDICAL HISTORY

Other than mild hypertension, Mr. B. has no significant medical or surgical history. He is independent and active, walking approximately 1 mi a day when his arthritis is not bothering him. He has never smoked cigarettes, cigar, or pipe. He denies allergies to food, medications, and inhalants. Mr. B. has osteoarthritis affecting his knees and hips, for which he takes ibuprofen 400 mg two or three times a day as needed. Monopril and ibuprofen are the only medications he takes. At his last visit, vital signs were: temperature 36.8°C (98.4°F), blood pressure (BP) 132/84, pulse 82, respirations 18, and weight 150 lb (68 kg).

## PHYSICAL FINDINGS

Mr. B. is alert, oriented to person and place, unsure of today's day and date.

| | |
|---|---|
| Vital signs: | Weight 146 lb (66 kg), supine BP 104/68 and pulse 106, sitting BP 88/60 and pulse 120, respiratory rate 22, temperature 100°F. |
| Skin: | Warm and dry, with tenting; dry mucous membranes. |
| Cardiac: | Apical pulse is 106 and regular, with no murmurs, $S_3$, or $S_4$ auscultated. No ankle edema noted. |
| Lungs: | Clear to auscultation bilaterally. |
| Abdomen: | Hyperactive bowel sounds are auscultated throughout the abdomen, which is soft with mild diffuse tenderness upon palpation, no guarding or rebound tenderness, and negative iliopsoas and obturator signs. |
| Rectal exam: | Negative for pain, hemorrhoids, or mass. Stool is negative for blood by Hemoccult testing. |

## LABORATORY FINDINGS

| | |
|---|---|
| Urinalysis dipstick: | Specific gravity is 1.030, pH is 7.0, 3+ ketones and trace protein. Glucose, blood, bilirubin, urobilinogen, leukocyte esterase, and nitrites are all negative. |
| Stool: | Negative for leukocytes by methylene blue stain. |

QUESTION 1. What additional historical information would be useful in formulating a diagnosis and plan of care? (Select all that apply.)
A. Prior stool pattern
B. History of diabetes
C. Ingestion of contaminated food
D. Contact with anyone with similar symptoms
E. Alcohol intake

QUESTION 2. Which one of the following signs is *strongly* indicative of dehydration in the elderly? (Select all that apply.)
A. Poor skin turgor
B. Orthostatic (postural) hypotension
C. Confusion

   D. Dry tongue with furrows and/or coating
   E. Lethargy

QUESTION 3. What is (are) the most likely diagnosis(es)? (Select all that apply.)
   A. Colon cancer
   B. Appendicitis
   C. Dehydration
   D. Viral gastroenteritis

QUESTION 4. What additional laboratory tests should be done today? (Select all that apply.)
   A. Complete blood count
   B. Serum electrolytes
   C. Stool cultures
   D. Urine cultures

QUESTION 5. What is the plan of treatment for this patient? (Select all that apply.)
   A. Refer to the emergency department (ED).
   B. Initiate gradual oral rehydration.
   C. Send home under supervision.
   D. Call the patient at home in 24 h.
   E. Hold Monopril the next day.

QUESTION 6. What is appropriate instruction for Mr. B. at this time? (Select all that apply.)
   A. Refrain from driving now.
   B. Rehydrate with clear liquids.
   C. Continue Monopril.
   D. Increase fluid intake if urine becomes dark.

QUESTION 7. What psychosocial factors need to be considered for Mr. B. to prevent dehydration and subsequent injury? (Select all that apply.)
   A. Income and other financial resources
   B. Local family and social support systems
   C. His wife's recent death
   D. Family obligations

## ANSWERS

QUESTION 1. What additional historical information would be useful in formulating a diagnosis and plan of care?
   A. YES. Prior stool pattern would help to rule out inflammatory bowel disease, obstruction, bleeding due to nonsteroidal anti-inflammatory drugs (NSAIDs), and other etiologies.
   B. YES. Diabetics may develop a bacterial overgrowth, resulting in diarrhea.
   C. YES. Mr. B. may have eaten contaminated food. Since his wife's death, he may be lax about refrigeration and food handling.
   D. YES. Recent exposure to others with similar symptoms would suggest infectious etiology.

E. *YES.* Mr. B. may be abusing alcohol in an attempt to cope with depression resulting from his wife's death 6 months ago.

**QUESTION 2.** Which one of the following signs is strongly indicative of dehydration in the elderly?

A. *NO.* Poor skin turgor is a common effect of normal aging on the skin. Thus, in older adults turgor may not be a reliable or valid estimate of hydration status.

B. *NO.* While orthostatic (postural) hypotension may be found in many dehydrated elderly patients, it is also a common side effect of many medications, especially antihypertensives. Many other factors of normal aging, such as decreased elasticity of the vascular system and impaired baroreflex function, may also affect postural changes in blood pressure.

C. *NO.* Again, while confusion may be found in the dehydrated elderly patient, it is only moderately correlated with dehydration, and many well-hydrated elderly have some degree of confusion. Confusion may be caused by many factors, including medications or other disease processes.

D. *YES.* Dry tongue with furrows and/or coating seems to be very highly associated with dehydration in the elderly. Mouth breathing and medications should be taken into consideration as the cause of dry oral mucosa, but furrows or coating of the tongue is most likely related to dehydration.

E. *NO.* Lethargy is only weakly indicative of dehydration, and has many other causes. To diagnose dehydration in an elderly patient, all the signs and symptoms, as well as the severity of the findings, must be taken into account.

**QUESTION 3.** What is (are) the most likely diagnosis(es)?

A. *NO.* Although tumors of the descending colon may cause diarrhea, cancer is less likely to present with vomiting and diarrhea. However, in view of a positive family history, it may be recommended that Mr. B. have a flexible sigmoidoscopy or colonoscopy sometime after the symptoms are resolved, unless he has had one recently.

B. *NO.* Appendicitis is unlikely because Mr. B.'s abdominal cramping is associated with a diarrhea stool and is generalized over the lower abdomen. His pain is not accentuated with movement. His tenderness is mild and diffuse, not specific over McBurney's point, and the iliopsoas sign is negative. He did not experience tenderness on rectal exam.

C. *YES.* Dehydration is likely in view of Mr. B.'s decreased blood pressure, increased pulse, 4-lb weight loss, and dry mucous membranes and skin. Factors that contribute to dehydration and volume depletion may include fever, diarrhea, vomiting, decreased vascular elasticity, hypodipsia, low-sodium diet, use of an angiotensin-converting enzyme (ACE) inhibitor, alcohol abuse, or NSAID use. Overuse of laxatives can also induce diarrhea and dehydration.

D. *YES.* Abrupt onset with 1-day duration of diarrhea and vomiting associated with headache, fatigue, and fever suggest viral infectious etiology. The absence of blood, mucus, and white cells in the stool support this diagnosis.

QUESTION 4. What additional laboratory tests should be done today?
A. *YES*. An increased hematocrit will assist in evaluating the degree of dehydration. An elevated white blood cell count could be indicative of infectious processes. Ibuprofen may cause gastrointestinal bleeding and anemia.
B. *YES*. Serum levels show the degree of electrolyte imbalances, allowing for rapid intervention in severe or life-threatening situations. Although the dehydration of vomiting and diarrhea tends to be isotonic, vomiting and diarrhea may cause excessive loss of sodium as well as loss of potassium.
C. *NO*. Stool cultures are not indicated in acute diarrhea until it has persisted for at least 48 h, or occult blood or leukocytes are present in the stool.
D. *NO*. A urinalysis (UA) was done, and it did not show any signs of urinary tract infection (UTI), such as leukocyte esterase, nitrites, or blood. In this case the UA is sufficient to rule out UTI.

QUESTION 5. What is the plan of treatment for this patient?
A. *NO*. Only after attempts to rehydrate the patient in the office have failed should he be referred to the ED.
B. *YES*. Gradual oral rehydration should be initiated in the office, with the vital signs monitored. Oral rehydration is the easiest and most cost-effective treatment. Electrolyte-balanced solution such as Pedialyte or the World Health Organization Oral Rehydration Solution may be used, but other liquids may be substituted. Water, in combination with diluted fruit or vegetable juices, flat nondiet sodas, broth, and decaffeinated tea with a half teaspoon of honey or a teaspoon of sugar are all good choices.
C. *YES*. A friend or family member should stay with Mr. B. for the next 24 h. The diarrhea and orthostatic hypotension put him at risk of falling. The dehydration and potential electrolyte imbalance put him at risk of injuries resulting from possible confusion. Any worsening of the symptoms should be reported immediately to the health care provider.
D. *YES*. Call the patient within 24 h to reevaluate symptoms and orientation. Persistence or worsening of symptoms may indicate a more serious problem that would necessitate a reevaluation in person.
E. *YES*. Monopril should not be taken tomorrow. Mr. B.'s blood pressure is below his normal baseline pressure as a result of the dehydration. The ACE inhibitor will furthur decrease the blood pressure and blunt the kidneys' ability to compensate for fluid losses and decreased BP. This mechanism will exacerbate the orthostatic hypotension, putting him at increased risk of falls and hypotensive crisis.

QUESTION 6. What is appropriate instruction for Mr. B. at this time?
A. *YES*. It is unsafe for Mr. B., other drivers, and pedestrians for him to be driving when he is feeling lightheaded.
B. *YES*. Even small amounts of liquids will be absorbed. However, if vomiting and diarrhea continue, Mr. B. should call the office.

**C.** *NO*. Monopril decreases total peripheral resistance and the reabsorption of water. Monopril may be resumed in 2 days if symptoms improve.
**D.** *YES*. Mr. B.'s urine may become more concentrated from several causes, including inadequate fluid intake—48 to 64 oz of fluids per day is recommended. Particular attention should be paid to fluid intake in hot and/or humid weather because aging may diminish the sensation of thirst as a result of malfunction of osmoreceptors in the hypothalamus.

**QUESTION 7.** What psychosocial factors need to be considered for Mr. B. to prevent dehydration and subsequent injury?
**A.** *YES*. Fixed and limited income may inhibit purchase of adequate foods and fluids. It is important to make sure he currently has and can maintain utilities such as gas and electricity (for safe food preparation and storage) and telephone (to be able to summon help if necessary).
**B.** *YES*. Mr. B.'s family and social support system are vital to his survival in the event of an emergency. It is important that he identify people who live close by and can check on him routinely. It is also important that he have a way to contact someone in the event of an emergency.
**C.** *YES*. The recent loss of his wife may predispose him to depression and put him at risk for alcohol and drug abuse, which can lead to dehydration as well as other health problems. Depression may affect his intake of foods and fluids.
**D.** *YES*. Mr. B. is the main support for his brother, who has been diagnosed with colon cancer. The sense of responsibility to his brother may make him neglect himself and his own health care, thereby putting him at increased risk. He also may worry about his own risk for colon cancer, contributing to anxiety and/or depression.

## REFERENCES

Goldstein, M. K., Oliveira, J. (1993). Constipation, diarrhea and fecal impaction. In T. Yoshikawa, E. Cobbs, K. Brummel-Smith (eds.), *Ambulatory Geriatric Care*, 476–484. St. Louis: Mosby-Yearbook.

Goroll, A. H. (1995). Evaluation of nausea and vomiting. In A. H. Goroll, L. A. May, A. G. Mulley, Jr. (eds.), *Primary Care Medicine: Office Evaluation and Management of the Adult Patient*, 3d ed., 334–338. Philadelphia: J. B. Lippincott.

Gross, C., Lindquist, R., Woolley, A., Granieri, R., Allard, K., Webster, B. (1992). Clinical indicators of dehydration severity in elderly patients. *J Emerg Med 10*, 267–274.

Richter, J. M. (1995). Evaluation and management of diarrhea. In A. H. Goroll, L. A. May, A. G. Mulley, Jr. (eds.), *Primary Care Medicine: Office Evaluation and Management of the Adult Patient*, 3d ed., 357–368. Philadelphia: J. B. Lippincott.

Sansenero, A. (1997). Dehydration in the elderly: Strategies for prevention and management. *Nurse Pract 22*(4), 41–72.

Weinberg, A., Mensher, K., The Council on Scientific Affairs, American Medical Association. (1995). Dehydration evaluation and management in older adults. *JAMA 274*, 1552–1556.

# 35

# Cough

*Patricia A. Furnace*
*Arlene Miller*

George S., an 82-year-old Caucasian male, comes to the office complaining of fatigue and a cough, which he has had for 2 weeks. He was last seen 2 months ago for a follow-up visit for stable hypertension.

## CHIEF COMPLAINT

"I've been coughing for 2 weeks, bringing up phlegm for about a week."

## HISTORY OF PRESENT ILLNESS

When the cough symptoms began, Mr. S. thought he had a common cold. Though his cough was nonproductive initially, it became productive of mucopurulent sputum about 1 week ago. He has had no hemoptysis.

**QUESTION 1.** Which of the following information would contribute to his history of present illness? (Select all that apply.)
   **A.** Recent travel
   **B.** Fever and chills
   **C.** Pneumococcal and yearly influenza vaccine
   **D.** Past history of similar symptoms
   **E.** Presence of a rash

## PAST MEDICAL HISTORY

Mr. S. has no known allergies. He has been treated for stable hypertension for 26 years, and is presently taking hydrochlorothiazide 25 mg each morning. He smoked one pack of cigarettes daily for 40 years but stopped 20 years ago. He drinks alcohol only on holidays, and drinks two cups of coffee each morning. He walks 2 miles three or four times a week. He denies ever using street/recreational drugs.

**QUESTION 2.** Which of the following would differentiate bronchitis from pneumonia? (Select all that apply.)
  A. Anorexia
  B. Burning sensation in the chest
  C. Diarrhea
  D. Presence of thick dark or bloody sputum
  E. Sudden onset of symptoms

## FAMILY HISTORY

There is no family history of tuberculosis (TB), diabetes mellitus, cancer, cardiovascular disease, or thyroid problems. Mr. S.'s parents died in their 80s from "old age, both had hypertension." He has an 85-year-old brother with hypertension. He has two children, 60 years and 57 years old, who are in good health.

## SOCIAL HISTORY

Mr. S. has been retired for the past 17 years from his job as an electrical engineer. His hobbies include fishing and activities with his five grandchildren, whom he sees weekly. His wife is 80 years old and in good health.

## OBJECTIVE DATA

| | |
|---|---|
| Vital signs: | Temperature 36.8°C (98.2°F), pulse 82, respirations 20, blood pressure 134/86, right arm sitting. Appears ill and coughing. |
| Head: | Normocephalic without tenderness. |
| Eyes: | Pupils equal and reactive to light and accommodation. Funduscopic examination within normal limits. |
| Ears: | Canals are patent without exudate. Tympanic membranes are pearly gray, with light reflex visualized bilaterally. |
| Nose: | Nares patent, erythematous and moist. |
| Sinuses: | Nontender. |
| Mouth/throat: | Pharynx injected, no tonsillar exudate. |
| Neck: | Supple, nontender, no palpable nodes. |
| Lungs: | Expiratory wheezing, bilaterally. Percussion sounds resonant. Vocal resonance is normal. No friction rub. |
| Cardiovascular: | Regular rate and rhythm, without $S_3$, $S_4$, murmurs, or clicks. |
| Extremities: | No pedal edema. |

**QUESTION 3.** What physical examination findings would be expected with acute bronchitis?
  A. Injected pharynx
  B. Pleural friction rub
  C. Pulmonary consolidation
  D. Tachypnea
  E. Wheezing

**Question 4.** Which of the following laboratory tests would be appropriate to confirm a diagnosis for this patient? (Select all that apply.)
A. Blood glucose
B. Chest x-ray
C. Oxygen saturation
D. Pulmonary function testing
E. Tuberculin skin test

## ASSESSMENT

**Question 5.** Which of the following are likely diagnoses for this patient? (Select all that apply.)
A. Acute bronchitis
B. Bacterial pneumonia
C. Chronic bronchitis
D. Influenza
E. Tuberculosis

## PLAN

**Question 6.** Management of acute bronchitis would include which of the following? (Select all that apply.)
A. Antibiotics
B. Bronchodilator
C. Smoking cessation
D. Strict bed rest

**Question 7.** Management of chronic bronchitis would include which of the following? (Select all that apply.)
A. Immunizations for influenza and pneumococcal pneumonia
B. Smoking cessation
C. Long-term use of bronchodilators, corticosteroids, and mucokinetics
D. Yearly TB skin tests

## ANSWERS

**Question 1.** Which of the following information would contribute to his history of present illness?
A. *YES.* A careful travel history is essential for identifying potential sources of this problem. For example, states that border the Ohio and Mississippi Rivers have a higher incidence of *Histoplasma capsulatum,* and there are geographic differences in the occurrence of other community-acquired bacterial pneumonias.
B. *YES.* A fever is present with bacterial, mycoplasmal, *Pneumocystis carinii,* and viral pneumonias. It may also be present in acute bronchitis. Sudden onset of chills is a hallmark sign of bacterial pneumonia. Chills usually do not occur with bronchitis. Atypical pneumonia may cause chills, but not a sudden onset of chills.
C. *YES.* Information about these vaccines will facilitate the differential diagnosis. Underutilization of the influenza and pneumococcal vaccines causes needless morbidity and mortality each year.

D. *YES.* Asking if the client has previously had any of these symptoms can help to differentiate among acute, recurrent, and chronic problems. Chronic bronchitis is defined as a productive cough that has been present for at least 3 months for 2 consecutive years. Management decisions and follow-up would be different for acute and chronic bronchitis.

E. *NO.* Asking about the presence of a rash would probably not help in establishing a diagnosis for this problem.

**QUESTION 2.** Which of the following would differentiate bronchitis from pneumonia?

A. *YES.* Anorexia and abdominal pain are frequently seen in clients with bacterial pneumonia. Anorexia is not frequently seen in clients with bronchitis.

B. *YES.* Burning in the chest is frequently present in bronchitis. Chest *pain* is a common complaint in clients with pneumonia.

C. *NO.* Diarrhea is not usually seen in clients with either bronchitis or pneumonia.

D. *YES.* Thick dark or bloody sputum is present with bacterial pneumonia. Bronchitis usually produces mucopurulent sputum after an initially nonproductive cough.

E. *YES.* Sudden onset of symptoms occurs with bacterial pneumonia. A gradual onset of symptoms occurs with bronchitis and nonpneumococcal pneumonias.

**QUESTION 3.** What physical examination findings would be expected with acute bronchitis?

A. *YES.* An injected pharynx is one of the physical examination findings present with acute bronchitis.

B. *NO.* A pleural friction rub is a common finding in pneumonia, especially in bacterial pneumonia.

C. *NO.* Pulmonary consolidation is found in pneumonia, not bronchitis. It is characterized by bronchophony, egophony, dullness on percussion, and rales. However, rales, rhonchi, and/or wheezing can occur with bronchitis.

D. *NO.* Tachypnea is not part of the clinical presentation for acute bronchitis. Tachypnea is observed with pneumococcal pneumonia. Nonpneumococcal pneumonia is more varied in its presentation, and the client usually appears less acutely ill.

E. *YES.* Wheezing is more likely to be present in acute bronchitis than in either pneumococcal or other types of pneumonia.

**QUESTION 4.** Which of the following laboratory tests would be appropriate to confirm a diagnosis for this patient?

A. *NO.* Mr. S. does not have diabetes mellitus, and blood glucose will not assist in diagnosing his problem or managing his care. However, if a person who has diabetes mellitus develops a respiratory infection, regular monitoring of the blood glucose will assist in the management of the diabetes. Blood glucose frequently increases with infectious diseases.

B. *YES.* A chest x-ray should be ordered when there is a suspicion of acute pneumonia. Pulmonary infiltrates are present with pneumonia. Bronchitis does not produce chest x-ray changes. If the clinical presentation favors acute bronchitis, a chest x-ray would not be necessary.

C. *YES.* Oxygen saturation would be normal in bronchitis. It may be either decreased or normal with acute pneumonia.

D. *NO.* Pulmonary function testing would be helpful in assessing pulmonary function status in a client with chronic bronchitis. It would not, however, differentiate between acute bronchitis and acute pneumonia.

E. *NO.* There is no information that suggests that Mr. S. has an increased risk for TB infection. For individuals over age 65, risk factors indicating a need for routine TB screening include institutionalization, contact with persons infected with TB, alcoholism, drug abuse, HIV infection, and immigration from countries with a high prevalence of TB. Symptoms that would increase the suspicion of active TB include a chronic cough, low-grade fever, and weight loss.

**Question 5.** Which of the following are likely diagnoses for this patient?

A. *YES.* Mr. S. initially had symptoms of a common cold and a nonproductive cough that is now productive of mucopurulent sputum. Physical examination reveals an injected pharynx and wheezing, but no signs of pulmonary consolidation.

B. *NO.* Mr. S. has no signs of pulmonary consolidation, which would be expected with a 2-week history of pneumonia. Also, patients with bacterial pneumonia generally have an acute onset of symptoms.

C. *NO.* There is no information that indicates that he has had this problem for at least 3 months for 2 consecutive years. However, smoking one pack of cigarettes per day for 40 years does increase his risk for chronic bronchitis.

D. *NO.* Influenza usually presents with a sudden onset of symptoms, including systemic symptoms of myalgia and malaise, and the client appears acutely ill.

E. *NO.* Tuberculosis would be a likely diagnosis if Mr. S. presented with a chronic cough, low-grade fever, and weight loss.

**Question 6.** Management of acute bronchitis would include which of the following?

A. *NO.* Bronchitis is usually viral in origin, and use of antibiotics would not change the course of the disease. Some practitioners prescribe an antibiotic if the patient has underlying chronic lung disease to prevent development of secondary pneumonia.

B. *YES.* Use of a bronchodilator, preferably in aerosol form, would help relieve the wheezing experienced by Mr. S.

C. *YES.* Smoking cessation should be encouraged for all clients who smoke. Asking about smoking and recommending smoking cessation during this type of office visit can be an important motivator for the patient.

D. *NO.* Strict bed rest will not assist in the resolution of acute bronchitis. However, rest will help keep the patient from feeling more fatigued.

**QUESTION 7.** Management of chronic bronchitis would include which of the following?
**A.** *YES.* Immunization for influenza should be done yearly in the fall. The polyvalent pneumonia vaccine should be administered to all patients who are at risk for pneumonia. This includes individuals with chronic bronchitis and those over 65 years of age. There currently is no consensus on the frequency of revaccination of individuals who have received the pneumococcal vaccine.
**B.** *YES.* Smoking cessation is important in the management of chronic bronchitis. The Transtheoretical Model of Behavior Change identifies five stages—precontemplation, contemplation, preparation, action, and maintenance—through which individuals pass or to which they relapse. Assessing an individual's current stage can be helpful for targeting interventions. Most individuals make more than one attempt to stop smoking before they are able to quit. This model, which has been used to understand smoking cessation, underscores the difficulties encountered when attempting to make lifestyle changes. Mr. S. quit "cold turkey" 20 years ago. This is the most effective method, followed by combining other methods with a behavioral program. Using nicotine gum or patches without a behavioral program is the least successful method. Smoking cessation is a difficult but not impossible endeavor.
**C.** *NO.* The ability of mucokinetic agents to facilitate expectoration has not been well documented. Systemic hydration, effective cough methods, and postural drainage are more effective in facilitating expectoration.
**D.** *NO.* Yearly TB skin tests are not recommended in patients with chronic bronchitis unless they belong to a high-risk group for TB. High-risk groups would include residents of long-term-care facilities, persons with HIV infection, and persons who are alcoholic, homeless, or intravenous drug abusers.

## REFERENCES

American Thoracic Society. (1995). Standards for the diagnosis and care of patients with chronic obstructive pulmonary disease. *Am J Respir Crit Care Med 152*(5), 77–121.

Glezen, W. A. (1997). Influenza: How to prepare for the 1997–1998 season. *J Respir Dis 18*, 721–736.

Griffith, H. W. (1997). *5 Minute Clinical Consult—1997.* Philadelphia: Lea & Febiger.

Komaiha, H., Jordan, G. W. (1997). Vaccination update: Safer agents, revised guidelines. *J Respir Dis 18*, 773–783.

Lipchik, R. J. (1996). Pneumonia. In J. Noble (ed.), *Textbook of Primary Care Medicine*, 2d ed., 1531–1540. Philadelphia: W. B. Saunders.

Prochaska, J. O., DiClemente, C. C., Norcross, J. C. (1992). In search of how people change: Applications to addictive behavior. *Am Psychologist 47*, 1102–1113.

Quenzer, R. W. (1996). Bronchitis and pneumonia. In R. H. Rubin, C. Voss, D. J. Derksen, A. Gately, R. W. Quenzer (eds.), *Medicine: A Primary Care Approach*, 123–127. Philadelphia: W. B. Saunders.

Rigotti, N. A. (1995). Smoking cessation. In A. H. Goroll, L. A. May, A. G. Mulley (eds.), *Primary Care Medicine*, 3d ed., 300–308. Philadelphia: J. B. Lippincott.

Rubin, R. H. (1996). Chronic cough. In R. H. Rubin, C. Voss, D. J. Derksen, A. Gately, R. W. Quenzer (eds.), *Medicine: A Primary Care Approach*, 107–111. Philadelphia: W. B. Saunders.

# 36

# Dementia/Depression

*Arlene Miller*
*Laina M. Gerace*

Mrs. V., a 72-year-old Hispanic woman, is accompanied to a rural clinic by her daughter, who is concerned about changes in her mother's behavior. Mrs. V. was seen 1 week ago by another health provider, who ordered laboratory tests to evaluate her complaints of fatigue and poor appetite. Mrs. V. does not speak English well, so she is assigned to a bilingual health care provider for her visit. During the interview, Mrs. V. appears discouraged and despondent, and does not make eye contact.

## CHIEF COMPLAINT

From Mrs. V.'s daughter: "My mother has stopped preparing meals, and hasn't left her house for the past few weeks. Last week she didn't take a bath, and this is very unusual for her."

## HISTORY OF PRESENT ILLNESS

Mrs. V. began to have periods of depressed mood about 2 years ago. Around that time, she stopped working as a babysitter because her arthritis became too painful, and she had some difficulty getting around. During the past year, she seemed to lose interest in some of her favorite activities, including cooking and visiting with friends. She admits to feeling fearful about leaving home, and does not leave the house without her husband or daughter. She denies having mental health problems in the past.

**QUESTION 1.** The presenting symptoms suggest which of the following as differential diagnoses? (Select all that apply.)
   **A.** Dementia
   **B.** Major depressive episode
   **C.** Panic disorder with agoraphobia
   **D.** Schizophrenia

## PAST MEDICAL HISTORY

Mrs. V. has been taking indomethacin (Indocin) for 2 years, with some relief of her joint pain. She denies symptoms of gastric irritation. She has no other chronic diseases. She does not drink alcohol or smoke.

## PHYSICAL FINDINGS

Physical examination within normal limits, with some stiffness and decreased range of motion in lower extremities. Mental status results are shown in this table:

**Mini-Mental Status Examination (Conducted in Spanish)**

|  | Patient Score | Possible Score |
| --- | --- | --- |
| Orientation | 7 | 10 |
| Immediate recall | 2 | 3 |
| Attention and calculation | 2 | 5 |
| Recall | 1 | 3 |
| Language | 5 | 9 |
| Total | 17 | 30 |

## ASSESSMENT

QUESTION 2. Which of the following information obtained from Mrs. V.'s history suggests the presence of depression? (Select all that apply.)
A. History of arthritis
B. Use of nonsteroidal anti-inflammatory drugs (NSAIDs)
C. Age over 70
D. Past history of depression

QUESTION 3. Which of the following statements is true regarding depression in older adults? (Select all that apply.)
A. Older adults with depression usually seek help by complaining of multiple physical symptoms rather than of depressed mood.
B. An older adult with depression who does not know the answer to a question on a mental status examination will usually prevaricate (make up an answer) rather than admit to ignorance or to forgetting the answer.
C. Older adults who are depressed are less likely than young adults to attempt or commit suicide.
D. Depression in older adults is usually self-limited, and intervention is not recommended.

QUESTION 4. Information from Mrs. V.'s mental status examination indicates which of the following? (Select all that apply.)
A. Changes associated with normal aging
B. Possible dementia
C. Clear signs of early-onset dementia
D. Changes associated with depression

**QUESTION 5.** Assessment of which of the following can assist in differentiating dementia from depression? (Select all that apply.)
A. Onset and course of functional decline
B. Ability to use language
C. Type of memory impairment
D. Patient's own perceptions of mental impairment

## PLAN

**QUESTION 6.** Considering Mrs. V.'s current status, which general treatment modalities are indicated? (Select all that apply.)
A. Trial of antidepressant pharmacotherapy
B. Prescribing a neuroleptic medication
C. Counseling regarding home safety and social support
D. Follow-up visit within 1 month

**QUESTION 7.** Which of the following factors is (are) particularly important to consider when treating older adults with antidepressant medications? (Select all that apply.)
A. Dosage of antidepressant medication for older adults is the same as for younger adults, and most treatment failures result from inadequate doses.
B. The anticholinergic effects of tricyclic antidepressants are particularly troubling for older adults.
C. Assessing plasma levels of antidepressants may be advisable to ensure optimal pharmacotherapy in older adults.
D. Newer antidepressants, such as selective serotonin reuptake inhibitors (SSRIs), may be better suited for older adults than tricyclic medications.

## ANSWERS

**QUESTION 1.** The presenting symptoms suggest which of the following as differential diagnoses?
A. *YES.* Dementia is a possible diagnosis, in view of slowly progressing cognitive deficits, including memory, personality, and behavior changes. Mrs. V. is experiencing changes that reflect impairment of social functioning and a decline in prior abilities.
B. *YES.* Mrs. V.'s vegetative symptoms of fatigue and poor appetite and her despondency and loss of interest in previously pleasurable activities are symptoms of depression.
C. *NO.* Although persons suffering from agoraphobia feel fearful about leaving their homes alone, Mrs. V. does not have the sympathetic nervous system symptoms that characterize panic attacks, such as palpitations, sweating, and dizziness.
D. *NO.* Although Mrs. V. does not maintain eye contact with the examiner and has evidence of diminished social and self-care functioning, she does not have evidence of thought disorder, such as delusions, hallucinations, or grossly disorganized speech or behavior.

**Question 2.** Which of the following information obtained from Mrs. V.'s history suggests the presence of depression?

    **A.** *YES.* Depression is often associated with chronic diseases, including arthritis, and may be present in individuals with chronic pain.

    **B.** *YES.* Depression is a side effect of several of the NSAIDs, including indomethacin.

    **C.** *NO.* Depression is not a normal or inevitable occurrence as one ages. Major depressive disorder has a lower prevalence in the elderly than in younger adults, which suggests that the physical aging process alone is not an etiologic factor. In fact, first onset of primary major depressive disorder after age 50 is uncommon.

    **D.** *YES.* A past history of depressive episodes may contribute to a diagnosis of major depressive disorder. The onset of a period of depression coinciding with Mrs. V.'s retirement as a day care provider is suggestive of adjustment disorder at that time, but more information regarding the course of depressive episodes since then should be obtained.

**Question 3.** Which of the following statements is true regarding depression in older adults?

    **A.** *YES.* Many older adults were raised during a time in which society viewed depression as a sign of weakness rather than a biologically based disease. Perhaps because they are not educated in the signs and symptoms of depression and are unable to articulate what they are experiencing, older people tend to present with vague symptoms such as somatic complaints, guilt or loss of self-worth, and impaired memory and concentration. Tearfulness and complaining of feeling "down" or "blue" are less frequent in the elderly. In addition, people from some ethnic backgrounds hesitate to seek help from mental health professionals, and first present in primary health settings. Many illnesses experienced by older adults produce functional decline and predispose them to depression. It is critical for primary care providers to be alert to symptoms that suggest depression that may be concomitant to other health problems.

    **B.** *NO.* Depressed persons tend to have decreased concentration and motivation to answer questions, and may either have delayed responses or simply answer that they do not know. They are aware of memory deficits, and will often complain about them to their health care provider. Prevarication is more likely to be used by people with dementia, who may be less aware that they have a memory problem.

    **C.** *NO.* Among depressed people from all age groups, the elderly have the highest suicide rate.

    **D.** *NO.* Evidence is accumulating regarding the efficacy of treating depression in the elderly. Psychotherapy alone may be effective for less severely ill, nonpsychotic outpatients, although there is little research in this area. Pharmacotherapy with antidepressant medications can be successful if the medication is chosen carefully.

QUESTION 4. Information from the Mrs. V.'s mental status examination indicates which of the following?

A. NO. The changes seen in Mrs. V. are not within normal limits. The mean score for persons aged 65 and over is 26. Mrs. V.'s score (17 out of 30 possible points) on the mental status examination falls into the 5th percentile for age 65 and over and indicates the need for further assessment.

B. YES. The changes seen in Mrs. V. may be early signs of dementia. However, since the mini-mental status examination is a screening tool, not a diagnostic instrument, further assessment is needed.

C. NO. While the changes seen in Mrs. V. may indicate dementia, some of her memory and cognitive deficits could be due to depression.

D. YES. The changes on the mini-mental status examination could also be due to depression. Because depression can occur concomitantly with dementia and has similar signs and symptoms, further assessment is needed to differentiate the two conditions.

QUESTION 5. Assessment of which of the following can assist in differentiating dementia from depression?

A. YES. Although there are exceptions, the onset and course of functional decline tends to be insidious in dementia and more rapid in depression. Furthermore, a psychosocial stressor such as a significant loss may precede the onset of depression. Functional decline in depression reverses when the mood disorder improves.

B. YES. In depression, while attention and concentration tend to show impairment, language abilities (e.g., vocabulary, use of sentences) are not affected. In dementia, use of language tends to deteriorate and become gradually more impoverished.

C. YES. In depression, the memory impairment tends to be sporadic and transitory, whereas in dementia, memory loss is progressive over time.

D. YES. In depression, the patient's own perception of mental impairment tends to exceed what others would observe. In dementia, the patient is more likely to deny impairment and invent (confabulate) stories to fill in memory gaps. Table 36-1 presents a clinical comparison of depression and dementia.

QUESTION 6. Considering Mrs. V.'s current status, which general treatment modalities are indicated?

A. YES. Because Mrs. V. has a recent history of depression (beginning 2 years ago), and depression often accompanies dementia, an antidepressant may improve both her mood and her cognitive functioning. At this stage, it may be difficult to differentiate whether her impairment is related to depression, dementia, or both. In the case of coexisting dementia and depression, it is advisable to treat the depression.

B. NO. There is no evidence that Mrs. V. has psychotic symptoms, and therefore neuroleptic medications are not indicated. In addition, there is some evidence that neuroleptics hasten cognitive decline in

TABLE 36-1   Clinical Comparison of Depression and Dementia

|  | Depression | Dementia |
|---|---|---|
| Onset | Abrupt/rapid | Chronic/slow |
| Duration | 2 weeks to months | Years |
| Prognosis | Reversible | Irreversible |
| Factors |  |  |
| Memory | Transitory loss | Progressive loss |
| Cognition | Intact, retarded | Impaired |
| Orientation | Oriented | Disoriented |
| Hallucinations | Uncommon | Common |
| Delusions | Uncommon | Common |
| Precursor | Loss, stress | Unknown |
| Emotions | Flat or distressed | Labile |
| Response to treatment | Usually significant | Little change |

SOURCE: Buschmann, M. T., Rossen, E. K. (1993). Depression in older women. Journal of Women's Health 2(3), 317–322. Reproduced with permission.

dementia patients who develop psychotic symptoms. The newer atypical neuroleptics, such as risperidone and olanzapine, are possible choices in the event that pharmacotherapy for psychotic symptoms is needed.

C. *YES.* Mrs. V. has declining cognitive and social functioning. Nonpharmacologic interventions are very important and should include counseling to improve safety, as well as strengthening the social support system for the patient and her caregivers. Patients with dementia need familiar and stable surroundings. Daily routines often increase their sense of security. The presence of clocks, calendars, newspapers, night lights, and checklists and frequent visits from caring individuals all enhance the patient's functioning. Education and counseling about the nature of Mrs. V.'s condition will help her family understand and deal with the changes they see.

D. *YES.* It is important to monitor Mrs. V.'s progress. Establishing a diagnosis of dementia can be problematic. The history and assessment of ongoing changes provide the most important data upon which to evaluate the patient. Ongoing assessment relies on corroborating observations of significant others, in this case Mrs. V.'s husband and daughter. If Mrs. V. improves on antidepressant medications, but still shows cognitive decline, then it is likely that she has coexisting depression and early dementia. Furthermore, if her cognitive decline is progressive and unrelenting, it is most likely due to Alzheimer's disease. If her cognitive decline is characterized by a more sudden onset and an incremental, stepwise decline, it may be multi-infarct dementia. Multi-infarct dementia is estimated to account for 10 to 20 percent of dementias in the elderly.

**TABLE 36-2** Confounds in the Diagnosis and Treatment of the Elderly

A. Concurrent nonpsychotropic medications may:
(1) Cause depression.
(2) Change antidepressant blood levels.
(3) Increase antidepressant side effects.
(4) Biochemically block antidepressant effects.
(5) Call for modifying the oral dosage.
B. Concurrent medical illnesses may:
(1) Cause depression biologically.
(2) Reduce the efficacy of antidepressant medication or psychotherapy.
(3) Change antidepressant drug metabolism.
(4) Impair ability to participate in psychotherapy.
(5) Create disability contributing to both chronicity and reduced treatment efficacy.
(6) Increase the need for simplified medication dosing schedules (e.g., once daily)
C. Concurrent nonmood psychiatric conditions may:
(1) Cause depression (e.g., early Alzheimer's).
(2) Call for different medications.
(3) Impair participation in psychotherapy.
(4) Reduce response to antidepressant medications (e.g., personality disorders).
(5) Worsen prognosis of the depression (e.g., alcoholism).
D. Other issues:
(1) Slower metabolism with age often requires lower dosages.
(2) Transportation difficulties may restrict access to care.
(3) Increased interview time needed.
(4) Fixed income may limit availability of therapy and nongeneric antidepressant medications due to cost.

SOURCE: Depression Guideline Panel (1993). *Depression in Primary Care,* vol. 2. Treatment of Major Depression. Clinical Practice Guidelines, No. 5. Rockville, MD. U.S. Department of Health and Human Services.

**QUESTION 7.** Which of the following factors is (are) particularly important to consider when treating older adults with antidepressant medications?

  A. *NO.* Antidepressant medication for older adults should be initiated at approximately half the dosage for younger adults. The decreased ratio of lean body mass to body fat, reduced total body water, and decreased plasma protein found in older adults lead to an increased risk of toxicity as a result of prolonged half-life and more active medication at receptor sites. In addition, depending on metabolic pathways and liver and kidney function, excretion of drugs may be less efficient.

  B. *YES.* Anticholinergic effects of tricyclic antidepressants, such as dry mouth, blurred vision, urinary hesitancy, and constipation, may be particularly troubling to older adults. These side effects may cause decreased adherence. In addition, certain other side effects, such as orthostatic hypotension, are particularly dangerous in the elderly because of the increased likelihood of falling and the concomitant risk of fractures. Orthostatic hypotension is especially likely to occur in individuals who are also taking antihypertensive medications. Since the medications within a class tend to be equally effective, the choice of antidepressant for the elderly should be based on minimizing the anticholinergic, central nervous system (e.g., drowsiness, insomnia/ agitation), and cardiovascular (e.g., orthostatic hypotension, arrythmias) effects.

**C.** *YES.* Assessing plasma levels of antidepressants may be advisable to ensure optimal pharmacotherapy in older adults, especially if they are taking other medications or have concurrent medical problems. Either of these can alter antidepressant absorption or metabolism, as can the natural metabolic slowing associated with aging. Therapeutic and toxic levels that have been established for younger adults are not appropriate for use as guidelines for older adults. Other factors that confound diagnosis and treatment of depression in the elderly are presented in Table 36-2.

**D.** *YES.* Newer antidepressants, especially SSRIs such as fluoxetine and sertraline, may be better suited for older adults than tricyclic medications because they are associated with fewer anticholinergic, cardiovascular, and sedative effects. Since they can be administered in daily doses, compliance and tolerability are enhanced. These drugs, which usually do not interfere with cognitive functioning, are especially preferred for patients with coexisting depression and dementia.

## REFERENCES

American Psychiatric Association. (1994). *Diagnostic and Statistical Manual of Mental Disorders (DSM-IV)*, 4th ed. Washington, DC: Author.

Buschmann, M. T., Rossen, E. K. (1993). Depression in older women. *Journal of Women's Health 2*(3), 317–322.

Depression Guideline Panel. (1993). *Depression in Primary Care*, vol. 2, Treatment of Major Depression. AHCPR Publication No. 93-0551. Rockville, MD: U.S. Department of Health and Human Services.

McShane, R., Keene, J., Gedling, K., Fairburn, C., Jacony, R., Hope, T. (1997). Do neuroleptic drugs hasten cognitive decline in dementia? Prospective study with necropsy follow up. *Br Med J 31*(14), 266–270.

Molloy, D. W., Alemayehy, E., Roberts, R. (1991). Reliability of a standardized mini-mental state examination compared with the traditional mini-mental state examination. *Am J Psychiatry 148*(1), 102–105.

Spratto, G., Woods, A. (1997). *Delmar's Therapeutic Class Drug Guide for Nurses.* New York: Delmar Publishers.

Terpstra, T. L., Terpstra, T. L. (1997). Treating geriatric depression with SSRIs: What primary care practitioners need to know. *The Nurse Practitioner 22*(9), 118–123.

Yoshikawa, T., Cobbs, E., Brummel-Smith, K. (1993). *Ambulatory Geriatric Care.* St. Louis: Mosby.

# 37

# Arthritis

*Eugenie F. Hildebrandt*
*Linda Ehrlich*

Mrs. J. is a married, 68-year-old Caucasian woman who is a patient in an urban clinic. She had previously been a patient at this clinic, but because of a change in her insurance carrier, she has not had health care for 2 years. A recently retired store clerk, Mrs. J. is enjoying needle work and gardening with her new-found free time. She is being seen today for joint discomfort.

## CHIEF COMPLAINT

"My joints have been getting more and more stiff and achy over the past 6 months."

## HISTORY OF PRESENT ILLNESS

Mrs. J. indicates that her joint discomfort has gradually increased over the last 4 years, but she does not recall when it first started. She currently has stiffness and aching in her hands, right hip, and left knee. Stiffness is present for about 15 min in the morning, but improves after a warm shower. Walking, standing, and gardening for prolonged periods of time cause increased pain in her hip and knee. Needlework aggravates the pain in her hands. She takes ibuprofen to relieve the discomfort in all her joints and uses a heating pad for the pain in her hip. Approximately 1 year ago she began to notice "bumps" on her fingers. She is concerned that these may be tumors.

## PAST MEDICAL HISTORY

Mrs. J.'s medical records indicate that she was seen 2 years ago for an upper respiratory infection that did not require medication. She denies trauma to the affected joints, or occupational repetitive motions during the 20 years she

worked as a clerk in a gift shop. She has no known food, drug, or environmental allergies. In addition to the ibuprofen for joint pain, Mrs. J. takes
Premarin 0.625 mg on days 1 to 25 of the month and Provera 5 mg on days
14 to 25 to prevent osteoporosis.

QUESTION 1. What additional historical information is needed for assess-
ment of the joint pain? (Select all that apply.)
 A. History of warmth or swelling of the affected joints
 B. Presence of fatigue
 C. The degree to which the joint symptoms affect activities of daily living
 D. Gastric/abdominal discomfort or any rectal bleeding
 E. Specific location of hand joint involvement

## PHYSICAL FINDINGS

Vital signs:        Temperature 37.1°C (98.7°F); pulse 88; respirations 12;
                    blood pressures—left arm sitting 135/88, right arm sitting
                    134/86, and left arm standing 130/86; height 5 ft 4 in.
                    (162.5 cm); weight 160 lb (72.6 kg).
General:            Moderately overweight, well-nourished older adult female
                    who ambulates with normal gait and exhibits mild
                    discomfort when sitting or rising
                    from a chair.
Musculoskeletal:    Full range of motion of all joints. No muscle atrophy or
                    asymmetry noted. Strength equal bilaterally.
                    Hands: Bilateral joint tenderness of the distal inter-
                    phalangeal (DIP) and proximal interphalangeal (PIP) joints
                    of the 2nd and 3rd digits with no redness or swelling;
                    2-mm Heberden's nodes on the DIP joints of both 4th
                    digits and right 3rd digit; 3-mm Bouchard's node on the
                    PIP joint of left 2nd digit. Hips: Discomfort on flexion and
                    internal rotation of right hip. Full range of motion (ROM)
                    in both hips. Extensor and flexor strength sym-metrical.
                    No redness, warmth, or edema.
                    Knees: Negative drawer signs bilaterally. Crepitus on
                    extension of left knee. Full ROM in both knees and
                    symmetrical extensor and flexor strength. No redness,
                    warmth, or edema. Left knee discomfort with weight
                    bearing.

QUESTION 2. What findings would warrant diagnostic testing? (Select all
that apply.)
 A. Joint pain without inflammation of weight-bearing and DIP hand joints
 B. Morning stiffness lasting several hours
 C. Fatigue, weakness
 D. Painful swelling with warmth and stiffness of joints

## ASSESSMENT

**QUESTION 3.** Based upon the history and objective findings, which is the most likely diagnosis for Mrs. J.?
- **A.** Gout
- **B.** Osteoarthritis
- **C.** Rheumatoid arthritis
- **D.** Psychosomatic illness

**QUESTION 4.** If Mrs. J. had presented with signs and symptoms of an inflammatory joint disease, which of the following blood tests would be useful in establishing a differential diagnosis? (Select all that apply.)
- **A.** Erythrocyte sedimentation rate (ESR) or C-reactive protein (CRP)
- **B.** Rheumatoid factor (RF)
- **C.** Antinuclear antibodies (ANA)
- **D.** Uric acid level

## PLAN

**QUESTION 5.** What should a plan for Mrs. J. include? (Select all that apply.)
- **A.** Patient education concerning proper body mechanics, exercise, and weight loss
- **B.** Complete rest of the hip joint until the pain subsides
- **C.** An immobilizer for the right knee
- **D.** Referral for surgery for removal of the phalangeal nodules
- **E.** Comfort measures, such as moist heat or cold applied to the joints

**QUESTION 6.** Which pharmacological measures would be appropriate in the management of Mrs. J.'s symptoms? (Select all that apply.)
- **A.** Nonsteroidal anti-inflammatory drugs (NSAIDs)
- **B.** Acetaminophen
- **C.** Oral corticosteroids
- **D.** Vitamins
- **E.** Topical analgesics

**QUESTION 7.** What would subsequent follow-up visits for Mrs. J. include? (Select all that apply.)
- **A.** Update of her history and a physical examination, including a Papanicolaou smear (Pap test) and mammogram
- **B.** Discussion of surgery to remove the bony nodules on her fingers
- **C.** Patient education regarding osteoarthritis
- **D.** Evaluation of the effectiveness of her management plan

## ANSWERS

**QUESTION 1.** What additional historical information is needed for assessment of the joint pain?
- **A.** *YES.* Warmth and swelling of the affected joints are considered to be characteristic features of inflammatory rheumatic diseases such as

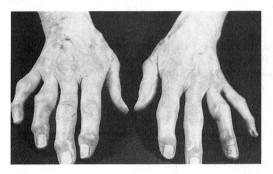

FIGURE 37-1. Degenerative joint disease: Heberden nodes at the distal interphalangeal joints and Bouchard nodes at the proximal interphalangeal joints (see Color Plate 7). (Reprinted from the Clinical Slide Collection on the Rheumatic Disease, copyright 1995, 1991. Used by permission of the American College of Rheumatology.)

rheumatoid arthritis, gout, and pseudogout. Heat and joint swelling are less characteristic of osteoarthritis, although both occasionally occur in some patients. The heat of osteoarthritis is usually of a much milder form, and the swelling is of insidious onset, feeling hard and bony compared to that of inflammatory arthritis, which presents more suddenly and feels soft and fluid-like.

B. *YES.* Fatigue is a systemic symptom commonly seen with rheumatoid arthritis, but not characteristic of osteoarthritis or gout.

C. *YES.* The degree to which the joint pain and stiffness affect activities of daily living is an indication of both the severity of the problem and the effectiveness of treatment.

D. *YES.* Gastrointestinal (GI) symptoms, including heartburn, dyspepsia, abdominal cramps or pain, nausea, vomiting, increased or decreased appetite, diarrhea, constipation, or stomatitis, are side effects of NSAIDs such as ibuprofen. Furthermore, GI bleeding secondary to NSAIDs may indicate peptic, duodenal, or intestinal ulceration or perforation, as well as intestinal obstruction and stenosis.

E. *YES.* The location of hand joint involvement can help in differentiating rheumatoid arthritis from osteoarthritis. Rheumatoid arthritis tends to affect the wrist, the metacarpophalangeal (MCP) joints, and the PIP joints, whereas osteoarthritis tends to involve the PIP and DIP joints, as well as the first carpometacarpal (CMC) joint of the thumb (see Fig. 37-1).

QUESTION 2. What findings would warrant diagnostic testing?

A. *NO.* In the absence of evidence of an inflammatory process, laboratory testing is not warranted. Furthermore, radiologic testing would be warranted only if the clinical picture could not be explained by a thorough history and physical examination or if surgical options were being explored.

B. *YES.* Morning stiffness that lasts less than a hour is associated with osteoarthritis, whereas stiffness lasting several hours supports a diagnosis of rheumatoid arthritis. If an inflammatory process is suspected, laboratory blood work can help aid in the diagnosis. Radiographs can be useful in ambiguous clinical presentations, but signs and symptoms that strongly suggest osteoarthritis mitigate the

need for diagnostic x-rays. In the case of rheumatoid arthritis, radiographic changes are usually not apparent during the first 6 months.
- C. *YES.* Fatigue and weakness can be general symptoms of systemic disease. Investigation of the cause of these symptoms is important in order to rule out significant illness.
- D. *YES.* Painful swelling with warmth and stiffness of joints is consistent with inflammatory joint diseases such as gout, pseudogout, and rheumatoid arthritis. It may also signal an infection in the joint from causes such as gonococcal arthritis, which usually affects the knee joint, or Lyme disease. Joint aspiration with subsequent culture of the fluid may be indicated for definitive diagnosis.

QUESTION 3. Based upon the history and objective findings, which is the most likely diagnosis for Mrs. J.?
- A. *NO.* Gout is usually associated with monoarticular joint involvement, most often of the great toe. Deposits of uric acid crystals cause intermittent, painful inflammation of the affected joint. Gout occurs most commonly in men over the age of 30 (90 percent), but can affect women, typically after menopause.
- B. *YES.* Mrs. J.'s history and physical examination strongly suggests a diagnosis of osteoarthritis: absence of systemic symptoms, insidious onset with progressive worsening, morning stiffness of short duration, increase of pain with joint use, involvement of weight-bearing joints, Heberden's and Bouchard's nodes, and an absence of inflammation of the involved joints. It is a common disorder, assumed to be related to overuse of the joints. Studies have found it to be radiographically evident in 80 to 100 percent of people over 60 years of age, 40 percent of whom exhibit symptoms.
- C. *NO.* Mrs. J. does not have the joint inflammation, systemic symptoms, symmetrical joint involvement, and pattern of pain associated with rheumatoid arthritis.
- D. *NO.* The presence of joint tenderness and Heberden's and Bouchard's nodes are indications of true organic joint pathology. The client's distress about "tumors" may stem from a lack of knowledge about her arthritic changes and represent an understandable concern that needs to be addressed.

QUESTION 4. If Mrs. J. had presented with signs and symptoms of an inflammatory joint disease, which of the following blood tests would be useful in establishing a differential diagnosis?
- A. *YES.* Erythrocyte sedimentation rate is a nonspecific indication of the presence and intensity of an inflammatory process. Using the Westergren method, normal ESR values in women are 0 to 20 mm/h for those <50 years of age, <30 mm/h for those 50 to 85 years of age, and <42 mm/h for those >85 years of age. Normal ESR values in men are 0 to 15 mm/h for those <50 years of age, <20 mm/h for those 50 to 85 years of age, and <30 mm/h for those >85 years of age. However, ESR elevations do not always rise in proportion to the inflammatory

process, and many healthy individuals have an elevated ESR. C-reactive protein may be a more useful test in rheumatoid arthritis (<8 mg/dL is normal). Like the ESR, CRP is helpful for monitoring the course and effect of therapy for inflammatory disorders. However, in any acute inflammatory change, CRP shows an earlier, more intense rise than the ESR, and with recovery, disappearance of CRP precedes the return to normal of the ESR. Furthermore, unlike the ESR, CRP is not influenced by anemia, congestive heart failure, or other pathologies.

B.  *YES.* High RF titers can be found in 80 to 90 percent of people with long-term rheumatoid arthritis. However, RF can be detected in only 33 percent of patients in the first 3 months of disease and in only 60 percent during the first 6 months. Also, RF can be found in other connective-tissue and chronic inflammatory diseases, such as sarcoidosis, tuberculosis, liver disease, and syphilis. Furthermore, 1 percent of the "normal" population can be positive for RF and about 10 to 20 percent of rheumatoid arthritis patients never develop RF. But the presence of RF along with correlating physical findings can be diagnostic of rheumatoid arthritis.

C.  *YES.* The specificity of an ANA profile is approximately 50 percent in detecting rheumatic disease in general, but it detects up to 95 percent of systemic lupus erythematosus (SLE). It is most useful for excluding SLE as a diagnosis.

D.  *YES.* Serum uric acid levels can be helpful in diagnosing gout. If a patient presents physical findings that correlate, an elevated uric acid level suggests the diagnosis of gout. A level greater than 7.5 mg/dL is considered elevated.

**QUESTION 5.** What should a plan for Mrs. J. include?

A.  *YES.* The use of proper body mechanics will decrease joint stress. Muscle-strengthening exercises will strengthen the supporting structures around the joint to preserve function, decrease pain, and retard joint deterioration. Range of motion exercises will increase flexibility and reduce stiffness. A referral to physical or occupational therapy can be useful for instruction concerning an exercise program, joint protection maneuvers, the use of assistive devices, if necessary, and gait training. Furthermore, Mrs. J.'s overweight status puts mechanical stress on her hip and knee joints. Therefore, she should be advised how to safely undertake an aerobic exercise program and maintain a lower-calorie, but well-balanced diet. Even modest degrees of weight loss can achieve substantial reductions in such mechanical stress.

B.  *NO.* Complete rest of a joint would result in loss of ROM, strength, and function. But since pain and joint damage may be exacerbated by use, short periods of rest throughout the day are appropriate.

C.  *NO.* Immobilization of the knee is inappropriate and would also result in loss of ROM, strength, and function.

D.  *NO.* Surgical intervention for the removal of these harmless nodules is usually not warranted. However, for seriously afflicted hip or knee joints, surgical replacement may be indicated. These surgeries usually provide very good symptomatic relief and functional improvement.

E.  *YES.* Moist heat or a hot shower can also be used to relieve morning stiffness. Use of heating pads should be discouraged, and they should be used only at the lowest temperature setting to decrease the potential for burns. Application of cold has also been found to relieve discomfort. Cold should not be applied for longer than 20 min at a time to prevent skin damage. Applying a towel or clothing between the skin and the source of heat or cold helps prevent burns or other skin damage.

QUESTION 6. Which pharmacological measures would be appropriate in the management of Mrs. J.'s symptoms?

A.  *YES.* Nonsteroidal anti-inflammatory drugs, such as aspirin, ibuprofen, and naproxen, are effective analgesics for arthritic pain, and many are available without a prescription at a low cost. Since osteoarthritis is not an inflammatory disease, the value of using NSAIDs has been questioned; furthermore, there is *theoretical* concern that NSAIDs might even be injurious, because they depress proteoglycan synthesis, which is needed for cartilage repair. However, it is also possible that they reduce a secondary inflammation that may be present in osteoarthritis. There is consensus, however, that a major side effect with these drugs is gastric upset or bleeding. The use of enteric-coated NSAIDs and taking the drug on a full stomach can help alleviate this problem.

B.  *YES.* Acetaminophen, 500 mg, three or four times a day, p.r.n., may provide pain relief without the higher cost or side effects of NSAIDs. Acetaminophen is used for its analgesic properties, as it does not have any anti-inflammatory effects. Caution should be exercised in its use with patients who have decreased liver function.

C.  *NO.* While corticosteroid medications are used for short-term anti-inflammatory therapy, they have no place in osteoarthritis management. These drugs have many adverse side effects, such as immune system suppression, adrenal suppression, behavior changes, and osteoporotic changes. Intra-articular injection of steroids into large joints, such as the knee, has been shown to provide some relief of pain, however. If long-term results (i.e., several months) are not achieved with one or two injections, this therapy should not be continued. Serious side effects of multiple steroid injections include joint destruction and infection.

D.  *NO.* Vitamins may be taken by the patient, but they are not specific for treating or reversing the effects of this disease. Patients should be urged to eat a well-balanced diet as their source of vitamins and other nutrients, and to avoid fad foods or diets that claim to cure arthritis.

E.  *YES.* The topical analgesic capsaicin may be useful in the treatment of osteoarthritis. Capsaicin has the ability to deplete and prevent the reaccumulation of substance P at the sensory nerve terminals, thus reducing pain. It is usually applied four times a day. Local burning may occur initially, but this side effect generally ceases with continued usage.

QUESTION 7. What would subsequent follow-up visits for Mrs. J. include?

A. *YES*. The client has not been seen on a regular basis, and preventive care such as a physical examination, Pap test, mammogram, and lipid screening has not been done for 2 years. It is appropriate to do a baseline Pap test if there is no documentation of previous Pap screening in which smears have been consistently normal. Annual mammography screening is recommended for women beginning at age 50. Lipid screening as an evaluation of cardiovascular disease risk is also recommended if it has not been done within the past 5 years or if the patient has had elevated levels in the past.

B. *NO*. Surgery for the removal of Heberden's and Bouchard's nodules is usually inappropriate. If deformity, pain that interferes with activities of daily living, or loss of function occur in the future, surgery may be considered at that time.

C. *YES*. Education should include information regarding the pathophysiology and prognosis of the disease, an exercise program, diet, medication, and comfort measures.

D. *YES*. Because of the chronicity of arthritis, intermittent follow-up appointments should be scheduled to monitor the progression of the disease. During return visits, effectiveness of the management plan, coping strategies, and support systems should be evaluated.

## REFERENCES

Bellamy, N. (1986). *Colour Atlas of Clinical Rheumatology*. Boston: MPT Press Limited.

Glaser, V. (1997). Rheumatoid arthritis: What's new in treatment? *Patient Care 31*(5), 81–99.

Goroll, A. H. (1995). Management of osteoarthritis. In A. H. Goroll, L. A. May, A. G. Mulley, Jr. (eds.), *Primary Care Medicine: Office Evaluation and Management of the Adult Patient*, 3d ed., 790–794. Philadelphia: J. B. Lippincott.

Goroll, A. H. (1995). Management of rheumatoid arthritis. In A. H. Goroll, L. A. May, A. G. Mulley, Jr. (eds.), *Primary Care Medicine: Office Evaluation and Management of the Adult Patient*, 3d ed., 780–789. Philadelphia: J. B. Lippincott.

Hellmann, D. (1996). Arthritis and musculoskeletal disorders. In L. Tierney, Jr., S. McPhee, M. Papadakis (eds.), *Current Medical Diagnosis and Treatment*, 35th ed., 719–767. Stamford, CT: Appleton & Lange.

Jarvis, C. (1996). *Physical Examination and Health* Assessment. Philadelphia: W. B. Saunders.

Pincus, T. (1993). A pragmatic approach to cost-effective use of laboratory tests and imaging procedures in patients with musculoskeletal symptoms. *Prim Care 20*, 795–813.

Uphold, C. R., Graham, M. V. (1994). *Clinical Guidelines in Family Practice*, 2d ed. Gainesville, FL: Barmarrae Books.

Wallach, J. (1996). *Interpretation of Diagnostic Tests*. Boston: Little, Brown.

# 38

# Prostate Disease

*Bernard P. Tadda*
*Marie Lindsey*

Lou G., a 66-year-old Caucasian male, has been seen regularly at this rural clinic for health maintenance. He was last seen at his annual examination 10 months ago, and was deemed healthy. Routine laboratory tests, including a complete blood count, lipid profile, stool for occult blood, and urinalysis, were normal, as were his electrocardiogram and tuberculin skin test. He told the triage nurse that the reason for this visit was for "personal problems," and that he wants to see his regular health care provider.

## CHIEF COMPLAINT

"I've been having some problems urinating for about 6 months."

## HISTORY OF PRESENT ILLNESS

Mr. G. reports that he has been having some problems with urination over the past 6 months that seem to be getting worse. He has been "leaking urine" at times and needing to get up in the night to urinate. Sometimes he has difficulty initiating urination, and the stream of urine seems to be weaker than it was previously. Mr. G. denies any pain or burning on urination, abdominal pain, gastrointestinal problems, discharge from the penis, fever, or sexual dysfunction.

## PAST MEDICAL HISTORY

Mr. G. has been married for 47 years and states that he has always been monogamous. He is a retired farmer and the father of two sons, who now work on the family farm. His only chronic problem is mild degenerative joint disease of the knees, for which he takes ibuprofen as needed. He does not smoke. He has no known allergies, and he has never had surgery or been hospitalized. The rest of the review of systems is unremarkable.

**QUESTION 1.** What further history would help in the assessment? (Select all that apply.)
- A. Use of over-the-counter medications
- B. Alcohol use
- C. Frequency of sexual relations
- D. Back pain

**QUESTION 2.** Which of the following observations would be helpful in establishing a differential diagnosis? (Select all that apply.)
- A. Presence or absence of genital lesions or penile discharge
- B. Abdominal masses
- C. Rectal tone
- D. Enlarged prostate

## PHYSICAL FINDINGS

Abdomen: Soft, nontender, no masses or organomegaly. Bowel sounds are active in all quadrants. No costovertebral angle tenderness.

Genitalia: Normal external male with circumcised penis. Testicles descended bilaterally without masses or tenderness. No hernia or regional lymphadenopathy.

Rectal: Good sphincter tone. Prostate is slightly enlarged, palpable, firm, and nontender with no bogginess or masses. Hemoccult is negative.

**QUESTION 3.** Which of the following laboratory tests would be most helpful to order at this time? (Select all that apply.)
- A. Serum creatinine
- B. Serum testosterone
- C. Urinalysis
- D. Glucose tolerance test

**QUESTION 4.** Which of the following would be the most accurate information to give the patient regarding his probable diagnosis? (Select all that apply.)
- A. He has normal symptoms of aging and should learn to adapt to his physiologic changes.
- B. His symptoms strongly suggest that he has prostate cancer.
- C. The enlargement of his prostate indicates that further tests will be needed.
- D. His symptoms may be related to a sexually transmitted disease (STD) requiring future evaluation.

## ASSESSMENT

The review of history, physical findings, and laboratory results leads to a tentative diagnosis of benign prostatic hyperplasia (BPH).

## PLAN

**QUESTION 5.** Which of the following options should be discussed for the treatment of BPH? (Select all that apply.)
A. Oral medications
B. Surgery
C. No treatment
D. Antibiotics

**QUESTION 6.** Mr. G. has heard about the medication finasteride (Proscar) and wants to know about possible side effects. What should he be told? (Select all that apply.)
A. Symptomatic relief may not be noticed for 6 to 12 months.
B. There is a possibility of sexual dysfunction/impotence with this drug.
C. The medication may cause some hair loss.
D. The medication may interfere with the action of ibuprofen.

**QUESTION 7.** If a firm nodule on the prostate was palpated, a serum prostate-specific antigen (PSA) should be drawn. Which of the following is true regarding PSA results? (Select all that apply.)
A. A low level suggests the diagnosis of BPH.
B. Benign prostatic hyperplasia may cause an elevation of the PSA.
C. The PSA is a useful tool to monitor treatment response for BPH.
D. An elevated PSA means that prostate cancer is present.

## ANSWERS

**QUESTION 1.** What further history would help in the assessment?
A. *YES.* Over-the-counter medications, such as "cold" preparations, have the potential to cause an exacerbation of bladder outflow problems.
B. *YES.* Alcoholic beverages can increase the volume of urine by suppressing antidiuretic hormone (ADH), and thus contribute to voiding difficulties.
C. *NO.* The *frequency* of his sexual relations has no bearing on his complaint.
D. *YES.* Back pain can be related to prostate disease in two ways: either as a result of renal calculi caused by bladder outlet obstruction or as a result of prostate cancer that has metastasized to the spine. Furthermore, back pain is often a symptom of several neurologic diseases that also result in bladder or bowel dysfunction, and can be a symptom of pyelonephritis.

**QUESTION 2.** Which of the following observations would be helpful in establishing a differential diagnosis?
A. *YES.* Genital lesions and penile discharge are symptoms of an STD. Mr. G. stated that he had been monogamous throughout his marriage, and there is no reason to doubt his honesty. However, as STDs can cause urinary symptoms, it is important to examine the genitalia for any signs of such infections.

B. *YES.* Abdominal masses, specifically a percussible or palpable bladder, indicate urinary retention, sometimes referred to as postvoid residual (PVR). A large PVR may be the result of a bladder outlet obstruction caused by an enlarged prostate.

C. *YES.* Lack of rectal tone suggests an underlying neurological condition rather than specific diseases of the prostate or could be a result of repeated anal intercourse.

D. *YES.* An enlarged prostate could be contributing to Mr. G.'s symptoms. However, examination of several large BPH clinical databases has demonstrated unequivocally that no *direct* relationship exists between prostate size and symptom severity or between prostate size and degree of bladder outlet obstruction. The self-administered International Prostate Symptom Score (I-PSS) is a validated tool for assessing the baseline severity, response to therapy, and disease progression of prostatism, which collectively refers to the following symptoms: frequency, hesitancy, urgency, straining to initiate urination, diminished caliber and interrupted urinary stream, incontinence, posturination dribbling, nocturia, and dysuria (see Table 38-1). Despite the usefulness of the I-PSS, it is not unusual for patients with identical symptom scores to report very different perceptions of the extent of aggravation resulting from the symptoms.

**QUESTION 3.** Which of the following laboratory tests would be most helpful to order at this time?

A. *YES.* The serum creatinine will indicate if there is any obstructive uropathy present.

B. *NO.* The serum testosterone will not add any valuable information in this case.

C. *YES.* A urinalysis is needed to check for any signs of infection that may contribute to the presenting symptoms.

D. *NO.* It is true that an enlarged prostate can lead to symptoms similar to those of diabetes mellitus (e.g., daytime and nighttime urinary frequency), and that diabetes can cause a neurogenic bladder; however, Mr. G. does not present with any other symptoms typical of diabetes. Furthermore, ruling out diabetes is better accomplished with a fasting plasma glucose than with a glucose tolerance test.

**QUESTION 4.** Which of the following would be the most accurate information to give the patient regarding his probable diagnosis?

A. *NO.* Although BPH is very common in older men (50 percent of men will have it by age 50 and 90 percent by age 85), it is inappropriate to suggest that his symptoms are merely due to aging.

B. *NO.* It is inappropriate to suggest a work-up for cancer at this time given the history and physical examination information. While prostate cancer cannot be ruled out at this point of the assessment, Mr. G.'s symptoms do not support this diagnosis any more than they support a diagnosis of BPH.

C. *YES.* The history and physical suggest BPH, but further testing will be needed to confirm the diagnosis.

D. *NO.* He has no history, signs, or symptoms suggestive of an STD.

TABLE 38-1   International Prostate Symptom Scores (I-PSS)

| Patient name: | Not at all | Less than 1 time in 5 | Less than half the time | About half the time | More than half the time | Almost always | Your score |
|---|---|---|---|---|---|---|---|
| 1. Incomplete emptying<br>Over the past month, how often have you had a sensation of not emptying your bladder completely after you finished urinating? | 0 | 1 | 2 | 3 | 4 | 5 | |
| 2. Frequency<br>Over the past month, how often have you had to urinate again less than two hours after you finished urinating? | 0 | 1 | 2 | 3 | 4 | 5 | |
| 3. Intermittency<br>Over the past month, how often have you found you stopped and started again several times when you urinated? | 0 | 1 | 2 | 3 | 4 | 5 | |
| 4. Urgency<br>Over the past month, how often have you found it difficult to postpone urination? | 0 | 1 | 2 | 3 | 4 | 5 | |
| 5. Weak stream<br>Over the past month, how often have you had a weak urinary stream? | 0 | 1 | 2 | 3 | 4 | 5 | |
| 6. Straining<br>Over the past month, how often have you had to push or strain to begin urination? | 0 | 1 | 2 | 3 | 4 | 5 | |

QUESTION 5. Which of the following options should be discussed for the treatment of BPH?

A. *YES.* There are several classes of medications that may relieve prostatic hypertrophy symptoms. One such therapy consists of alpha adrenergic antagonists, which may decrease the resistance along the prostatic urethra by relaxing the smooth muscle component of the prostate. Examples of alpha adrenergic antagonists include prazosin, alfuzosin, indoramin, terazosin, doxazosin, tamsulosin, and phenoxybenzamine. A second choice is Proscar, a drug that acts as a form of medical castration in that it blocks the production of dihydrotestosterone (DHT) androgen, upon which the prostate is dependent for its development. Proscar lowers serum and prostatic levels of DHT without lowering serum testosterone levels and may prevent further enlargement of the prostate, whereas alpha blockers do not. It is also the only hormonal therapy that is approved by the Food and Drug Administration for BPH. Alternative therapies, such as the saw palmetto berry, have also been shown to be effective in the treatment of BPH.

**TABLE 38-1** (*continued*)   **International Prostate Symptom Scores (I-PSS)**

| | None | 1 time | 2 times | 3 times | 4 times | 5 or more times | |
|---|---|---|---|---|---|---|---|
| **7. Nocturia** Over the past month, how many times did you most typically get up to urinate from the time you went to bed at night until the time you got up in the morning? | 0 | 1 | 2 | 3 | 4 | 5 | |
| Total I-PSS Score = | | | | | | | |

| Quality of Life due to Urinary Symptoms | Delighted | Pleased | Mostly satisfied | Mixed—about equally satisfied & dissatisfied | Mostly dissatisfied | Unhappy | Terrible |
|---|---|---|---|---|---|---|---|
| If you were to spend the rest of your life with your urinary condition just the way it is now, how would you feel about that? | 0 | 1 | 2 | 3 | 4 | 5 | 6 |

The International Prostate Symptom Score (I-PSS) is based on the answers to seven questions concerning urinary symptoms. Each question allows the patient to choose one out of five answers indicating increasing severity of the particular symptom. The answers are assigned points from 0 to 5. The total score can therefore range from 0 to 35 (asymptomatic to very symptomatic).

Furthermore, the International Consensus Committee (ICC) recommends the use of only a single question to assess the quality of life. The answers to this question range from "delighted" to "terrible" or 0 to 6. Although this single question may or may not capture the global impact of BPH symptoms or quality of life, it may serve as a valuable starting point for a doctor-patient conversation.

The ICC strongly recommends that all physicians who counsel patients suffering from symptoms of prostatism utilize these measures not only during the initial interview but also during and after treatment in order to monitor treatment response.

SOURCE: Noble, J. (ed.). (1996). *Textbook of Primary Care Medicine*, 2d ed. St. Louis: Mosby-Year Book. With permission.

B. *YES.* Removal of the obstruction by surgical means is one of the options for treating BPH. Symptom improvement is high following surgery, with low morbidity and complication rates. However, the occurrence of retrograde ejaculation can be significant after surgery as compared to its occurrence with medical treatment.

C. *YES.* Based on the severity of symptoms and the evaluation of relief from available treatment alternatives, sometimes "watchful waiting," for 6 to 12 months, is a viable option. Behavior changes may also be added to this regimen, such as encouraging patients to avoid fluid intake after 7:00 P.M. and to decrease caffeine (none after 12:00 noon) and alcohol intake.

D. *NO.* As Mr. G.'s symptoms do not suggest an infection, antibiotics are not indicated.

QUESTION **6.** Mr. G. has heard about the medication finasteride (Proscar) and wants to know about possible side effects. What should he be told?
A. *YES.* At least 6 to 12 months may be required to determine whether a beneficial response has been achieved using Proscar. This is compared to the 4 to 6 weeks that may be needed to realize a beneficial response using alpha adrenergic antagonists.
B. *YES.* Although the incidence is low, there is a possibility of sexual dysfunction with finasteride.
C. *NO.* This medication does not promote hair loss; in fact, the drug in lower doses is being used as a treatment for baldness.
D. *NO.* This medication does not interfere with the action of ibuprofen.

QUESTION **7.** If a firm nodule on the prostate was palpated, a serum prostate-specific antigen (PSA) should be drawn. Which of the following is true regarding PSA results?
A. *NO.* The significant finding is an elevation of a PSA, not a lower result. Elevations of the PSA suggest possible prostatic cancer, but are not diagnostic of BPH. However, BPH may cause elevations of the PSA without prostatic cancer involvement.
B. *YES.* Persons with BPH may have modest elevations of the PSA.
C. *NO.* The PSA is a useful tool to monitor treatment of prostatic cancer, not of BPH.
D. *NO.* An elevated PSA is only a screening tool for prostate cancer. Further testing would be needed to diagnose prostatic cancer.

## REFERENCES

Balch, J., Balch, P. (1993). *Prescription for Nutritional Healing: A Practical A to Z Reference to Drug-Free Remedies using Vitamins, Minerals, Herbs and Food Supplements.* Garden City Park, NY: Avery Publishing.

Burton Goldberg Group. (1994). *Alterative Medicine: The Definitive Guide.* Puyallup, WA: Future Medicine Publishing.

Goodson, J., Barry, M. (1995). Management of benign prostatic hyperplasia. In A. H. Gorall, L. A. May, A. G. Mulley (eds.), *Primary Care Medicine: Office Evaluation and Management of the Adult Patient,* 3d ed., 705–708. Philadelphia: J. B. Lippincott.

Goodson, J., Barry, M. (1995). Screening for prostate cancer. In A. H. Gorall, L. A. May, A. G. Mulley (eds.), *Primary Care Medicine: Office Evaluation and Management of the Adult Patient,* 3d ed., 657–659. Philadelphia: J. B. Lippincott.

Guthrie, R. (1997). Benign prostatic hyperplasia in elderly men. What are the special issues in treatment? *Postgrad Med 101,* 141–143, 148, 151–154.

Hollander, J. B., Diokno, A. C. (1996). Prostatism: Benign prostatic hyperplasia. *Urol Clin North Am 23*(1),75–86.

Morton, A. R., Lepor, H. (1996). Prostate disorders—Benign and malignant. In J. Noble (ed.), *Textbook of Primary Care Medicine,* 1782–1791. St. Louis: Mosby.

*Physicians' Desk Reference: Nurse's Handbook.* (1996). Montvale, NJ: Medical Economics Company.

Tchetgen, B., Oesterling, J. (1995). The role of prostate-specific antigen in the evaluation of benign prostatic hyperplasia. *Urol Clin North Am 22,* 333–344.

Weinstock, M., Neides, D. (1996). *The Resident's Guide to Ambulatory Medicine,* 2d ed. Columbus, OH: Anadem.

# VIII

## FAMILY

# Introduction

## Arlene Miller

A family is characterized by emotional bonds and commitment, mutual identity and goals, and specific, shared behaviors and rituals. The family life cycle considers normal processes in the multigenerational system over time, and reflects individual developmental transitions among family members. A systems orientation considers family functioning in terms of basic norms and belief systems that are expressed through implicit and explicit relationship rules. These rules organize family interaction and optimally serve to maintain the system in a stable but flexible way. Norms govern individual roles and behaviors, and their consequences within the system. Belief systems include shared values and assumptions that guide behavior within the family and the larger social systems in which the individual and family may be embedded.

Competent family functioning includes cohesiveness, fostering autonomy among members, shared negotiation of power, support for family members, capacity for change, and effective communication patterns. Functional communication includes clear, dynamic transmission and reception of both the meaning and the intent of a message. A family may participate in behavior that is dysfunctional, referring to patterns that are unworkable and associated with symptoms of distress. Factors that affect individual family members have an impact on the entire family as a system, and patterns that may be functional at the individual or family level may have dysfunctional consequences at another level.

Within the context of a broad, national cultural pattern, significant variations exist. The traditional view of a nuclear family consisting of married parents and their children has broadened in recent years to include blended families or stepfamilies, same-sex or single-parent families, grandparents as primary caregivers to their grandchildren, and other alternative family compositions. Families transmit the cultural patterns of their own ethnic background and class, as well as their attitudes toward others of different backgrounds. Cultural and religious values can have a tremendous impact on family relationships by enforcing or approving family norms. These values also influence beliefs regarding health and illness.

Family health is a dynamic process that includes the activities a family uses to promote and protect the well-being of the family unit as well as its individual members. In dysfunctional systems, the opportunity for abuse and neglect can occur, either from family members or from nonrelated caretakers. Interventions must be family-oriented rather than focused solely on the victim. Family violence is a serious public health problem. Children, pregnant women, and the frail elderly are at highest risk, but screening methods are problematic and uncertain. Although the U.S. Preventive Services Task Force found insufficient evidence to recommend either for or against specific screening instruments to detect family violence, it does recommend that clinicians be alert to the various presentations of child, spouse/partner, and elder abuse, and to include questions about physical abuse when taking a history. The American Medical Association Guidelines for Adolescent Preventive Services recommend that teenagers should be asked annually about emotional, physical, and sexual abuse.

Family interviews are not always an option in busy primary care settings, but planning health care interventions that use either a family-as-patient or family-as-context approach may greatly enhance and ensure successful treatment. Family-oriented health promotion interventions can be developed throughout the life cycle. Constructing a family genogram can facilitate the process of family assessment, and provides a useful diagram that can include communication patterns and relations, family members' health status, health practices, and support systems.

The case studies in this chapter utilize a systems approach to selected problems that involve and have an impact on the whole family. Sometimes problems in family functioning are overlooked when health care providers focus only on individuals, as demonstrated by the case study of a family in transition, in which a woman's plan for weight loss is influenced by her family dynamics. The case study of family communication during adaptation to chronic illness illustrates the importance of health care providers' using competent interviewing skills for effective intervention at a family level. The two other cases in this chapter focus on family violence: child abuse and elder abuse and neglect. Often, the primary health care provider is in the best position to detect early cases of family dysfunction, and plays an important role in documentation, intervention, reporting, and/or referral.

## REFERENCES

Friedman, M. (1986). *Family Nursing: Theory and Assessment.* Norwalk, CT: Appleton-Century-Crofts.

McCarthy, N. C. (1994). Health promotion and the family. In C. Edelman, C. Mandle (eds.), *Health Promotion throughout the Lifespan,* 3d ed., 179–201. St. Louis: Mosby.

McGoldrick, M., Heiman, M., Carter, B. (1996). The changing family life cycle: A perspective on normalcy. In F. Walsh (ed.), *Normal Family Processes,* 2d ed., 405–443. New York: Guilford Press.

Murray, R. B., Zentner, J. P. (1996). *Nursing Assessment and Health Promotion: Strategies through the Life Span,* 6th ed. Norwalk, CT: Appleton & Lange.

U.S. Preventive Services Task Force. (1996). *Guide to Clinical Preventive Services,* 2d ed. Baltimore: Williams & Wilkins.

Walsh, F. (1996). Conceptualization of normal family processes. In F. Walsh (ed.), *Normal Family Processes,* 2d ed., 3–69. New York: Guilford Press.

# 39

# Child Injury versus Abuse

*Dorothy Kent*

*Marie L. Talashek*

Tommy is a 3-year-old Caucasian boy who is in day care, and the day care teacher noticed bruising on the child's arm. When asked about his "owey," the child reportedly said, "Daddy whupped me." The day care center director called Child Protective Service (CPS) and the child is in temporary custody of a CPS caseworker, who is bringing Tommy to the primary care clinic of a military base for bruising suspected to be due to child abuse. The CPS worker has spoken with the child's mother, a lieutenant in the Navy. The mother is on her way to the clinic to meet her child and the caseworker.

## CHIEF COMPLAINT

The CPS caseworker wants to know the severity of the injuries and whether they could be the result of child abuse. The mother is clearly agitated, and the child is clinging to her leg.

QUESTION 1. What are the responsibilities of the primary health care provider for the family at this visit? (Select all that apply.)
A. Obtain a history and physical examination.
B. Decide if it is safe for the child to go home with his mother.
C. Question the child's father about what happened.
D. Protect the family's privacy regarding prior treatment for spouse abuse injuries when talking with the CPS caseworker.

QUESTION 2. What steps might be helpful for completing an accurate evaluation? (Select all that apply.)
A. Talk with the caseworker privately first.
B. Remind the child and mother that your job is to help them stay healthy and safe.
C. Talk privately with the mother before talking with the child.

   **D.** Offer the child juice and provide a supervised play opportunity.
   **E.** Talk with the child separately from the parent and caseworker.

## HISTORY OF PRESENT ILLNESS

The child and mother both say that the father grabbed the little boy by the arm when he cried after being told to finish his dinner. The mother claims that her husband came home late from work and was upset about an altercation with his boss; he has been experiencing a lot of work-related stress recently. They began arguing as she served him dinner, because he had been drinking. When Tommy cried, the father forcefully grabbed him by the arm, jerking him up in the air, and spanked him hard on the bottom with his hand several times. The father stormed out of the house, returning home after the mother and Tommy were asleep. After the incident, the mother checked Tommy's buttocks and arm, which were red but did not seem to need further care. She lay down with him as he cried himself to sleep. This morning they left for the day care center and work before the father got out of bed. The mother has been seen twice for injuries sustained when her husband hit her; she has done nothing about this abuse. She is now concerned that her husband seems to be losing control, as this is the first time that he has hit Tommy. The mother's perspective is that the father is under a lot of stress at work and "takes it out" on her. She is frightened for both herself and Tommy, but she loves her husband. Tommy denies any pain except at the area of the bruise and states that his mother has never hit him and that his daddy must have been "really mad" at him because he never got hit before. The husband has never received treatment for alcohol or drug abuse. They see their families only once or twice a year because they live in another part of the country. Tommy's mother has several good friends in the military, but she does not think her husband has made any really good friends since they moved here about 4 years ago.

QUESTION 3. Parental risk factors associated with child abuse include which of the following? (Select all that apply.)
   **A.** Preexisting spouse abuse
   **B.** Alcoholism or other substance use
   **C.** Domestic violence in the homes where the parents grew up
   **D.** Lack of interest in controlling the child's behavior

QUESTION 4. Child risk factors associated with child abuse injury include which of the following? (Select all that apply.)
   **A.** Young age
   **B.** Physical disability or chronic illness
   **C.** Adolescence
   **D.** Social isolation

## PAST MEDICAL HISTORY

Tommy has received care at this facility since birth. His mother is in the Navy and received prenatal care here. The father is also a patient at the facility. Tommy has never been hospitalized or received care at the emergency room. His immunizations and health maintenance are in compliance with the American Academy of Pediatrics recommendations.

## PHYSICAL EXAMINATION

**QUESTION 5.** The physical assessment should include which of the following? (Select all that apply.)
  A.  Comprehensive examination of all skin
  B.  Head, eyes, ears, nose, and throat (HEENT)
  C.  Observation, percussion, and palpation of the abdomen
  D.  Growth and developmental screening
  E.  Neurological and musculoskeletal system

Physical findings including growth and development are normal except for a bruise on the upper right arm and one in the shape of a hand on the buttocks (see Fig. 39-1).

## ASSESSMENT

**QUESTION 6.** What assessment and/or recommendations are appropriate?
  A.  No indication of abuse
  B.  Removal from home
  C.  Hospitalization for Tommy
  D.  Recent abuse without permanent damage

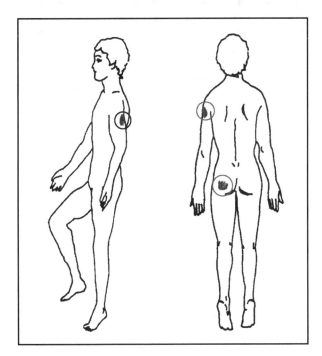

**FIGURE 39-1.**
Physical findings:
bruises.

## PLAN

QUESTION 7. The Naval Family Service Center on the base offers the following programs. Which program(s) should be recommended for this family? (Select all that apply.)
A. Parenting classes
B. Alcoholism evaluation and treatment as indicated
C. Classes in anger management for the father and assertiveness training for the mother
D. Referral to military social service department
E. Family therapy

## ANSWERS

QUESTION 1. What are the responsibilities of the primary health care provider for the family at this visit?
A. YES. A history and physical examination specific to abuse etiology is necessary to determine whether or not abuse has occurred. In cases of suspected abuse, evaluating the injury is the unique contribution of the primary care provider.
B. NO. It is the responsibility of the CPS caseworker to determine the safety of the child and whether removal from the home is necessary. Health care professionals are an integral part of the decision to remove a child from the home, but are not ultimately responsible for that decision. Health care professionals are mandated to report all suspected cases of abuse to CPS. Civil and criminal immunity are guaranteed to health care providers acting within their professional capacity.
C. NO. It is the responsibility of the CPS caseworker to interview all involved parties.
D. NO. Any available information relevant to family abuse must be revealed during the investigation. Spousal abuse has been associated with an increased likelihood of child abuse. Child Protective Services can also be involved in the protection of the mother. Children of victimized mothers are eight times more likely to be victimized than are children of mothers who have never been victimized.

QUESTION 2. What steps might be helpful for completing an accurate evaluation?
A. NO. It is best to talk with the caseworker and the mother together. If the caseworker is initially interviewed without the mother present, this may alienate the mother. Cooperation of the mother with the primary care provider and caseworker will facilitate problem solving.
B. YES. The mother and child should be told that their safety and health are very important. In addition, the mother should be told that she will be apprised of each step in the procedure, and that nothing will be done without her knowledge. A caring approach will facilitate both her trust and her cooperation in the assessment of the situation.
C. YES. Since the mother has a relationship with the health care provider, she can facilitate gaining the cooperation of the child. The mother

should be asked to provide details about why, how, and when the bruising happened, whether there were any other injuries at the time, and her role during the incident.

D. *YES.* Tommy is frightened, and placing him in a nonthreatening environment while the provider talks with his mother is important.

E. *YES.* It is important that Tommy be interviewed separately after he has calmed down. He should be asked to provide details about why, how, and when the bruising happened and whether this has happened before. He should be asked about whether he is afraid and who hits him. Observations during this clinic visit seem to indicate that a good relationship exists between Tommy and his mother. However, in other cases abused children may avoid their parents and appear surprisingly cooperative and affectionate with the examiner. Other behavioral signs of abuse include exaggerated fearfulness and apprehension, excessive complaining, clinginess, mood swings and behavior lability, fearfulness of adult caretakers, sleeping or eating disorders, and withdrawal from adult physical contact. In an older child, depression, aggression, and suicidal ideation or attempts may indicate abuse.

**QUESTION 3.** Parental risk factors associated with child abuse include which of the following?

A. *YES.* Preexisting spouse abuse has been associated with child abuse. Violence against a spouse often spills over to abuse of the children.

B. *YES.* Alcoholism and use of other drugs are associated with child abuse.

C. *YES.* An association has been found between being abused as a child and becoming abusive as an adult. It is important to note, however, that not all abused children will grow up to become abusing adults. Differences between abused children who go on to be abusive parents and abused children who do not are not well understood.

D. *NO.* Usually the opposite is true. Abuse often occurs because the adult is attempting to control the child's behavior. Parental characteristics that may play a part in abuse are poor impulse control, limited coping skills in the presence of high stress levels, lack of parenting skills, and poor understanding of child development and age-appropriate behavior.

**QUESTION 4.** Child risk factors associated with child abuse injury include which of the following?

A. *YES.* Because of their smaller physical size and development level, children between 3 months and 3 years of age are more vulnerable to serious injury and fatality from abuse. Battered-child syndrome, shaken infant syndrome, and nonorganic failure to thrive are common manifestations in younger children who are abused.

B. *YES.* Infants or children of any age with disabilities or chronic illnesses may be perceived as different by their parents, and thus are at risk for abuse. Also at risk are children who are difficult to console or who are unresponsive to parental nurturing.

C. *NO.* Adolescents, by virtue of their size and maturity, are better able to protect themselves and thus are less likely to sustain physical injuries.

D.  *YES.* Social isolation is often concomitant with abuse. Socially isolated children are less likely to tell someone about the abuse or have some-one ask about an injury. The abuse can continue and has the potential of escalating in severity.

**QUESTION 5.** The physical assessment should include which of the following?
A.  *YES.* The color, pattern, and location of all bruises are useful in differ-entiating accidental from inflicted bruising. The most typical area of abuse is the back from the neck to the knees. Bruises in different states of healing over the body are indicative of a pattern of continuous child abuse. However, care must be taken because preschool children often have multiple bruises on their extremities that occur during active playing. Dermatological conditions can also be mistaken for child abuse. As Tommy is examined, supplemental historical data can be gathered by asking the child about any additional bruising.
B.  *YES.* Examination of the HEENT should include a careful assessment of the fundi for bleeding, the oral mucosa for lacerations, and the mouth for missing or chipped teeth.
C.  *YES.* Observation, percussion, and palpation of the abdomen are impor-tant elements of the physical examination of a suspected case of child abuse. Child abuse can lead to organ damage and internal bleeding which must be ruled out by careful examination for abdominal tenderness.
D.  *YES.* Changes in patterns of growth and development may be important indicators of abuse or neglect. A drop in the growth curve is indicative of a problem that could be related to undernutrition. Lags in developmental progress may be related to the stress and fear associated with violence. Mothers who are abused may be so preoccupied with their own situa-tion that they fail to provide a nurturing environment for their children.
E.  *YES.* A neurological examination is needed to identify head or nerve injuries. A musculoskeletal examination is required to rule out frac-tures and injuries to muscles. A complete range of motion of all joints should be done.

**QUESTION 6.** What assessment and/or recommendations are appropriate?
A.  *NO.* The explanations given about Tommy's bruises indicate abuse.
B.  *NO.* The mother is quite concerned and cooperative with the provider and the social worker, and removal from the home is the last resort. Reporting, identification, treatment, evaluation, and follow-up of the child and his mother should be sufficient in this case. If military per-sonnel are perpetrators of abuse, they can be moved to military bar-racks and be required to undergo evaluation and treatment for all identified problems. The local CPS will turn the case over to the mili-tary if adequate programs are offered. Otherwise, the local CPS man-ages the case and arranges for services until the referral agencies report that the family is no longer considered at risk.
C.  *NO.* Hospitalization is not needed because Tommy's injuries do not require additional medical follow-up. In extreme cases hospitalization may be used for safety in the event that adequate protective custody is not available for the child.

**D.** *YES.* The child's version of the "spanking" incident and subsequent bruising supports the assessment of recent abuse. At this examination, no old injuries were found.

**QUESTION 7.** The Naval Family Service Center on the base offers the following programs. Which program(s) should be recommended for this family?

**A.** *YES.* Parenting classes are important for both parents. They should attend together so that they can develop mutual patterns of parenting. Abusive parents may have distorted perceptions or unrealistic expectations of their child. Parenting classes provide education about child development and age-appropriate behavior, as well as specific skills to deal with child behavior.

**B.** *YES.* Tommy's father should be required to undergo alcohol and drug evaluation. Child abuse is highly correlated with substance use. In this case, a contract would be made with the father to be evaluated for substance abuse as part of the care plan.

**C.** *YES.* Tommy's father can be taught appropriate alternative methods for dealing with his anger. Tommy's mother can gain the skills needed to take action, such as removing herself and her son from danger when necessary. Assertiveness can help her develop competence in using needed community resources.

**D.** *YES.* Referral to a case manager on the base is important because the caseworker can coordinate all of the referrals and take responsibility for monitoring the family. The military Family Advocacy Program (FAP) addresses prevention.

**E.** *YES.* Family therapy may help this family because they have sufficient verbal skills, and the level of anger and frustration has not escalated to an overwhelming degree. Tommy's mother expresses love for her husband and commitment to the family. Therapy would allow them to confront the abuse openly and help them identify dysfunctional patterns within the family system. The family can set long- and short-term goals, develop consensus on family rules and tasks, and learn supportive interpersonal communication patterns, thereby enhancing family functioning and stopping abusive patterns.

## REFERENCES

Brady, M. (1996). Role relationships. In C. Burns, N. Barber, N. Brady, A. Dunn (eds.), *Pediatric Primary Care: A Handbook for Nurse Practitioners.* Philadelphia: W. B. Saunders.

DePanfilis, D., Salus, M. (1992). *Child Protective Services: A Guide for Caseworkers,* rev. Washington, DC: U.S. Department of Health and Human Services.

DePanfilis, D., Salus, M. (1992). *A Coordinated Response to Child Abuse and Neglect: A Basic Manual,* rev. Washington, DC: U.S. Department of Health and Human Services.

Reece, R. (1994). *Child Abuse: A Medical Diagnosis and Management.* Philadelphia: Lea & Febiger.

U.S. Navy. Medical and the Navy Family Advocacy Program: Medical Guidelines and Protocols.

# 40

# Family in Transition

*Arlene Miller*
*Laina M. Gerace*

Ms. H., a 45-year-old Caucasian woman, has been followed closely by a family nurse practitioner (FNP) in a private, fee-for-service group practice for 6 months. In spite of careful efforts to personalize an exercise and diet plan, her weight is slowly climbing upward after an initial 15-lb decrease. Her practitioner is puzzled by this situation, since she feels they have a good relationship and Ms. H. seemed so highly motivated. When Ms. H.'s 53-year-old husband and 18-year-old twin daughters, Mona and Mimi, accompany her to the office one day, the FNP invites Ms. H.'s family to meet with them after their usual individual session.

## CHIEF COMPLAINT

"I've been having trouble staying on my diet for the past few weeks, and my family isn't really helping me."

## HISTORY OF PRESENT
## HEALTH PROBLEM

Ms. H. came to the office 6 months ago for a routine physical examination and a request to start a weight loss diet. At that time, she was assessed to be approximately 50 lb overweight. She had no apparent medical etiology for obesity. She stated that her weight had steadily crept up over the past 20 years, and she now wanted to "gain control over her life." She also wanted to look better in the workplace, as she intended to get a new job. Ms. H. was started on a 1200-calorie, low-fat diet and initiated a four-day-a-week moderate-intensity aerobic walking plan supplemented by weight training and diet support group at the local health club. She initially averaged a weight loss of 2 to 3 lb/week, but over the past month she has been gaining weight back.

During the course of the 50-min family interview, it becomes apparent that although Mr. H., who is also obese, explicitly supported his wife's efforts to improve her appearance by encouraging her visits to the FNP, paying for her health club membership, and applauding her efforts to walk in the mornings, he frequently buys her favorite snack foods and leaves them on the kitchen counter. He rewards his wife's weight loss by taking her out for expensive dinners. Throughout the interview, whenever Ms. H. complained about her husband's behavior, Mona repeatedly took her father's side. Whenever her parents disagreed during the discussion, Mimi commented in a derogatory way about her own appearance.

## PAST MEDICAL HISTORY

Ms. H. has no acute or chronic health problems and is in good health except for obesity.

## FAMILY MEDICAL HISTORY

Ms. H.'s 72-year-old mother has high blood pressure, and her 75-year-old father, who is a "drinker," has angina pectoris.

## SOCIAL HISTORY

Ms. H. has not worked outside the home since her daughters were born. The girls are planning to leave for college in a month, and Ms. H. states that she is looking forward to working full-time. Mr. H. is obese, his hair is graying and thinning, he "drinks a little," and he reveals that he was recently passed over for a promotion at his job. Mona is very slender, but her sister Mimi is quite overweight. Mona and Mimi graduated from high school 3 weeks ago. They have both stopped going to church regularly, and this has been a disappointment to their parents.

QUESTION 1. Which of the following are potential health risks for members of this family? (Select all that apply.)
A. Obesity
B. Alcohol abuse
C. Obsessive-compulsive disorder
D. Hypertension
E. Anorexia nervosa

QUESTION 2. What *individual* life-cycle issues or developmental tasks may be affecting the H. family members? (Select all that apply.)
A. Mona and Mimi need to reconnect with each other and their parents to forge a closer tie during young adulthood.
B. Mr. and Ms. H. have to resolve personal issues of intimacy and mutual trust so that they can develop their marital relationship.
C. Mona and Mimi should be dealing with issues regarding their own autonomy and identity.
D. Mr. and Ms. H. may be responding to issues regarding generativity and reassessing life goals.

QUESTION 3. What *family* life-cycle issues or developmental tasks may be affecting the H. family? (Select all that apply.)
A. Maintaining constancy in intergenerational relationships
B. Releasing or launching young adults
C. Reconciliation of conflicting loyalties or philosophies of life
D. Experiencing menopause and loss of reproductive ability

## ASSESSMENT

QUESTION 4. Which of the following are possible interpretations of the behavior observed during this interaction? (Select all that apply.)
A. The girls' actions suggest that their relationship and communication patterns have been present for a long time.
B. This family's pathological communication patterns have led to significant delays in the daughters' psychological development.
C. Mr. and Ms. H. are both ambivalent about her potential weight loss and job.
D. Mimi and Mona are overly involved with Ms. H., causing her to withdraw her affection from her husband.
E. Mr. H.'s sabotage of his wife's diet plan is probably a cry for help and reflects a need for individual psychotherapy.

## PLAN

QUESTION 5. Which of the following health promotion interventions could be implemented by the primary care provider using a "family-as-patient" perspective? (Select all that apply.)
A. Explore the effects of Ms. H.'s weight loss that might have a negative impact on the family.
B. Place each member of the family on a diet plan that meets his or her optimal health needs.
C. Practice methods of communication that emphasize direct expression of feelings and intentions.
D. Discuss alternative solutions of the problem with the family as a whole.

## ANSWERS

QUESTION 1. Which of the following are potential health risks for members of this family?
A. *YES.* Obesity is often found among several family members, and this is evident in a genogram of the H. family (see Fig. 40-1). Overweight is rarely the result of endocrine, metabolic, or neurological disturbance. A genetic tendency to obesity exists, demonstrated by studies that correlate parental weight more closely with the weight of natural than with that of adopted children. However, weight status is more commonly related to lifelong food and physical activity habits that are transmitted and sustained by family eating and exercise patterns. The use and withholding of food for purposes other than nourishment, such as entertainment, reward, consolation, or punishment, are among the values and practices that are often transmitted across several generations.

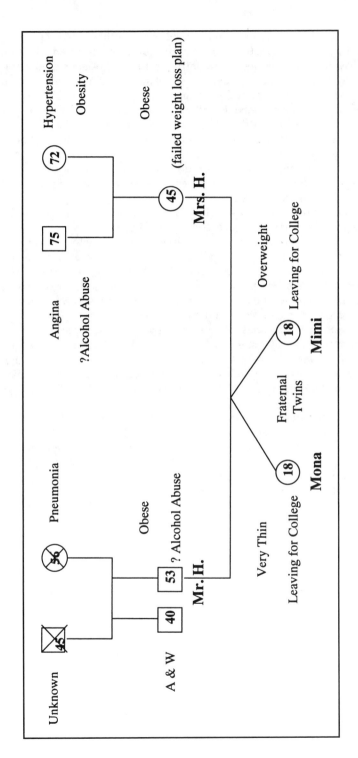

FIGURE 40-1.   Genogram.

**B.** *YES.* Alcohol abuse is frequently found in more than one member of a family. The combination of a genetic, biochemical predisposition and psychosocial factors may contribute to alcohol abuse. Alcoholism may occur during any developmental stage and may be a learned response or an effort at self-medication for feelings of depression or inadequacy. Drinking behavior often follows the pattern of one's parents. In addition, a pattern of alcoholism is frequently found in the families of origin of nonabusing spouses, who unconsciously choose husbands with characteristics similar to those of their fathers, brothers, or other family members. We do not know the extent of Mr. H.'s drinking behavior, but his comment regarding "drinking a little" requires further assessment.

**C.** *NO.* There are no data available that indicate that any of the H. family members has obsessive-compulsive disorder.

**D.** *YES.* The members of this family have several risk factors for cardiovascular disease (CVD). Ms. H. has a family history of obesity and hypertension. She is also at risk of CVD and hypertension because she is obese. Mr. H.'s obesity and possible alcohol abuse are risk factors for CVD and other health problems. These factors have potential health implications for Mona and Mimi as well.

**E.** *NO.* Although Mona is described as being very slender, there is no evidence at this time that she suffers from an eating disorder. Her weight status, however, may reflect conscious choices in eating behavior that are a reaction to her mother's and sister's obesity. Additional assessment regarding her weight history may be warranted.

QUESTION 2. What *individual* life-cycle issues or developmental tasks may be affecting the H. family members?

**A.** *NO.* This is a time for further individuation (psychological autonomy) from the family of origin. Mona and Mimi need to establish independence from their parental home, and to resolve inevitable changes in their relationships with each other and with their parents.

**B.** *NO.* Although they are always important, issues of intimacy and mutual trust are particularly salient during young adulthood. However, Mr. and Ms. H. may find that they will need to resolve intimacy issues in their relationship that did not become apparent until their children left home.

**C.** *YES.* Mona and Mimi should be dealing with issues regarding their own psychological autonomy and identity. These include accepting and stabilizing self-concept and body image, reassessing values and priorities, and establishing independence from the family of origin.

**D.** *YES.* Mr. and Ms. H. may be responding to issues regarding generativity and reassessing life goals. Reassessing life goals, including career, use of leisure time, and contribution to community, is an important task of midlife. As children gain independence and the family's need for nurturance is diminished, one may substitute community or career contributions as a way to remain creative and meaningfully engaged. Facing disappointment and lost opportunities can be particularly discouraging during this time, when adults begin to accept a change in time perspective and their own limitations.

**QUESTION 3.** What *family* life-cycle issues or developmental tasks may be affecting the H. family?

**A.** *NO*. This is a time for establishing more mature, reciprocal relationships with young adult children, while remaining available to them for support as needed. Inflexibility in intergenerational relationships makes it difficult for young adults to explore their own needs for independence and their newly developing identities as adult members of society (see Table 40-1).

**B.** *YES*. The releasing or launching of young adults is particularly difficult in families in which the members have been overly involved with each other, or in which children serve the function of keeping the parents focused on issues other than their own relationship. Fears regarding their parents' vulnerability may increase the conflict felt by young adults when exercising independence, and these fears may be acted out in immature or regressive behavior.

**C.** *YES*. Differences in lifestyle and philosophy are often a source of conflict for families. Although children's outward behavior may seem very different from their parents', some attempt to accept or understand young adult children is important. Though their children will not be exactly like them, parents will usually find that the basic values they instilled within their children will remain. Often, variations in lifestyle

TABLE 40-1   The Stages of the Family Life Cycle

| Stage | Stress |
|---|---|
| Forming the family | New living situation<br>Adjusting to partner's desires<br>Adjusting to partner's family<br>Finances |
| Birth of first child | Changes in work patterns<br>Child-rearing<br>Finances |
| Children in school | School performance<br>Behavioral problems |
| Children leave home | Redefining parental roles<br>Second career / mother's working |
| Retirement | Redefining self-worth<br>More time together<br>Adjusting to health problems<br>Finances |
| Death | Bereavement<br>Finances |

SOURCE: Enelow, A. J., Forde, D., Brummel-Smith, K. *Interviewing and Patient Care,* 4th ed. Copyright © 1996, 1986, 1979, 1972 by Oxford University Press. New York: Oxford University Press. Used by permission of Oxford University Press, Inc.

and behavior represent experimentation with behavioral options, and are part of the process of establishing a sense of individual identity.

D. *NO.* There is no evidence that experiencing menopause and loss of reproductive ability is a problematic issue for Ms. H., nor is there a suggestion that this has implications for the family system in this case.

**QUESTION 4.** Which of the following are possible interpretations of the behavior observed during this interaction?

A. *YES.* Some patterns of behavior observed during this visit have a repetitive quality, such as when Mimi manages to draw attention to herself when her parents argue. Certain relationship and communication patterns tend to be consistent in families over time, especially those that are used to avoid conflict. A family system will attempt to maintain equilibrium, and may continue to use coping strategies that are no longer effective or are in fact dysfunctional. Some mechanisms of avoiding conflict in families include scapegoating, forming coalitions, withdrawal of emotional ties, repetitive verbal or physical fighting, compromise, and designating a particular family member to take on a specific role, such as healer or protector. If these mechanisms are used exclusively in a family, the issues are unlikely to be resolved, and will continue to arise.

B. *NO.* There is as yet insufficient evidence that Mona and Mimi have significant psychopathology or are developmentally delayed in any way. If suspicions regarding the appropriateness of their behavior persist, however, the primary care provider should recommend additional evaluation as appropriate.

C. *YES.* It appears that Mr. and Ms. H. are both ambivalent about her potential weight loss and job. Mr. H.'s ambivalence is expressed through inappropriate "rewards" for her successful dieting behavior, and may be prompted by fears about her success given his own lack of advancement. By allowing Mr. H. to interfere in her diet plan, Ms. H. may be expressing her own ambivalence regarding the change in her role within the family and in the workplace, as well as a change in her appearance. We do not have enough information regarding their relationship and the way they each cope with change. Additional exploration regarding these issues is necessary and is within the scope of the primary care provider.

D. *NO.* There is not enough evidence to suggest that Mimi and Mona are overly involved with Ms. H., causing her to withdraw her affection from her husband. It is possible that Mona's seemingly protective behavior regarding her father reflects an alliance within the family system. Families have multiple subsystems, which may include shifting dyads or triads. Coalitions may form when some family members band together against other members, sometimes resulting in antagonism or anger. This is sometimes a dysfunctional way to avoid family conflict.

E. *NO.* Mr. H.'s sabotage of his wife's diet plan is not in itself evidence of depression or need for individual psychotherapy. Since the family is a system, change in one family member has an impact on others. Mr. H.

is responding to a change in the family system, and may not be responding in a functional way. Intervention at the family level may be more effective than at the individual level, however.

QUESTION 5. Which of the following health promotion interventions could be implemented by the primary care provider using a "family-as-patient" perspective?
A. *YES.* Exploring possible negative effects of Ms. H.'s weight loss may help to make some of the family members' fears more explicit, and allow more open discussion in a relatively "safe" environment. Even positive change reflects disruption of a previously stable system. Since the family as a whole is greater than the sum of its parts, a change in one member may threaten equilibrium and cause anxiety or conflict (see Table 40-2).

TABLE 40-2  Summary of Family Interventions

1. **Develop a therapeutic relationship.** Establish rapport and trust between yourself and the family by being open to the family structure or system and the cultural values and norms that are manifested. Use therapeutic communication principles. Use the family's language, but be a model for clear, effective communication. Remember the trust, influence, and impact that you have on the family unit. Be empathic, supportive, and impartial as you give feedback to the family. Thus you will enable the family members to identify and modify patterns that cause dysfunction and discomfort.

2. **Identify issues with the family.** Subjective issues are what the family members perceive as problem areas. Objective issues are what you see as limits or problems. Have each family member list or identify problems and areas for change. Refrain from challenging or questioning the accuracy of anyone's values or statements of problem areas. Do not side with any one particular member. Encourage family members also to explore those areas that you see as dysfunctional.

3. **Encourage and assist members in their communication skills,** to listen to one another, to talk kindly, and to clarify their own perceptions and the feelings, thoughts, and behaviors of the others. You gently confront and are a mirror for the family members so that they can gain increased understanding of themselves as a unit. As they learn to talk honestly to one another, members will have less need to deny the pain they feel or deny hurtful behaviors practiced in family living.

4. **Establish a teaching plan for the family unit if it is appropriate,** either for the client as a member of the family or for the family as a whole. Help each one to find appropriate resources in the external environment as well as to identify personal strengths for managing a situation. Encourage the family to find ways to adapt the life style or home situation to manage better an illness or crisis.

5. **Determine willingness of family members to participate in counseling and change.** Keep in mind that families, according to Systems Theory, strive to maintain

(*continued*)

**TABLE 40-2** (*continued*)  **Summary of Family Interventions**

their balance and are frightened and ambivalent about negotiating and enacting change. Have each member participate in defining the problem and in making the decision for change to enable family members to feel more in control of what is occurring and more willing to participate. Even so, some members may continue to be resistant to change during counseling or may choose not to participate at all. It is essential for you to remain objective, reassuring, and supportive. Considerable theoretical knowledge, communication skill, and supervised practice are necessary before you will be able to work with deep, long-term, or complex problems; resistant behavior; power struggles; or coalitions.

6. **Negotiate a contract as to the goals for treatment.** Identify with the family one or two goals that are crucial to work toward to begin to achieve some happiness and smoother function. Later, other goals may be added to the list. It is better to set small achievable goals that the family perceives as

worthwhile than to inhibit family change through an extensive list of statements. Remember that the behavior of any one family member is a symptom of a problem in the family system.

7. **Negotiate a contract about specific behavioral changes that can be accomplished** and that will encourage family members to interact or behave in ways that break dysfunctional patterns or rigid structures. Assist members to disagree constructively and to contract with one another for change. Help the family to anticipate problem areas, work through alternatives, and explore consequences of the alternatives.

8. **Be patient.** Do not expect great change. The family may change its behavior, but only to the point that is comfortable and tolerable to all. Regression to previous patterns will occur. Your consistent kindness and encouragement may be the main factors in the family coping with stressors or crises, adjusting daily routines to the needs of an ill member, or staying with therapy and trying to modify behavior.

SOURCE: Murray, R. B., Zentner, J. P. (1966). *Nursing Assessment and Health Promotion: Strategies through the Life Span,* 6th ed. Norwalk, CT: Appleton & Lange.With permission.

B. *NO.* Although each of the members of this family might benefit from a change in diet, individual interventions at this time would not address the family system issues. Exploring each family member's eating patterns in relation to the family's rituals surrounding food might be a useful intervention at the family level that would benefit each member indirectly.

C. *YES.* Sometimes interactions that were useful for families during earlier life-cycle stages become obsolete and dysfunctional at later times. New methods of communication that emphasize direct expression of feelings and intentions would be helpful for this family as the daughters become more mature and must renegotiate their relationships with their parents to reflect their change in status to "adult children." This kind of intervention is appropriate in a primary care setting if the provider feels comfortable with it and has ample opportunity. Otherwise, a referral for family counseling may be appropriate.

D. *YES.* By discussing alternative solutions of the problem with the family as a whole, new communication and problem-solving skills can be practiced, and family members can gain insight into their own behavior. Since Ms. H. seems to have difficulty confronting the inconsistencies in her husband's behavior regarding her diet, a family discussion session that makes this ambivalence explicit may be very useful if it is handled in a skillful way. Learning new ways to express feelings and opinions would be helpful for the parents in this family, and the primary care provider can serve as a role model for improved communication.

## REFERENCES

Enelow, A. J., Forde, D. L., Brummel-Smith, K. (1996). *Interviewing and Patient Care,* 4th ed. New York: Oxford University Press.

Friedman, M. (1986). *Family Nursing: Theory and Assessment.* Norwalk, CT: Appleton-Century-Crofts.

Like, R. C., Rogers, J., McGoldrick, M. (1988). *Reading and interpreting genograms: A systematic approach. J Fam Pract 26*(4), 407–412.

McCarthy, N. (1994). Health promotion and the family. In C. Edelman, C. Mandle (eds.), *Health Promotion throughout the Life Span,* 3d ed., 179–201. St. Louis: Mosby.

McGoldrick, M., Heiman, M., Carter, B. (1996). The changing family life cycle: A perspective on normalcy. In F. Walsh (ed.), *Normal Family Processes,* 2d ed., 405–443. New York: Guilford Press.

Murray, R. B., Zentner, J. P. (1996). Nursing Assessment and Health Promotion: *Strategies through the Life Span,* 6th ed. Norwalk, CT: Appleton & Lange.

Walsh, F. (1996). Conceptualization of normal family processes. In F. Walsh (ed.), *Normal Family Processes,* 2d ed., 3–69. New York: Guilford Press.

# 41

# Family Communication: Adjustment to Chronic Illness

*Arlene Miller*
*Laina M. Gerace*

Mr. M. is 72 years old and recently returned home after triple bypass surgery. He returns to the group practice clinic office for his first follow-up appointment accompanied by his wife and daughter. During initial discussion with his health care provider (HCP), he reveals that although he seems to be recovering well physically, he has not increased his activity as recommended, and has not begun to do things for himself. After his physical examination, his wife and daughter are invited into the office, with Mr. M.'s permission.

## CHIEF COMPLAINT

"I'm just not myself since I had my surgery."

## HISTORY OF PRESENT ILLNESS

Mr. M. experienced two myocardial infarctions (MIs) during the past 5 years. After the last one, arterial blockages were identified by angiography, and he was scheduled for triple bypass surgery. Mr. M. thought he had been in fairly good health prior to his heart attacks, and had stopped smoking after his first MI. The surgery was successful, and his first postoperative week was uneventful. He was described as cooperative during his hospital stay, and was given an ambulation schedule on discharge.

## SOCIAL HISTORY

Mr. M. lives with his 68-year-old wife and their 40-year-old daughter, Anna. Two older, married sons live in the suburbs of the same city. Mr. M. worked for the same company as a salesman for many years, and retired 3 years ago. His wife has never worked outside the home. Mr. and Mrs. M. immigrated to the United States from Eastern Europe 45 years ago. All of their children were born in this country.

## OBJECTIVE DATA

Excerpt of interview with the family:

1. HCP:     Mr. M., what activities have you participated in this week?
2. Mrs. M.: He's not following his exercise like he is supposed to. I tell him what to do, but he stays in bed all day.
3. Anna:    Yes, he isn't really following the doctor's orders. He never listens to what we say.
4. HCP:     (Looks at Mr. M.) What exercise program was recommended for you when you left the hospital?
5. Anna:    He should be walking four times a week. (She shows the HCP detailed information she has written regarding her father's exercise program. Mrs. M. looks through her purse, eventually taking out several bottles of medication and placing them on the desk in front of the HCP.)
6. Mr. M.:  I don't see how walking around the block is going to help me get my strength back. It just makes me more tired.
7. Anna:    Dad, you're just as stubborn as you always were!
8. Mrs. M.: Anna, don't talk that way to your father. We have to help him get better again.
9. Anna:    You don't help much by giving him all that rich food!

QUESTION 1. What additional information might be helpful for further assessing this family's interaction patterns and creating an opportunity for intervention?
   A. A 24-h diet recall for all three family members
   B. Each family member's perception of Mr. M.'s illness and prognosis
   C. Past history of psychotherapy in any of the family members
   D. A discussion of the way family members got along before Mr. M.'s surgery

## ASSESSMENT

QUESTION 2. Which of the following statements best describes the overall effectiveness of the M. family's communication during this interview?
   A. There is considerable interaction, during which individual family members express their feelings and views in a straightforward, empathic manner.
   B. The individuals in this family seem to be able to express their needs and obtain validation from one another.
   C. Several interactions demonstrate dysfunctional communication.
   D. The interactions seem very superficial and suggest that neither Mrs. M. nor Anna is really aware of the seriousness of Mr. M.'s medical condition.

QUESTION 3. Several times during this interview, two individuals in this family seem to form an alliance, leaving one family member out. Which of the following dyads are demonstrated? (Select all that apply.)
   A. HCP/Mr. M.
   B. Mrs. M./Anna
   C. Mrs. M./Mr. M.
   D. HCP/Mrs. M.


## MANAGEMENT

QUESTION 4. Which of the following seems to characterize the HCP's effectiveness during the interchange?
   A. The HCP maintains fairly tight control of the situation.
   B. The HCP alienates each of the family members by being unsupportive of Mr. M.
   C. The HCP acts as a role model for improving communication patterns.
   D. The HCP makes an attempt to focus on Mr. M.'s problem in this excerpt, but does not demonstrate effective interviewing skills.


QUESTION 5. When the HCP refocuses the conversation on Mr. M.'s exercise program (see line 4 of interview), what techniques might she have used instead to bring Mrs. M. and Anna into the conversation? (Select all that apply.)
   A. Confront Mrs. M.'s avoidance of the topic by asking her to sit down and pointing out that she is not being honest with herself about her fears for Mr. M.'s health.
   B. Address both Anna and Mrs. M. and ask them to talk about their impressions of Mr. M.'s illness.
   C. Validate the family's concern for Mr. M.'s welfare.
   D. Reassure the family that Mr. M.'s prognosis is very good if he adheres to his treatment plan.


QUESTION 6. Which of the following factors has implications for cross-cultural family interventions? (Select all that apply.)
   A. Immigrants usually acculturate to the dominant culture's health values within the first 5 years after resettlement.
   B. Family values and communication patterns are often transmitted intergenerationally, even if parents are born in a different country from their children.
   C. People from Eastern Europe tend to be self-effacing, avoid public contradiction or direct conflict, and appear to suppress feelings of anger or pain.
   D. Acceptable components of adopting the sick role differ among cultural groups, and this may have an impact on patients' adherence to medical advice.

## ANSWERS

**QUESTION 1.** What additional information might be helpful for further assessing this family's interaction patterns and creating an opportunity for intervention?

A. *NO.* Although a 24-h diet recall for Mr. M. might provide information that would be useful for nutrition counseling, focusing specific questions on individuals would not encourage discussion or demonstrate usual patterns of interaction among the members in this family.

B. *YES.* Eliciting each family member's perception of Mr. M.'s illness and prognosis might facilitate making some of their concerns or fears explicit, allowing the HCP to address them directly. Bringing their perceptions into the open may also help family members to set realistic goals, express their underlying support for Mr. M., and encourage him to express his ambivalence regarding his condition.

C. *NO.* Knowing about the past history of psychotherapy is not necessary for developing a plan for the family at this time.

D. *YES.* A group discussion of the way family members got along before Mr. M.'s surgery might provide an opportunity to elicit usual patterns of interaction. Often, very brief observations can contribute rich samples or snapshots of family communication patterns. These snapshots might provide insight into the family's usual methods of dealing with stress, roles and alliances within the family system, and strengths or weaknesses that can be utilized in later interventions by the HCP.

**QUESTION 2.** Which of the following statements best describes the overall effectiveness of the M. family's communication during this interview?

A. *NO.* Although it seems as though the individual family members express their feelings of anger toward each other directly, it is probable that by doing so they are also expressing their feelings of fear or anxiety indirectly.

B. *NO.* The individuals in this family seem to have difficulty expressing and validating their needs directly. Although they seem to respond to manifest or explicit information, they do not address the implicit meaning of the other family members' statements.

C. *YES.* Several interactions demonstrate dysfunctional communication. These include assuming that others share one's own feelings without validating them, interceding or speaking for another, being judgmental, using sarcasm, and cutting off communication as a means of defense against topics perceived as uncomfortable.

D. *NO.* Although the interactions seem very superficial, they do not suggest that either Mrs. M. or Anna is unaware of the seriousness of Mr. M.'s medical condition. Their anxiety or frustration about Mr. M.'s condition may be expressed by assigning blame to each other, which suggests that they do not feel in control of the situation.

**Question 3.** Several times during this interview, two individuals in this family seem to form an alliance, leaving one family member out. Which of the following dyads are demonstrated?
   A. *NO.* The HCP attempts to engage Mr. M. in the interview, but this does not represent an alliance.
   B. *YES.* In this family, there are shifting coalitions. Mrs. M. and Anna are aligned in saying that Mr. M. "isn't really following the doctor's orders" (see line 3 of interview), but this switches later when Anna accuses her mother of giving him food that is too rich (line 9). In some families, the spousal alliance is weakened when one parent (usually the mother) forms a coalition with the children, thereby relegating the other parent to a marginal, less involved role in the family. This situation may have occurred in this family, and may be reflected in Mr. M.'s lack of involvement in his own health care, although further substantiating data are needed.
   C. *NO.* There is not enough information to support an alliance between Mr. and Mrs. M.
   D. *NO.* The HCP does not engage Mrs. M. in direct conversation during this interview.

**Question 4.** Which of the following seems to characterize the HCP's effectiveness during the interchange?
   A. *NO.* In this brief interchange, the HCP has not controlled the situation. Instead of answering her question, the family members cast blame on one another for Mr. M.'s lack of participation in his own rehabilitation. More structure would provide better control of the situation. For example, the HCP could begin the interview by explaining the purpose for bringing the family together and what kind of information is being sought. An example might be: "We are here to discuss how things are going since Mr. M.'s heart surgery. This is a good time for us to identify any problems related to Mr. M.'s recovery that concern the whole family."
   B. *NO.* Although anger is expressed in the interview, the anger is not directed at the HCP. Indeed, the family is trying to please the HCP by providing information.
   C. *NO.* Although the HCP attempts to draw Mr. M. into the conversation, her approach does not model improved communication patterns. In order to act as a role model, the HCP needs to be more direct. For example, the HCP could say, "I appreciate everyone's information, but we also need to hear from Mr. M."
   D. *YES.* The HCP attempted to focus on Mr. M.'s problem in this excerpt, but she was unsuccessful. The HCP needs to be more assertive in eliciting a response from Mr. M.

**Question 5.** When the HCP refocuses the conversation on Mr. M.'s exercise program (see line 4 of interview), what techniques might she have used instead to bring Mrs. M. and Anna into the conversation?
   A. *NO.* This type of confrontation is highly interpretive and is inappropriate in this situation. A more caring, empathic comment should be used

TABLE 41-1   The Illness Trajectory for Anticipatory Family Guidance

| Phase | Potential Problems | Supportive Guidance |
|---|---|---|
| Illness onset | Denial of symptoms<br>Blaming the victim<br>Reluctance to accept diagnosis<br>  and treatment | Empathic listening<br>Define and validate situation<br>Offer support |
| Accepting illness | Imbalance in family system<br>Physical and/or emotional<br>  impairment<br>Disruption of lifestyle | Foster open discussion<br>Point out family strengths<br>Acknowledge seriousness<br>  of problems<br>Advocate for family resources |
| Beginning<br>  treatment | Family stress<br>Family role shifts<br>Financial concerns | Foster shared responsibilities<br>Facilitate instrumental<br>  support as needed |
| Recovery | Seeking secondary gains<br>Unwillingness to accept<br>  limitations | Set appropriate limits<br>Provide encouragement<br>  and education |
| Rehabilitation | Relapse (depending on illness)<br>Loss of role status<br>  and self-worth | Teach relapse prevention<br>Acknowledge role limitations<br>Facilitate new acceptance |

instead. For example, the HCP could say, "I can sense how concerned you are about Mr. M.'s health."

B.  YES. Discussing Anna's and Mrs. M.'s impressions of Mr. M.'s illness would be important. Illness in one family member has an impact on every family member, and can cause great stress and instability. In this family, dysfunctional communication can lead to additional disequilibrium if the family has difficulty adjusting to chronic illness. Family conferences, in which anticipatory and supportive guidance are provided, can be extremely helpful in resolving difficulties, particularly during the early stages of illness (see Table 41-1).

C.  YES. In addition to a general comment about the family's concern for Mr. M., this can also be done by eliciting each person's perspective on the situation, including the patient's and the family members'.

D.  NO. This response would constitute false reassurance. Mr. M. is an older man who has had two MIs and has undergone triple bypass surgery. While he may have many good years left, there is no guarantee regarding his prognosis.

QUESTION 6. Which of the following factors has implications for cross-cultural family interventions?

A.  NO. Acculturation is related to many factors, including age at immigration, gender, and education. Although people do tend to adopt more aspects of the dominant value system the longer they are in a country and the higher their social class, little is known regarding adoption of health-related values and behaviors. People who remain in an ethnic neighborhood, who socialize primarily with individuals from the same cultural background, and whose religion reinforces their values tend to maintain cultural norms longer than those who become integrated or assimilated into the dominant culture. Ethnic values and expectations regarding health and illness behavior may be maintained for many years, even when individuals appear to have acculturated to the language and cultural norms of the dominant culture.

B.  YES. Family values and communication patterns are often transmitted intergenerationally, and cultural factors can play a major role in the family life cycle. There is evidence that ethnic values and identification are retained for several generations after immigration, influencing family life-cycle patterns. Ethnic differences in values, role expectations, and interactions among family members persist in second-, third-, and even fourth-generation Americans.

C.  NO. While it may be inappropriate to generalize behaviors to specific cultures, being self-effacing, avoiding public contradiction or direct conflict, and appearing to suppress feelings of anger or pain tend to be more representative of people from Asian than from European cultures. In many Asian cultures, less value is placed on distinguishing oneself from the group than in Western cultures, in which great emphasis is placed on individual autonomy.

D.  YES. Acceptable components of adopting the sick role differ among cultural groups. Cultural norms vary widely regarding appropriate sick roles, kind of communication about the disease, who should be the primary caretaker, and normative rituals at different stages of health, such as healing, hospital visits, funerals, and mourning. In some families, particularly Jewish families and others from Eastern Europe, it is common and acceptable to discuss physical symptoms or health problems openly. In contrast, Irish families and White Anglo-Saxon Protestants tend to minimize ailments. Families in which great value is placed on being solicitous toward sick members may unknowingly interfere with patients' adherence to medical advice, and families that revere doctors and value medical care may facilitate treatment.

## REFERENCES

Berry, J. W., Kim, U., Minde, T., Mok, D. (1987). Comparative studies of acculturative stress. *International Migration Review* 21, 491–511.

Chang, K. (1995). Chinese Americans. In J. N. Giger, R. E. Davidhizar (eds.), *Transcultural Nursing: Assessment and Intervention,* 2d ed., 395–414. St. Louis: Mosby.

Enelow, A. J., Forde, D. L., Brummel-Smith, K. (1996). *Interviewing and Patient Care,* 4th ed. New York: Oxford University Press.

Hofer, J. (1996). Family communication. In P. J. Bomar (ed.), *Nurses and Family Health Promotion,* 94–106. Philadelphia: W. B. Saunders.

McGoldrick, M. (1996). Ethnicity, cultural diversity and normality. In F. Walsh (ed.), *Normal Family Processes,* 2d ed., 331–360. New York: Guilford Press.

Rolland, J. S. (1996). Mastering family challenges in serious illness and disability. In F. Walsh (ed.), *Normal Family Processes,* 2d ed., 444–473. New York: Guilford Press.

# 42

# Elder Abuse/Neglect

*Eugenie F. Hildebrandt*
*Arlene Miller*

Mrs. S. is a 78-year-old divorced woman who lives with her son, Bill. She has come to the clinic today on the recommendation of the parish nurse from Mrs. S.'s church, who sees Mrs. S. periodically. The parish nurse visited Mrs. S. at home last week, and called the health care provider after finding little food in the home, noting also that Mrs. S. had a bruise on the left side of her face. Bill accompanies his mother to the clinic, and seems reluctant to leave her alone during the encounter.

## CHIEF COMPLAINT

"That nurse from my church worries about me, but I'm feeling about right for someone who is 78 years old."

**QUESTION 1.** In light of the information provided by the parish nurse, which of the following issues should the primary care provider consider when conducting the encounter? (Select all that apply.)
  **A.** Does Mrs. S. want to be interviewed alone?
  **B.** Is it important to allow Bill to express his perception of the situation?
  **C.** Which side will the provider take?

Mrs. S. decides not to have her son participate in the interview with the primary care provider.

## HISTORY OF PRESENT ILLNESS

Mrs. S. is reluctant to talk about the fading bruise on her face, stating vaguely that she just hit herself on an open cabinet door one day. She denies vertigo, falling, general or episodic weakness, feeling faint, or losing consciousness. She denies use of alcohol or any prescription medications, including anticoagulants. She admits that her son has been frustrated with her lately because she has to "nag at him" to help with house and yard maintenance that she used to be able to do alone. She states that she does not always eat well because some months her social security income does not last through the end of the month and sometimes she has no transportation to a grocery store to purchase food. She denies weight loss of more than 5 lb over the last year.

Two months ago her son, Bill, started to eat alone at a diner after work several nights a week and therefore does not see the need to do much grocery shopping for Mrs. S. Mrs. S. stopped driving 3 years ago because of diminished visual acuity. She is now dependent on her son for transportation. She also needs some help with the household expenses, and finds it increasingly difficult to do the cooking, laundry, cleaning, and yard work that she has always done for the two of them. She feels she has no alternative to her living situation and does not want to do anything that will upset Bill.

## PAST MEDICAL HISTORY

Mrs. S. has no known food, drug, or environmental allergies. She has no chronic illnesses other than osteoarthritis. She uses acetaminophen for occasional headaches or joint discomfort.

## SOCIAL HISTORY

Mrs. S. was divorced from her husband 30 years ago, after 25 years of marriage. Her husband was employed most of the time during their marriage. However, during periods of unemployment, he often vented his frustration by shouting at his wife and son and striking them. Mrs. S. states that her 54-year-old son, Bill, doesn't get along with many people, has few friends, and never married. He is a long-time employee in a local factory, and he and Mrs. S. have always lived together in her small home 2 mi from the edge of town. She and her son have not had a close relationship; much of their time together is spent watching television. Mrs. S. has one sister who lives 600 miles away.

QUESTION 2. Which of the following are risk factors for elder abuse and neglect? (Select all that apply.)
   A. Financial dependence of the potential abuser on the elderly person
   B. Low socioeconomic status
   C. Substance abuse or psychological stress in the potential abuser
   D. Short-term caregiving to the older adult
   E. Poor health and cognitive or functional impairment in the elderly person

QUESTION 3. What statements in Mrs. S.'s history raise suspicions of neglectful behavior on the part of her son? (Select all that apply.)
   A. Bill's reluctance or refusal to assist with home maintenance tasks that she can no longer do alone
   B. Mrs. S.'s assertion that she has to "nag" at her son to take her to the grocery store for food
   C. Bill's eating at a restaurant without taking Mrs. S.
   D. Bill's reluctance to leave his mother alone with the nurse in the clinic

## OBJECTIVE DATA

Vital signs:   Temperature 36.9°C (98.5°F), pulse 84, respirations 12, blood pressure 134/86, weight 110 lb (49.9 kg), height 5 ft 5 in.

General:   Alert, pale, thin, older adult woman who appears subdued and ill at ease.

Cognition:   Mini-mental status examination within normal limits, with a score of 27/30.

Skin:   Dry with poor turgor. Bruise on left cheek is yellow-green, 3 cm × 4 cm. Purple, 4 cm × 5 cm bruise on left upper arm. Red-purple bruise with small skin tear on right forearm.

Laboratory:   Hemoglobin 12 g/dL. Hematocrit 36%.

In response to direct questioning during the physical examination, Mrs. S. admits that her son shouted at her and, on two occasions, struck her. The first time, 10 days ago, she sustained a bruise to her face. Her bruises on both arms resulted from similar behavior yesterday.

QUESTION 4. Which of the following factors are typical of abusive situations? (Select all that apply.)
A. Mrs. S.'s initial reluctance to talk about her bruises
B. Mrs. S.'s admission that Bill shouted at her and struck her
C. Bill's long-term employment in a factory job
D. Bill's witnessing and experiencing his father's physically abusive behavior as a young child

## ASSESSMENT

QUESTION 5. Which of the following are considered types of elder abuse? (Select all that apply.)
A. Physical abuse
B. Psychological abuse
C. Financial exploitation
D. Willful neglect

QUESTION 6. Based on the history and clinical findings, what is a likely assessment of Mrs. S.? (Select all that apply.)
A. Anemia
B. Old age
C. Senile dementia, Alzheimer's type
D. Physical abuse related to dysfunctional family relationship

## PLAN

QUESTION 7. Which of the following should be included in the short-range plan for this family? (Select all that apply.)
A. Mrs. S. and her son should be referred for counseling.
B. Mrs. S. should be removed from the home, with possible nursing home placement.

C. Bill should be reported to the local police department.
D. Mrs. S. should be given a follow-up appointment within 3 months.

QUESTION 8. What are the legal and ethical ramifications of this situation? (Select all that apply.)
A. If the competent older adult chooses to remain in an abusive situation, a provider must intervene anyway.
B. Laws in all states require reporting of suspected abuse of older adults.
C. Since this is a relatively low-risk situation, the health care provider should not interfere.
D. The legal system in most states mandates family therapy as the primary intervention for domestic violence.

## ANSWERS

QUESTION 1. In light of the information provided by the parish nurse, which of the following issues should the primary care provider consider when conducting the encounter?
A. YES. Mrs. S. is legally competent. Therefore, she may decide whether or not to have her son present during the encounter. She may fear retaliation from her son or fear that the home situation will get worse. If Mrs. S. refuses to include Bill at this time, a joint visit can be considered in the future.
B. YES. Bill should be given an opportunity to express his perception of the situation. Mrs. S. may be unaware of job-related or other stressors that may have reduced Bill's ability to cope with frustration.
C. NO. A nonjudgmental approach is important while gathering information regarding the situation.

QUESTION 2. Which of the following are risk factors for elder abuse and neglect?
A. YES. Financial dependence on the victim is a risk factor for elder abuse and neglect. Domestic violence has a multifactorial etiology that includes social conditions (usually social or physical isolation from neighbors, relatives, or friends), family conflict, cultural attitudes, and biological factors.
B. NO. Abuse occurs in families of every socioeconomic level.
C. YES. The influence of alcohol or drugs may serve to decrease inhibitions or lower a person's tolerance of frustration. Psychological stress makes caregivers less able to deal with the stresses inherent in the long-term care of another person.
D. NO. Long-term caregiving is more likely to generate abuse because of the stress of the work involved and the lack of respite for the caregiver.
E. YES. Persons who are psychologically or mentally impaired may require more intense supervision, may be overly dependent or physically or verbally abusive themselves, or may be less responsive to the efforts of the caregiver. These factors make caregiving more stressful and less rewarding to the caregiver and increase the likelihood of abuse.

**QUESTION 3.** What statements in Mrs. S.'s history raise suspicions of neglectful behavior on the part of her son?

**A.** *YES.* Indifference to sharing the workload in the home may be a result of her son's inflexibility and his difficulty in recognizing her decline.

**B.** *YES.* Neglect can reflect many types of problems in a wide range of situations. Not providing the opportunity to get food from the grocery store or refusal of other needed assistance with instrumental activities of daily living constitutes neglect. Other signs of neglect would include malnutrition or sudden weight loss, poor hygiene, inappropriate clothing, and lack of compliance with treatment in a formerly compliant patient.

**C.** *NO.* It is appropriate that adult children and their parents have time away from each other. Mrs. S.'s increasing dependence may place a greater strain on the relationship between mother and son; therefore, Bill's creating time away from the stressful situation may be a healthy coping behavior. This does not negate his responsibility, however, for ensuring adequate food for his mother in his absence.

**D.** *YES.* Bill's reluctance to leave his mother alone with the health care provider is a sign that raises suspicion, but is not diagnostic of abuse or neglect. It may be a way for him to continue to exert control over his mother, or to monitor possible accusations of abusive behavior.

**QUESTION 4.** Which of the following factors are typical of abusive situations? (Select all that apply.)

**A.** *YES.* Most older adults who are abused are reluctant or ashamed to discuss it. Spouses and adult children are the most common perpetrators of elder abuse or neglect. Mrs. S. may be afraid of community censure or legal ramifications for her son. She may be afraid that he will retaliate or that one of them might be made to leave their home.

**B.** *YES.* Shouting constitutes psychological abuse, and striking is physical abuse. It is estimated that at least 1 million older Americans are abused annually. Victims are most likely to be Caucasian women over 70 years of age with some mental or physical impairment.

**C.** *NO.* Bill's long-term employment indicates some economic stability. Even though he does not have many friends, long-term employment demonstrates his ability to function in some social situations. Financial dependence or unemployment is more typical of abusive situations.

**D.** *YES.* Witnessing and experiencing physically abusive behavior during childhood constitutes an important risk factor for later domestic violence, including elder abuse.

**QUESTION 5.** Which of the following are considered types of elder abuse?

**A.** *YES.* Physical abuse includes beating, shoving, slapping, sexually molesting, or restraining the older adult against his or her will.

**B.** *YES.* Psychological abuse includes isolating or excluding older adults from the family or outside activities, treating them like children, or verbally attacking them.

   C. *YES.* Financial exploitation or abuse includes taking money or re-sources from older adults without their consent, or forcing them to sign over the title to property or to submit to management of their affairs against their will.

   D. *YES.* Neglect occurs when basic needs—food, clothing, shelter, med-ical care, and other resources, including hearing aids and eyeglasses—are withheld. Benign neglect refers to situations in which the caregiver is ignorant of or unable to provide appropriate care. Willful neglect is deliberate and intended to harm. It should be treated in the same way as other forms of abuse.

**QUESTION 6.** Based on the history and clinical findings, what is a likely assessment of Mrs. S.?

   A. *NO.* The hemoglobin and hematocrit are in the low range of normal. However, Mrs. S. may be at risk for anemia and malnutrition because of her difficulty getting to the grocery store for food.

   B. *NO.* Old age is not a diagnosis. Many older adults accommodate to the functional decline associated with aging and lead relatively healthy, satisfying lives.

   C. *NO.* Mrs. S.'s ability to provide both recent and remote history and her performance on the Mini-Mental Status Exam indicate intact mental capacity.

   D. *YES.* The verbal and physical abuse by Bill are documented in the his-tory. The bruises on Mrs. S.'s arm indicate physical abuse. The history suggests elements of a dysfunctional family relationship.

**QUESTION 7.** Which of the following should be included in the short-range plan for this family?

   A. *YES.* Arrangements for counseling by a skilled mental health profes-sional should be made. Despite the limited success of interventions in family violence, benefits are substantial for families in which the cycle of violence can be interrupted. Since there have been few incidents so far, it is possible that family counseling can assist Bill and Mrs. S. to communicate better, find other ways to express frustration, learn more positive coping skills, and use community resources more effectively.

   B. *NO.* Removal from the home and placement in a nursing home would decrease Mrs. S.'s independence and probably result in a swifter decline in her functional status. Efforts should be made to increase the social support and resources for this family. Mrs. S.'s initial reluctance to confide in health care professionals may be related to fear that she might be removed from her home, as well as fear for her son.

   C. *NO.* Rather than reporting Bill to the police, the situation should be reported to an appropriate protective or social service agency. All indi-viduals who present to health care settings with multiple injuries and implausible explanations should be assessed for possible physical abuse, with pregnant women and the elderly given special considera-tion because of their increased vulnerability. Suspected cases of abuse should include appropriate documentation and treatment of physical injuries, and referrals should include telephone numbers for crisis centers, shelters, and protective service agencies.

**D.** *NO.* Follow-up needs to be more timely. It would be appropriate to call Mrs. S. the following day to check on how she and her son are relating, after they discuss their problems with an outside resource person. Close monitoring and support are needed, and efforts should be made to ensure that referral appointments are kept.

QUESTION **8.** What are the legal and ethical ramifications of this situation?

**A.** *NO.* Elder abuse raises ethical issues related to competency, privacy, and the right of an adult to refuse treatment. The provider should counsel the older adult about the danger, but must honor his or her decision. Unless the older adult is determined to be mentally incompetent after a formal competency hearing, social service workers may have no legal right to intervene or overrule a refusal of intervention.

**B.** *NO.* Reporting laws vary among states. In most states, however, professionals are protected from criminal or civil liability for reporting suspected elder abuse, and indeed in some states may be fined for failing to do so. Practitioners need to be familiar with the state laws where they practice.

**C.** *NO.* Real or potential neglect or abuse of clients warrants intervention by primary care providers. Counseling, information about community support services, and referral to appropriate social service agencies are appropriate.

**D.** *NO.* Although elder abuse may be most effectively treated by family therapy and social service interventions, it is considered a criminal matter as well. As such, it brings the victim and the abuser into the criminal justice system. Fear of becoming involved with the legal system and reluctance to risk having someone in their family incarcerated serve as powerful deterrents to older adults' reporting their own children or spouses as abusers.

## REFERENCES

Iris, M. (1997). Abuse and neglect. In J. R. Webster, C. E. Woodson (eds.), *Geriatrics Resource Guide*, 3d ed., 57–61. Chicago: Northwestern University. (Available from Buehler Center on Aging, Northwestern University Medical School, Chicago, IL.)

Jarvis, C. (1996). *Physical Examination and Health Assessment.* Philadelphia: W. B. Saunders.

Murray, R. B., Zentner, J. P. (1993). *Nursing Assessment and Health Promotion,* 5th ed. Norwalk, CT: Appleton & Lange.

Rathbone-McCuan, E. (1986). Elder abuse resulting from care giver overload in older families. In N. Datan, A. L. Greene, H. W. Reese (eds.), *Life Span Developmental Psychology: Intergenerational Relationships*, 245–264. Hillsdale, NJ: Erlbaum.

U.S. Preventive Services Task Force. (1996). *Guide to Clinical Preventive Services,* 2d ed. Baltimore: Williams & Wilkins.

Youngkin, E. Q., Davis, M. S. (1994). *Women's Health.* Norwalk, CT: Appleton & Lange.

# Index

# Index

Page numbers in *italics* refer to illustrations and those ending in *t* to tables.

ISBN 0-07-105487-1

90000

9 780071 054874